Eicosanoids and the Gastrointestinal Tract

ADVANCES IN EICOSANOID RESEARCH

Series Editor Keith Hillier

Eicosanoids and Reproduction
Edited by Keith Hillier

Eicosanoids in the Gastrointestinal Tract
Edited by Keith Hillier

Eicosanoids in Inflammatory Conditions of the Lung, Skin and Joints
Edited by Martin Church and Clive Robinson

Eicosanoids in the Cardiovascular and Renal Systems
Edited by Perry Halushka and Dale Mais

ADVANCES IN EICOSANOID RESEARCH

Series Editor Keith Hillier

Eicosanoids and the Gastrointestinal Tract

Edited by

Keith Hillier

Senior Lecturer
Clinical Pharmacology Group
Medical Faculty
University of Southampton
UK

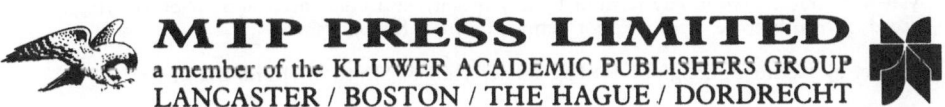

MTP PRESS LIMITED

a member of the KLUWER ACADEMIC PUBLISHERS GROUP

LANCASTER / BOSTON / THE HAGUE / DORDRECHT

Published in the UK and Europe by
MTP Press Limited
Falcon House
Lancaster, England

British Library Cataloguing in Publication Data

Eicosanoids and the gastrointestinal tract.
  1. Man. Gastrointestinal tract. Effects of eicosanoids
  I. Hillier, Keith, *1943–*
  616.3'3

ISBN-13: 978-94-010-7069-0   e-ISBN-13: 978-94-009-1281-6

DOI: 10.1007/978-94-009-1281-6

Published in the USA by
MTP Press
A division of Kluwer Academic Publishers
101 Philip Drive
Norwell, MA 02061, USA

Library of Congress Cataloging in Publication Data

Eicosanoids and the gastrointestinal tract/edited by Keith Hillier.
     p. cm.—(Advances in eicosanoid research)
  Includes bibliographies and index.

    1. Gastrointestinal system—Pathophysiology. 2. Arachidonic acid—
Derivatives—Physiological effect. I. Hillier, K. (Keith), 1943–
II. Series. III. Series: Advances in eicosanoid research series.
    [DNLM: 1. Eicosanoic Acids—pharmacology. 2. Gastrointestinal System—drug
effects. QU 90 E3452]
RC802.9.E33 1987
616.3'3—dc19
DNLM/DLC   88-1129
for Library of Congress   CIP

Copyright © 1988 MTP Press Limited

Softcover reprint of the hardcover 1st edition 1988

Typeset by Lasertext, Longford Trading Estate, Thomas Street, Stretford, Manchester

Contents

List of contributors

A. Allen
Department of Physiological Science
University of Newcastle
Framlington Place
Newcastle upon Tyne NE2 4HH
UK

A. Aly
Department of Medicine
Division of Gastroenterology
Karolinska Hospital
PO Box 60500
S-104 01 Stockholm
Sweden

N K Boughton-Smith
Department of Mediator Pharmacology
Wellcome Research Laboratories
Beckenham
Kent BR3 3BS
UK

C H Cho
Department of Pathology
Brigham & Womens' Hospital
Harvard Medical School
75 Francis Street
Boston, MA 02115
USA

G Flemström
Department of Physiology and Medical
  Biophysics
Uppsala University Biomedical Centre
PO Box 572
S-751 23 Uppsala
Sweden

A Garner
Biosciences Department
ICI Pharmaceuticals Division
Macclesfield SK10 4TG
UK

A C Hunter
Department of Physiological Science
University of Newcastle
Framlington Place
Newcastle upon Tyne NE2 4HH
UK

J P Keogh
Department of Physiological Science
University of Newcastle
Framlington Place
Newcastle upon Tyne NE2 4HH
UK

S J Konturek
Institute of Physiology
Academy of Medicine
ul. Grzegorzecka 16
31-531 Krakow
Poland

M Ligumsky
Department of Gastroenterology
Hadassah University Hospital
PO Box 12000
Jerusalem 91120
Israel

P K Moore
Department of Pharmacology
King's College
University of London
Manresa Road
London SW3 6LX
UK

G Pihan
Department of Pathology
Brigham & Womens' Hospital
Harvard Medical School
75 Francis Street
Boston, MA 02115
USA

D Rachmilewitz
Department of Gastroenterology
Hadassah University Hospital
PO Box 12000
Jerusalem 91120
Israel

K D Rainsford
Anti-inflammatory Research Unit
Strangeways Research Laboratory
Worts Causeway
Cambridge CB1 4RN
UK

EICOSANOIDS AND THE GASTROINTESTINAL TRACT

A Robert
Diabestes & GI Diseases Research
The Upjohn Company
Kalamazoo
MI 49001
USA

S Szabo
Department of Pathology
Brigham & Womens' Hospital
Harvard Medical School
75 Francis Street
Boston, MA 02115
USA

B J R Whittle
Department of Mediator Pharmacology
Wellcome Research Laboratories
Beckenham
Kent BR3 3BS
UK

Series Editor's Foreword

The original series, *Advances in Prostaglandin Research*, edited by Sultan M. M. Karim, was published by MTP Press in three volumes in 1975 and 1976. A glance at those books illustrates the progress that has been made since then. The thromboxanes were mentioned twice (first publication 1975) and prostacyclin not once (first publication 1976); leukotrienes were only on the horizon.

The amazing generation of research data in the last 10–15 years has given new, broad insights into many areas, including asthma, inflammation, renal, cardiovascular and gastrointestinal diseases and in reproduction, and has led in some instances to real clinical benefit.

This series, *Advances in Eicosanoid Research*, reflects the current understanding of prostaglandins, thromboxanes and leukotrienes. The aim is to provide an introductory background to each topic and the most up-to-date information available.

Although each book stands alone, the eicosanoids cut across many boundaries in their basic actions; selected chapters from each book in the Series will provide illuminating and productive information for all readers which will advance their education and research.

In the production of this series, I must acknowledge with pleasure my collaboration with editors and authors and the patient endeavours of Dr. Michael Brewis and the staff at MTP Press.

KEITH HILLIER
University of Southampton
England

Preface

Eicosanoids and the Gastrointestinal Tract is one of the series of books entitled *Advances in Eicosanoid Research*. An overview of the wealth of published literature in this area has not before been gathered together in the present form under one cover. Each area is dealt with in an extended manner by eminent authors in the field giving critical appraisals of results and problems that require solutions.

The wide range of biological effects of eicosanoids in the gastrointestinal tract gives rise to particular problems of interpretation and these have been dealt with in an admirable way by the authors. The book covers the gastrointestinal clinical uses of eicosanoids but also provides quite novel reviews on laboratory animal and *in vitro* models that have not been appraised in the recent past.

KEITH HILLIER

1
The role of eicosanoids in inflammatory bowel disease

M. Ligumsky and D. Rachmilewitz

INTRODUCTION

The aetiology and the pathogenesis of inflammatory bowel disease (IBD) are still obscure. Infective agents and immunological mechanisms, as well as environmental and dietary factors[1,2] have been and are extensively investigated.

Since a specific aetiological factor has yet to be identified, the non-specific features of IBD prevail: general symptoms of inflammation, pathological picture consistent with non-specific inflammatory reaction and a relatively favourable response to agents such as salazopyrin and corticosteroids. Arachidonic acid metabolites (eicosanoids) which, synergistically with mediators such as histamine and bradykinin, play a role in propagating the inflammatory signs[3] have attracted attention in regard to their possible role in the pathogenesis of IBD.

CHEMISTRY

Eicosanoids are derived from 20-carbon-chain unsaturated fatty acids, mainly from arachidonic acid. By the cyclo-oxygenase pathway, arachidonic acid is metabolized into prostaglandins (PG), prostacyclin (PGI_2) and thromboxane (Tx). An alternative lipoxygenase oxidative pathway metabolizes arachidonic acid into non-cyclized 20-carbon unsaturated fatty acids such as hydroperoxy-eicosatetraenoic acids (HPETEs), hydroeicosatetraenoic acids (HETEs) and leukotrienes.

BIOLOGICAL ACTIVITIES

Prostaglandins possess various biological activities. They induce and mediate the propagation of inflammatory signs such as oedema, pain and fever[3-5].

1

Prostanoids affect water and electrolyte transport in the gut[6], have vasoactive effects, and induce smooth muscle contraction. They decrease gastric acid secretion, increase mucus and bicarbonate production and provide cytoprotection[7]. Lipoxygenase metabolites such as leukotrienes contribute to the inflammatory process by acting as chemotactic factors for human neutrophils, induce lysosomal enzyme release from neutrophils and increase capillary permeability[8,9]. Several lipoxygenase metabolites also affect intestinal secretion[10].

EICOSANOIDS AND THE GUT

Occurrence and synthetic capacity

During the last two decades, data reported by many investigators suggest that the gastrointestinal tract in humans and in animals is able to synthesize and release arachidonic acid metabolites[11,12]. The major products of the cyclo-oxygenase pathway in the gut are PGE, PGI_2, PGD, PGF and thromboxanes. Prostanoid synthesis was determined in homogenates of gut mucosa and the stable metabolites could be detected in gut luminal fluid. Their release was shown *in vitro* in an organ culture system[13], and *in vivo* into dialysis bags placed in the rectum of human subjects[14]. Recently, lipoxygenase pathway metabolites such as 12-HETE and 15- and 5-lipoxygenase products including leukotriene B_4 have been reported to be present in the human colon as well as in animal models[15-17].

Determination of eicosanoids is, however, associated with methodological difficulties. A major concern regards the spontaneous synthesis of eicosanoids in response to trauma − such as tissue excision and homogenization. Thus the tissue content determination is the less accurate and valid method for studying the role of endogenously synthesized eicosanoids in various physiological and pathological mechanisms occurring in the gut.

The precise cellular origin of gut eicosanoids is not certain. Whereas epithelial cells are able to synthesize eicosanoids, most appear to be produced in the subepithelial layer by leukocytes, platelets and endothelial cells[18]. Their catabolism occurs mainly in the surface epithelial cells[19].

Effect of eicosanoids on intestine

1. Electrolytes and water transport
Several prostanoids have been shown to induce small intestinal secretion and to change gut motility[6]. The effect on the human colon is less established. In rat and rabbit models, high concentrations of PGE and PGA impaired colonic fluid transport and recently 5-HPETE and 5-HETE (but not LTB_4 or LTC_4) have been shown to stimulate short circuit current and active chloride secretion in rabbit colon[10]. These compounds however have not yet been shown to affect human colonic secretion. The possible mechanisms whereby these compounds affect colonic secretion are stimulation of adenylate cyclase

2

activity[20,21], effects on calcium flux[22], inhibition of Na^+-K^+-ATPase activity[23] and effects on mucosal blood flow or intestinal motility[12,24].

2. Blood flow

The effect of eicosanoids on splanchnic blood flow has been previously studied[25]. However, their effect on large intestinal blood flow is not well established. PGF and thromboxane A_2 generally induce mesenteric vasoconstriction, while PGE and PGI_2 induce vasodilatation. The physiological effects of the various eicosanoids including lipoxygenase metabolites on gut blood flow are still to be fully explored.

3. Mucus secretion

Prostanoids stimulate mucus secretion in the small and large intestine[26,27]. In organ culture of rat colonic mucosa, cyclic AMP increased glycoprotein synthesis[28]. This implies that the mechanism by which PGs increase mucus production may be mediated by cyclic AMP. As in the stomach, mucus secretion may play a role in intestinal protection against injurious agents.

4. Motility

Extensive work has been done on the effects of eicosanoids on intestinal smooth muscle[11,29,30]. Generally, the longitudinal muscle is contracted by PGE, PGF and leukotrienes, and the circular muscle relaxes to PGE and contracts to PGF. These effects depend upon the experimental conditions and animal species. In humans, administration of prostanoids may cause abdominal crampy pain. PGE may alter colonic motility waves.

Eicosanoids and IBD

1. Detection and characterization

Since IBD is characterized by local and systemic inflammatory signs and diarrhoea, the role of arachidonic acid metabolites in IBD has attracted many investigators and stimulated intensive research. Gould[31] was the first to report PGE levels in colonic secretions of patients with active ulcerative colitis. Further work was done in vitro on rectal mucosa of patients with ulcerative colitis[13,32]. Rectal mucosal biopsies were excised from patients with active ulcerative colitis, and incubated on a meshed grid in an organ culture dish. It was clearly shown that PGE_2, 6-keto-$PGF_{1\alpha}$ and thromboxane release from the diseased mucosa into the culture medium was significantly increased as compared to the release from control biopsies. There was about 100% increase of PGE_2 and thromboxane release, and about 50% increase in prostacyclin. Moreover, prostanoid release by biopsies obtained from patients in remission was similar to that found in controls. A similar increase in prostanoid release was also detected in colonic mucosa of patients with active Crohn's disease[33].

The trend of increased prostanoid production by the inflamed bowel was confirmed by other authors using different methodology. Rampton et al.[14] using the in vivo rectal dialysis technique showed that colonic PGE_2 release in untreated acute ulcerative colitis was 13 times higher than in controls. They also showed a linear correlation between increase of PGE_2 release, and decrease of rectal potential difference. This correlation is attributed to the inflammatory process which simultaneously alters epithelial permeability and increases PGE_2 release. These data sustain the notion that increased prostanoid production in IBD may account, at least in part, for the local and systemic inflammatory manifestations as well as for the diarrhoea. The lipoxygenase pathway products, 5-HETE and leukotrienes, were also shown to increase in IBD – to an even greater extent than PGE_2 and thromboxane[15]. From the cumulative data, it seems that activation of both arachidonic acid metabolic pathways in IBD occurs at the level of free arachidonic acid rather than activation of cyclo-oxygenase or lipoxygenase. It is plausible that both pathways are activated by enhanced phospholipase activity in the inflamed mucosa, where tissue damage is ongoing. This is in agreement with the notion that prostanoids and leukotrienes play a role in enhancing and propagating the inflammation rather than being its primary cause. Moreover, there is evidence that leukotrienes induce PG and thromboxane release from macrophages[34] and perhaps also from other inflammatory cells, thus further contributing to the inflammatory signs.

In studies performed with primary cultures of epithelial and mononuclear cells isolated from inflamed colonic mucosa of patients with active Crohn's disease[18], it was found that prostanoid synthesis by mononuclear cells was up to 3.5- and 6-fold higher than that of mononuclear and epithelial cells isolated from normal colon. Increased prostanoid synthesis was also found in mononuclear cultures isolated from Crohn's ileitis as compared to prostanoid synthesis by ileal epithelial cells. In active ulcerative colitis, cultures of isolated mononuclear and epithelial cells also synthesized more prostanoids than respective cells isolated from normal colon. However, the difference was not statistically significant, most probably because of the high dose steroid therapy all ulcerative colitis patients were receiving. The results imply that in active IBD, mononuclear cells are responsible for the bulk of the increased intestinal prostanoid synthesis. Apart from the monocyte–macrophage system, lymphoid cells of the lamina propria may also be responsible for PG production. This, in turn, may influence some cellular immune functions[35] contributing to the inflammatory state in IBD. It is known that monocytosis frequently accompanies IBD[36]. Peripheral blood mononuclear cells were isolated from patients with active IBD and from controls and incubated for 24 hours. Prostanoid release into the culture medium was determined[37]. In active Crohn's disease, accumulation of PGE_2 and thromboxane was 2–3 times higher than in controls or in patients in remission. In ulcerative colitis, the release of both prostanoids was not enhanced. The increased prostanoid release by peripheral blood mononuclear cells in Crohn's disease parallels the state of the inflammation in the gut wall.

The lipoxygenase pathway is active in neutrophils and monocytes. This pathway produces leukotrienes and monohydroxyfatty acids. Leukotriene B_4 (LTB_4) and 5-hydroxy-6,8,11,14-eicosatetraenoic acid (5-HETE) are products of this pathway and the major arachidonic acid metabolites in neutrophils. LTB_4 and 5-HETE have significant biological effects: LTB_4 is a potent neutrophil chemotactic factor, increases vascular permeability and causes aggregation and degranulation of neutrophils. 5-HETE, having less potent effects on

4

neutrophils also induces, at high concentrations, colonic chloride secretion. The histological features of the inflamed mucosa in IBD include neutrophil infiltration and oedema, suggesting that chemotactic and permeability inducing factors have a role in this process. Sharon and Stenson[15] investigated the possible role of lipoxygenase pathway metabolites as mediators of inflammation in IBD. Colonic mucosal scrapings from surgical specimens of patients with IBD and of normal mucosa derived from uninvolved areas of colonic resections for adenocarcinoma were incubated with radiolabelled arachidonic acid. In the normal mucosa, the majority of the arachidonate was not metabolized. In contrast, in the diseased mucosa of either Crohn's disease or ulcerative colitis, a significant portion of the arachidonic acid was converted to LTB_4 or to monohydroxyfatty acids including 5-HETE. Determination of mucosal content of lipoxygenase products by lipid extractions and HPLC revealed that LTB_4, 12-HETE, 15-HETE and 5-HETE were endogenously present in IBD mucosa. LTB_4 content averaged 254 ng/g mucosa whereas normal mucosal content was less than 5 ng/g mucosa. Several other investigators[38,39] confirmed that increased synthesis of lipoxygenase products exists in IBD. In one of the studies[39], a marked decline in LTB_4 concentration was reported following treatment of ulcerative colitis patients with prednisolone.

Further evidence for the possible role of lipoxygenase products in IBD is derived from studies performed in the rat acetic acid colitis model[17]. In this model, though it lacks resemblance to human colitis, inflammation was induced 24 hours following administration of dilute acetic acid into the rat colon. Histology showed ulcerations with pronounced neutrophil infiltration. In the inflamed mucosa in contrast to the undamaged mucosa, an increased capacity to synthesize LTB_4, 5-HETE, 12-HETE and 15-HETE as well as an increased mucosal content of these compounds was found. When acetic acid colitis was induced in neutropenic rats, a significant decrease in the production of LTB_4 and 5-HETE from arachidonic acid was noted[40]. This implies that the major source of these substances is in the neutrophils infiltrating the mucosa. It was also shown that LTB_4 is probably the major chemotactic factor in ulcerative colitis mucosal extracts.

Recently, evidence has been presented regarding certain factors which may modulate arachidonic acid metabolism[41]. Bradykinin tissue levels are suggested to be increased in IBD, and may have effects on the propagation of the inflammatory reaction and may also contribute to the diarrhoea. Bradykinin binds to receptors on the baso-lateral membrane of epithelial cells[42]. It activates phospholipase A_2 which forms free arachidonic acid from phospholipids of the cell plasma membranes[43]. In normal small intestine and colon, bradykinin predominantly affects arachidonic acid metabolism via the cyclo-oxygenase pathway. It increases the release of PGE_2 in the small intestine and colon and alters intestinal active electrolyte transport. Most of these effects are blocked by indomethacin: however, some effects are probably exerted through the lipoxygenase pathway. Most studies on the effect of bradykinin on eicosanoid formation were performed in normal tissue. The role of bradykinin in affecting arachidonate metabolism in inflamed mucosa has not been thoroughly investigated.

2. Mechanism of diarrhoea in IBD

Eicosanoids, either of the cyclo-oxygenase or the lipoxygenase pathway, may contribute to diarrhoea in IBD. *In vitro,* certain eicosanoids alter active chloride secretion, active sodium transport and chloride absorption as well as intestinal motility. PGE_2 decreases active sodium and chloride absorption and increases chloride secretion in small and large bowel[6,20–22]. Recently, it has been shown that lipoxygenase products such as 5-HETE may also alter intestinal electrolyte transport in the rabbit[10]. However, not all lipoxygenase products have a demonstrable effect on intestinal transport, and the effect on intestinal motility has yet to be explored. Alteration in intestinal motility may also contribute to the diarrhoeal state[44].

Arachidonic acid metabolites may induce their effect on active ion transport by affecting several possible cellular mediators[41]. PGE_2 alters active electrolyte transport in the small intestine by activation of the adenylate cyclase–CAMP system. Prostacyclin increases and thromboxane decreases adenylate cyclase activity. Several prostanoids also decrease intestinal $Na^+–K^+$-ATPase activity, the enzyme responsible for sodium absorption[45]. In patients with active proctitis, colonic $Na^+–K^+$-ATPase activity is decreased[46] and colonic adenylate cyclase activity was shown to be increased. This increase was induced by the enhanced endogenous prostanoid synthesis[47]. Whether this increase is associated with changes in electrolyte transport awaits further studies. Intracellular messengers for the effect of lipoxygenase products have not yet been identified. Some data suggest that Ca^{2+} may play a role as a messenger for these products[41] although firm data regarding this hypothesis are still lacking.

3. Eicosanoids and inflammatory signs

Cyclo-oxygenase and lipoxygenase products may be involved in the pathogenesis of the symptoms and signs which commonly prevail in IBD. These compounds may induce pain, fever, anorexia, weight loss and leukocytosis. Leukotrienes were shown to decrease the threshold for pain and to amplify many aspects of the inflammatory response. However, the role of eicosanoids in producing any of these clinical manifestations in IBD has not yet been established.

Eicosanoids and treatment of IBD

In the upper GI tract, inhibition of prostanoid synthesis by non-steroidal anti-inflammatory drugs (NSAIDs) is associated with mucosal damage in humans and animals[7,48]. Exogenous prostanoids prevent or diminish this damage. In the lower GI tract, indomethacin suppositories induced a change in rectal mucosal potential difference and potassium transport which reverted towards normal on indomethacin withdrawal[49]. Moreover, Rampton *et al.* found that several patients with ulcerative colitis relapsed following ingestion of analgesics such as paracetamol[50]. From our own experience, application of flufenamic acid enemas to ulcerative colitis patients in remission caused relapse of the inflammation and urged us to stop this trial. These data suggest that

6

colonic prostanoid deficiency may, as in the stomach and duodenum, predispose to mucosal damage and disease relapse.

On the other hand, the firm observation that in active IBD colonic prostanoid and leukotriene synthesis is increased and may mediate the inflammatory response was confirmed by many groups in studies performed on big populations. It is also difficult to explain, on the basis of prostanoid synthesis inhibition, the effect of paracetamol in induction of disease relapse. Paracetamol is a very weak cyclo-oxygenase inhibitor *in vitro*, and does not affect mucosal cyclo-oxygenase in the upper GI tract. Moreover, since huge quantities of NSAIDs are consumed by large populations, the prevalence of relapses of IBD would be expected to be much higher than the present rates. Thus evidence for prostanoid deficiency as a factor in induction of the disease is not firmly substantiated.

Goldin and Rachmilewitz[51] performed the only study in which direct evidence of colonic 'cytoprotection' by exogenous prostanoid administration was evaluated. Twenty-four patients with ulcerative colitis in complete remission maintained by sulphasalazine were allocated to receive either abraprostil (Upjohn) 15(R)-15-methyl-PGE_2 200 μg/day, previously used successfully in a higher dose for the treatment of peptic ulcer disease, or to continue with sulphasalazine 2.0 g/day for 28 weeks. Of the 12 patients who discontinued sulphasalazine and received the prostaglandin preparation five flared up within the first four weeks and three others had to stop the trial because of severe diarrhoea. In contrast, only two of the 12 sulphasalazine-treated patients flared up during the 28 weeks' trial. The adverse response to the synthetic prostaglandin indicates that the inflammatory and the diarrhogenic effect of this specific prostanoid are readily expressed in patients with ulcerative colitis overcoming the potential cytoprotective effects. However, it may very well be that a smaller dose or a different prostanoid will be found useful for maintaining remission in ulcerative colitis.

The role of eicosanoids has been of interest also in regard to the therapeutic effects of the conventional drugs applied in IBD – steroids and sulphasalazine. Glucocorticoids, the most potent drugs available for the treatment of active IBD, prevent the formation of free arachidonic acid from arachidonate bound to membrane phospholipids by inhibiting phospholipase A activity and thus blocking both cyclo-oxygenase and lipoxygenase pathways. Prednisolone was shown, *in vitro*, to inhibit prostanoid synthesis by colonic mucosa[52] as well as to inhibit the release of arachidonate from cell membranes by induction of the inhibitory protein macrocortin. However, it is difficult to evaluate whether the prompt beneficial effect of glucocorticoids can be exclusively related to their effect on arachidonic acid metabolism, or whether this effect is shared by other eicosanoid-independent mechanisms, such as alteration of the immune response. The effect of a non-glucocorticoid drug in the active disease state which inhibits phospholipase A activity thus compromising substrate availability for eicosanoids formation would help to clarify the mechanism whereby glucocorticoids exert their beneficial effects and may also prove to be an alternative treatment modality.

Several *in vitro* studies have shown that sulphasalazine and its breakdown product, 5-aminosalicylic acid (5-ASA), decrease prostanoid synthesis, probably by inhibition of microsomal cyclo-oxygenase. We have reported that sulfasalazine and 5-ASA inhibit PGE_2 release by cultured colonic mucosa[13]. 5-ASA also decreases PGI_2 and thromboxane release[32]. 5-ASA is a less potent inhibitor of prostanoid synthesis as compared to indomethacin or fenamates but, with respect to inhibition of prostanoid synthesis, is the active moiety in sulphasalazine. Other observations indicated that in lower concentrations sulphasalazine, but not 5-ASA or sulphapyridine, inhibited the degradation of colonic prostanoids *in vitro*[53,54]. Prostanoid degradation is an important factor in the determination of net prostanoid tissue levels. The decreased colonic prostanoid synthesis noted following application of sulphasalazine may represent the net effect of the induced inhibition of prostanoid synthesis and the degradation. Recently, it was reported that 5-ASA could act as a co-factor for prostanoid synthesis in human rectal mucosa. The finding that sulphasalazine decreases prostanoid degradation led to the hypothesis that it may act by promotion of colonic prostanoid levels, thereby enhancing cytoprotection and thus maintaining remission. This hypothesis is not well substantiated especially in view of the fact that treatment with exogenous prostanoid failed to maintain remission and even induced exacerbation of IBD.

Lipoxygenase products may also mediate the inflammatory response especially via their chemotactic effect, thus inducing accumulation of inflammatory cells in the affected area of the gut[41]. Sulphasalazine, 5-ASA, and its metabolite N-acetyl-5-ASA may inhibit the lipoxygenase pathway in human colonic mucosa and other tissues[17,40] thus providing an additional explanation for their mode of action. This effect, however, is weak and its correlation with the clinical state awaits further evaluation. Potent inhibitors of the cyclo-oxygenase pathway, such as indomethacin or fenamates, cause experimental enterocolitis and may aggravate colitis in the human. This deleterious effect on the gut may be explained by inhibition of the synthesis of 'protective' prostaglandins or by a shift in the arachidonic acid metabolism from the cyclo-oxygenase to the lipoxygenase pathway thus increasing the levels of leukotrienes and maintaining the signs of inflammation. In order to further evaluate the role of lipoxygenase products, patients with active ulcerative colitis were treated with benoxoprofen, a cyclo-oxygenase and lipoxygenase inhibitor, but no beneficial effect was achieved[55]. On the other hand, in experimental colitis induced by acetic acid in the rat[56], administration of indomethacin intrarectally was associated with decreased severity of inflammation and decreased PGE_2 content of the colonic mucosa. In conclusion, the evidence that the mechanism responsible for the therapeutic effect of the drugs used in IBD is directed towards inhibiting either the cyclo-oxygenase or the lipoxygenase pathway or both is still inconsistent, controversial and deserves further prompt evaluation.

It is also difficult to attribute the beneficial effect of sulphasalazine and 5-ASA only to their modification of arachidonic acid metabolism by either pathway. During clinical relapse, treatment with sulphasalazine or 5-ASA alone is usually not sufficient to induce remission. Moreover, withdrawal of the drug from patients in remission did not change either the disease state or rectal mucosa PGE_2 content. Differential effects of sulphasalazine on eicosanoid synthesis were noted *in vitro* where low concentrations of the drug selectively inhibited thromboxane production[57]. This selectivity may contribute to an effect on immune function or render increased resistance to injury, since thromboxane is regarded as a vasoconstrictor and ulcerogenic agent in the gastric mucosa[58]. Inhibiting thromboxane synthesis or applying thromboxane antagonists may also promote the release of cytoprotective prostanoids such as prostacyclin[59].

The combination of glucocorticoids and NSAIDs was also tested in regard to their effects on colonic prostanoid synthesis. *In vitro*, the combination of prednisolone and flufenamic acid has a synergistic effect on inhibiting PGE_2 formation by colonic mucosa[32]. This may suggest that combination therapy with corticosteroids and certain NSAIDs when administered in low doses may have a favourable role in reducing the inflammatory signs. The effect of this combination should be tested on the lipoxygenase pathway as well.

REFERENCES

1. Donaldson, R.M. Jr. (1983). Crohn's disease. In Sleisenger, M.H. and Fordtran, J.S. (eds.) *Gastrointestinal Disease*, pp. 1088–1121. (Philadelphia: W. B. Saunders Co.)
2. Cello, J.P. (1983). Ulcerative colitis. In Sleisenger, M.H. and Fordtran, J.S. (eds.) *Gastrointestinal Disease*, pp. 1123–1168. (Philadelphia: W. B. Saunders Co.)
3. Vane, J.R. (1976). Prostaglandins as mediators of inflammation. *Adv. Prostgl. Thromboxane Res.*, **2**, 791–801
4. Lewis, G.P. (1983). Immunoregulatory activity of metabolites of arachidonic acid and their role in inflammation. *Br. Med. Bull.*, **39**, 243–248
5. Malmsten, C.L. (1985). Prostaglandins, thromboxanes and leukotrienes in inflammation. *Semin. Arthritis Rheum.*, **15** (Suppl. 1), 29–35
6. Rachmilewitz, D. (1980). Prostaglandins and diarrhea. *Dig. Dis. Sci.*, **25**, 897–899
7. Miller, T. (1983). Protective effects of prostaglandins against gastric mucosal damage: current knowledge and proposed mechanisms. *Am. J. Physiol.*, **245**, G 601–623
8. Ford-Hutchinson, A.W., Bray, M.A., Doig, M.V., Shipley, M.F. and Smith, J.H. (1980). Leukotriene B, a potent chemotactic and aggregating substance released from polymorphonuclear leukocytes. *Nature*, **286**, 264–265
9. Dahlen, S.E., Bjork, J., Hedquist, P., Arfors, K.E., Hammarstrom, S., Lindgren, J.A. and Samuelsson, B. (1981). Leukotrienes promote plasma leakage and leukocyte adhesion in postcapillary venules: *in vivo* effects with relevance to the acute inflammatory response. *Proc. Natl. Acad. Sci. USA*, **78**, 3887–3891
10. Musch, M.W., Miller, R.J., Field, M. and Siegel, M.I. (1982). Stimulation of colonic secretion by lipoxygenase metabolites of arachidonic acid. *Science*, **217**, 1255–1256
11. Bennett, A., Stamford, I.F. and Stockley, H.L. (1977). Estimation and characterisation of prostaglandins in the human gastrointestinal tract. *Br. J. Pharmacol.*, **61**, 579–586
12. Robert, A. (1976). Prostaglandins and the digestive system. In Ramwell, P.W. (ed.) *The Prostaglandins*, pp. 225–266. (New York: Plenum Press)
13. Sharon, P., Ligumsky, M., Rachmilewitz, D. and Zor, U. (1978). Role of prostaglandins in ulcerative colitis. *Gastroenterology*, **75**, 638–640
14. Rampton, D.S., Sladen, G.E. and Youlten, L.J.F. (1980). Rectal mucosa prostaglandin E_2 release and its relation to disease activity, electrical potential difference and treatment in ulcerative colitis. *Gut*, **21**, 591–596
15. Sharon, P. and Stenson, W. (1984). Enhanced synthesis of leukotriene B_4 by colonic mucosa in inflammatory bowel disease. *Gastroenterology*, **86**, 453–460
16. Boughton-Smith, N.K., Hawkey, C.J. and Whittle, B.J.R. (1983). Biosynthesis of lipoxygenase and cyclo-oxygenase products from (^{14}C)-arachidonic acid by human colonic mucosa. *Gut*, **24**, 1175–1182

17. Sharon, P. and Stenson, W.F. (1985). Metabolism of arachidonic acid in acetic acid colitis in rats. *Gastroenterology*, **88**, 55–63
18. Zifroni, A., Treves, A.J., Sachar, D.B. and Rachmilewitz, D. (1983). Prostanoid synthesis by cultured intestinal epithelial and mononuclear cells in inflammatory bowel disease. *Gut*, **24**, 659–664
19. Smith, S.S., Warhurst, G. and Turnberg, L.A. (1982). Synthesis and degradation of prostaglandin E_2 in the epithelial and subepithelial layers in the rat intestine. *Biochem. Biophys. Acta*, **713**, 684–687
20. Matuchansky, C. and Coutrot, S. (1978). The role of prostaglandins in the study of intestinal water and electrolyte transport in man. *Biomedicine*, **28**, 143–148
21. Racusen, L. and Binder, H.J. (1980). Effect of prostaglandin on ion transport across isolated colonic mucosa. *Dig. Dis. Sci.*, **25**, 900–904
22. Rask-Madsen, J. and Bukhave, K. (1983). Prostaglandins and intestinal secretion. In Turnberg, L.A. (ed.) *Intestinal Secretion*. Proceedings of the 3rd BSG/SK&F International Workshop, pp. 76–83 (Knapp, Drewett & Sons)
23. Sharon, P., Karmeli, F. and Rachmilewitz, D. (1981). Celiac disease, pernicious anemia, colchicine therapy and ulcerative colitis: a common role for Na–K-ATPase in decreased intestinal water absorption (Abstract). *Gastroenterology*, **80**, 1282
24. Bennett, A. (1972). Effects of prostaglandins on the gastrointestinal tract. In Karim, S.M.M. (ed.) *Prostaglandins: Progress in Research*, pp. 205–21 (Lancaster: MTP)
25. Gallavan, R.H. and Jacobson, E.D. (1982). Prostaglandins and the splanchnic circulation. *Proc. Soc. Exp. Biol. Med.*, **170**, 391–397
26. Cassidy, M.M. and Lightfoot, F.G. (1980). Effects of prostaglandin E_1 administered by gastric intubation, on mucus secretory patterns in rat small intestine. *Adv. Prostagl. Thromboxane Res.*, **8**, 1589–1593
27. Rampton, D.S., Breuer, N.F., Vaja, S.G., Sladen, G.E. and Dowling, R.H. (1981). Role of prostaglandins in bile salt-induced changes in rat colonic structure and function. *Clin. Sci.*, **61**, 641–648
28. Lamont, J.T. and Ventola, A. (1977). Stimulation of colonic glycoprotein synthesis by dibutyryl cyclic AMP and theophylline. *Gastroenterology*, **72**, 82–86
29. Bennett, A. and Fleschner, B. (1970). Prostaglandins and the gastrointestinal tract. *Gastroenterology*, **59**, 790–800
30. Waller, S.L. (1973). Prostaglandins and the gastrointestinal tract. *Gut*, **14**, 402–417
31. Gould, S.R. (1976). Assay of prostaglandin-like substances in faeces and their measurement in ulcerative colitis. *Prostaglandins*, **11**, 489–497
32. Ligumsky, M., Karmeli, F., Sharon, P., Zor, U., Cohen, F. and Rachmilewitz, D. (1981). Enhanced thromboxane A_2 and prostacyclin production by cultured rectal mucosa in ulcerative colitis and its inhibition by steroids and sulphasalazine. *Gastroenterology*, **81**, 444–449
33. Rachmilewitz, D., Karmeli, F., Zifroni, A., Hawkey, C.J. and Sachar, D.B. (1982). Enhanced prostanoid synthesis in Crohn's disease (Abstract). *Gastroenterology*, **82**, 1154
34. Feuerstein, N., Foegh, M. and Ramwell, P.W. (1981). Leukotrienes C_4 and D_4 induce prostaglandin and thromboxane release from rat peritoneal macrophages. *Br. J. Pharmacol.*, **72**, 389–391
35. Droller, M.J., Schneider, M.U. and Perlman, P. (1978). A possible role of prostaglandins in the inhibition of natural and antibody-dependent cell-mediated cytotoxicity against tumor cells. *Cell. Immunol.*, **39**, 165–177
36. Auer, I.O., Wechsler, W. and Ziemer, E. (1978). Immune status in Crohn's disease. Leukocyte and lymphocyte subpopulations in peripheral blood. *Scand. J. Gastroenterology*, **13**, 561–571
37. Rachmilewitz, D., Ligumsky, M., Haimovitz, A. and Treves, A.J. (1982). Prostanoid synthesis by cultured peripheral blood mononuclear cells in inflammatory disease of the bowel. *Gastroenterology*, **82**, 673–679
38. Peskar, B.M., Dreyling, K.W., May, B., Thieves, M., Morgenroth, K., Goebell, H. and Peskar, B.A. (1985). Increased formation of leukotriene B_4 and sulphidopeptide-leukotrienes by rectal mucosa of patients with Crohn's disease and ulcerative colitis (Abstract). *Gut*, **26**, A 252–253
39. Lauritsen, K., Laursen, L.S., Bukhave, K. and Rask-Madsen, J. (1985). Effects of systemic

prednisolone on arachidonic acid metabolites determined by equilibrium *in vivo* dialysis of rectum in severe relapsing ulcerative colitis (Abstract). *Gastroenterology*, **88**, 1466

40. Stenson, W.F. (1986). Role of lipoxygenase products as mediators of inflammation in IBD. In Rachmilewitz, D. (ed.) *Inflammatory Bowel Diseases 1986*. Proceedings of the 2nd International Symposium on IBD in Jerusalem. pp. 95—103 (Dordrecht: Martinus Nijhoff)
41. Donowitz, M. (1985). Arachidonic acid metabolites and their role in inflammatory bowel disease. *Gastroenterology*, **88**, 580—587
42. Manning, D.C., Snyder, S.A., Kachur, J.F., Miller, R.J. and Field, M. (1982). Bradykinin receptor-mediated chloride secretion in intestinal function. *Nature*, **299**, 256—259
43. Schremmer, J.M., Blank, M.L. and Wykle, R.L. (1979). Bradykinin-stimulated release of ^{3}H-arachidonic acid from phospholipids of $HSDM_1C_1$: comparison of diacyl phospholipids and plasmalogens as sources of prostaglandin precursors. *Prostaglandins*, **18**, 491—505
44. Konturek, S.J., Thor, P., Pawlik, W., Gustaw, P. and Dembinski, A. (1982). Role of prostaglandins in myoelectric, motor and metabolic activity of the small intestine in the dog. In Weisbeck, M. (ed.) *Motility of the Digestive Tract*, pp. 437—44. (New York: Raven Press)
45. Matsukawa, R., Terao, N., Hayakawa, M. and Takiguchi, H. (1981). Effect of prostaglandin A_2 on Na^+-K^+-ATPase activity in basolateral plasma membrane of rat intestine *in vitro*. *Biochem. Biophys. Res. Commun.*, **101**, 1305—1310
46. Rachmilewitz, D., Karmeli, F. and Sharon, P. (1984). Decreased colonic Na-K-ATPase activity in active ulcerative colitis. *Isr. J. Med. Sci.*, **20**, 681—684
47. Rachmilewitz, D., Karmeli, F. and Selinger, Z. (1983). Increased colonic adenylate cyclase activity in active ulcerative colitis. *Gastroenterology*, **85**, 12—16
48. Hawkey, C.J. and Rampton, D.S. (1985). Prostaglandins and the gastrointestinal mucosa: are they important in its function, disease or treatment? *Gastroenterology*, **89**, 1162—1188
49. Rampton, D.S. and Barton, T.P. (1984). Are prostaglandins cytoprotective in the human large intestine? The effect of indomethacin on rectal mucosal function and prostaglandin E_2 release *in vivo*. *Agents Actions*, **14**, 715—718
50. Rampton, D.S., McNeil, N.I. and Sarner, M. (1983). Analgesic ingestions and other factors preceding relapse in ulcerative colitis. *Gut*, **24**, 187—189
51. Goldin, E. and Rachmilewitz, D. (1983). Prostanoids cytoprotection for maintaining remission in ulcerative colitis. *Dig. Dis. Sci.*, **28**, 809—811
52. Hawkey, C.J. and Truelove, S.C. (1981). Effect of prednisolone on prostaglandin synthesis by rectal mucosa in ulcerative colitis: investigation by laminar flow bioassay and radioimmunoassay. *Gut*, **22**, 190—193
53. Hoult, J.R.S. and Moore, P.K. (1978). Sulphasalazine is a potent inhibitor of prostaglandin 15-hydroxydehydrogenase: possible basis for therapeutic action in ulcerative colitis. *Br. J. Pharmacol.*, **64**, 6—8
54. Kolassa, N., Becker, R. and Wiener, H. (1985). Influence of sulphasalazine, 5-aminosalicylic acid and sulphapyridine on prostanoid synthesis and metabolism in rabbit colonic mucosa. *Prostaglandins*, **29**, 133—142
55. Hawkey, C.J. and Rampton, D.S. (1983). Benoxoprofen in the treatment of active ulcerative colitis. *Prostagl. Leukotrienes Med.*, **10**, 405—410
56. Mann, N.S., Demers, L.M. (1983). Experimental colitis studied by colonoscopy in the rat: effect of indomethacin. *Gastrointest. Endosc.*, **29**, 77—82
57. Boughton-Smith, N.K., Hawkey, C.J. and Whittle, B.J.R. (1983). Sulphasalazine and the inhibition of thromboxane synthesis in human colonic mucosa (Abstract). *Br. J. Pharmacol.*, **80**, 604P
58. Whittle, B.J.R., Kauffman, G.L. and Moncada, S. (1981). Vasoconstriction with thromboxane A_2 induces ulceration of the gastric mucosa. *Nature*, **292**, 472—474
59. O'Keefe, E.H., Edward, C.K., Liu, Greenberg, R. and Ogletree, M.L. (1985). Effects of a thromboxane synthetase inhibitor and a thromboxane antagonist on release and activity of thromboxane A_2 and prostacyclin *in vitro*. *Prostaglandins*, **29**, 785—797

2
Laboratory methods for studying the role of eicosanoids in inflammatory bowel disease

N. K. Boughton-Smith and B. J. R. Whittle

INTRODUCTION

Since Gould first described an increase in the level of prostaglandin-like substances in the faeces of patients with active ulcerative colitis[1], considerable research work has centred on the role of prostaglandins and other eicosanoids in inflammatory bowel disease (IBD). The results of these studies have been considered elsewhere in this book. The present chapter describes the laboratory methods that have been used to study the role of eicosanoids in IBD.

Eicosanoids

The term eicosanoid can be used to describe any 20-carbon (eicosa means 20) fatty acid. However, since the major fatty acids formed by mammalian tissues are derived from arachidonic acid (eicosatetraenoic acid), the term eicosanoid is generally used to describe this fatty acid and the family of metabolites formed from it.

The concentration of free arachidonic acid in cells is very low, as most of it is incorporated into the phospholipids of cell membranes. The liberation of arachidonic acid from phospholipids by the hydrolytic action of phospholipases, particularly phospholipase A_2, is the rate-limiting step in the biosynthesis of the eicosanoids[2]. Early investigations demonstrated that mechanical and chemical stimuli or immunological challenge of tissues led to the biosynthesis of prostaglandins. Therefore, manipulation of tissue can lead to mechanical stimulation of membranes and hence to prostaglandin formation, and this must be considered in all *in vitro* studies with intestinal tissues[3].

The metabolism of arachidonic acid can be brought about by two distinct types of enzyme, cyclo-oxygenase and lipoxygenase (Figure 2.1).

Cyclo-oxygenase products

Cyclo-oxygenase catalyses the oxidation of arachidonic acid via unstable endoperoxide intermediates to the prostaglandins and thromboxane. These prostanoids have potent biological activity. There is considerable evidence to suggest that the vasodilation produced by prostaglandin E_2 (PGE$_2$) and prostacyclin (PGI$_2$) is important in the erythema and oedema of acute inflammation[3,4]. Inhibition of cyclo-oxygenase, and therefore prostaglandin formation, by non-steroid anti-inflammatory drugs is considered to be the mechanism of their anti-inflammatory activity[3-5]. The prostaglandins also have potent effects on intestinal function[6]. The vasodilator prostaglandins increase intestinal blood flow, while PGE$_2$ and PGF$_{2\alpha}$ stimulate intestinal motility in a variety of species including man. Prostaglandins of the E and F series and their analogues also evoke a watery diarrhoea in experimental animals and man, probably mediated by changes in mucosal water and electrolyte secretion[7,8].

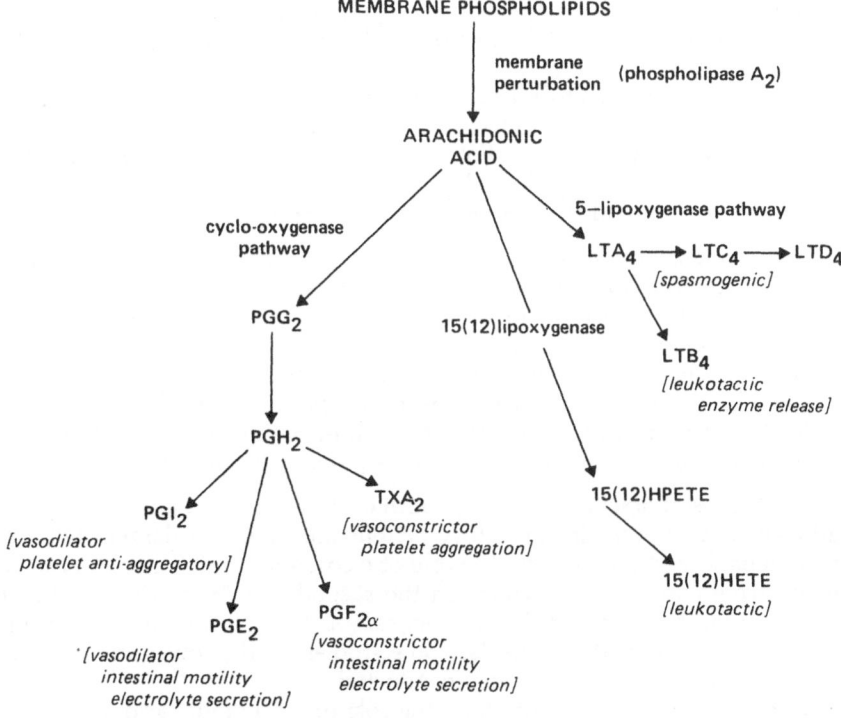

Figure 2.1 Major pathways of arachidonic acid metabolism, showing the biological activity of individual eicosanoids. (PG – prostaglandin; TX – thromboxane; HPETE – hydroperoxyeicosatetraenoic acid; HETE – hydroxyeicosatetraenoic acid; LT – leukotriene)

Lipoxygenase products

The major lipoxygenase enzymes are the 12-, 15- and 5-lipoxygenases, which convert arachidonic acid to unstable monohydroperoxy acids (HPETEs) from which are formed the more stable monohydroxy acids (HETEs)[5]. Further transformation of 5-HPETE leads to the formation of an unstable intermediate leukotriene (LT), A_4, which can be enzymically transformed[9] to the dihydroxy acid LTB_4 or to the sulphidopeptidyl leukotrienes, LTC_4, LTD_4 and LTE_4.

The lipoxygenase-derived metabolites of arachidonic acid have potent effects in activating leukocytes[3,4,10]. The original finding that 12-HETE was chemotactic for human polymorphonuclear leukocytes has been extended to include the other monohydroxy and hydroperoxy acids. The dihydroxy metabolite, LTB_4, is one of the most potent chemotactic agents known and also induces aggregation, lysosomal enzyme release and superoxide production in polymorphonuclear leukocytes.

Role of eicosanoids in inflammatory bowel disease

Many of the effects of the prostaglandins on the intestine are similar to the clinical manifestations of active IBD[11]. These intestinal actions, combined with the proinflammatory effects of both cyclo-oxygenase and lipoxygenase products, suggest that metabolites of arachidonic acid may be important in IBD.

The eicosanoids therefore have many biological activities which may be expected of a mediator of inflammation. However, for a substance to be considered as a mediator, several other criteria have to be fulfilled. The criteria for the identification of a physiological mediator were originally described by Sir Henry Dale and have been modified to apply to inflammation:

(1) The proposed mediator should have the appropriate biological activity.
(2) The mediator should be recoverable from the site of inflammation.
(3) The mediator must be identified by appropriate pharmacological and physicochemical techniques.
(4) Antagonists of the action or inhibitors of the release of the mediator should reduce the inflammatory response produced by the mediator.
(5) Inhibition of destruction (or metabolism) of the mediator should increase the magnitude of the inflammatory response attributed to it.

Metabolites of arachidonic acid of both cyclo-oxygenase and lipoxygenase pathways have potent inflammatory actions and therefore largely fulfill the first criteria. Investigations into the role of eicosanoids in inflammatory bowel disease have concentrated mainly on the second and third criteria, with the identification, by appropriate techniques, of their formation in inflamed intestinal tissue from IBD patients. Some studies on the fourth criteria, using enzyme inhibitors, have also been conducted.

In order to understand more fully the role of arachidonic acid metabolites, it is important to know the profile of products that can be formed by intestinal tissue and whether they are altered in IBD. Several investigations have assessed the metabolites of arachidonic acid formed by normal and inflamed human and animal intestinal tissues. In addition, the effect of drugs, used in the treatment of IBD, on arachidonic acid metabolism in both human and animal colonic tissues, and in animal models of inflammatory bowel disease have also been studied.

The methods used in these investigations are outlined below, with a more detailed description of the methodology used in some of our own studies.

EICOSANOID FORMATION IN INFLAMMATORY BOWEL DISEASE

Methods *in vivo*

The first reported increase of prostaglandins in ulcerative colitis was in the faeces of patients with active disease[1]. The prostaglandins were extracted from stools and bioassayed for prostaglandin-like activity using the rat stomach strip. The results were later confirmed[12] by specific radioimmunoassay (RIA) of $PGF_{2\alpha}$ and PGE_2. An increase in the level of prostaglandin metabolites has also been measured in the plasma and in the urine of patients with ulcerative colitis[12,13].

More recently, investigators have used dialysis bags to measure the *in vivo* formation of prostaglandins and other eicosanoids. The dialysis bags were either placed in the rectum of patients or control subjects[14], or taken orally (equilibrium dialysis) and collected after passage through the entire gastrointestinal tract[15]. The use of dialysis bags also allows the measurement of changes in electrolytes and facilitates the recording of potential difference across the colonic mucosa[14]. Samples from the rectal dialysis are relatively clean and eicosanoids can be assayed directly or further purified by lipid extraction before estimation. Using this technique, increases in PGE_2 and other eicosanoids, including LTB_4, were measured in the dialysate from patients with IBD, the levels of which were dependent on the disease activity[14,15]. Rectal dialysis as used in man could also be adapted for use in experimental models of inflammatory bowel disease.

These relatively non-invasive *in vivo* methods of assessing eicosanoid synthesis have the advantage of enabling a continuous monitoring of eicosanoid levels in patients during relapse and remission of disease. However, they do not define the source of the eicosanoids measured. While in rectal dialysis most of the material is undoubtedly from local tissue, it does not provide a direct measurement of arachidonic acid metabolism by the intestinal tissue.

Methods *in vitro*

Most investigations into eicosanoid formation in IBD have utilized *in vitro* techniques. Various tissue preparations have been used to evaluate the metabolism of either endogenous or exogenous arachidonic acid (Table 2.1). A number of studies have also investigated the *in vitro* effects of drugs used in the treatment of IBD on eicosanoid synthesis.

Table 2.1 Preparations of colonic tissue used to measure eicosanoid formation

Tissue preparation	Eicosanoids	
	Cyclo-oxygenase	Lipoxygenase
In vivo dialysate	14,15	15
Organ culture	18,19,20,21	–
Fragments	22,24,29	29,34,37
Homogenate	25,26,35,38	26,29,35
Cell culture	30	

Eicosanoid formation from endogenous arachidonic acid has been measured in vivo dialysate, organ and cell culture. In studies on the metabolism of [^{14}C]arachidonic acid, homogenates and tissue fragments of colon were used. Citations as in reference list

Intestinal tissue
In the majority of studies, human intestinal tissue has been used. Biopsy samples of rectal mucosa, obtained during sigmoidoscopy, have been a common source of tissue. Bowel tissue removed at operation for severe IBD has also been a source of inflamed tissue. Control tissue has either been obtained as biopsy specimens from healthy volunteers or as macroscopically and histologically normal tissue obtained at operation for carcinoma. In some studies, tissue from patients with intestinal disorders other than IBD, such as irritable bowel syndrome, have been used.

Tissue preparation and incubation
The metabolism of arachidonic acid is a dynamic process. The metabolites are not stored preformed but synthesized on demand when a particular stimulus occurs. The tissue preparations and incubation procedures used to study eicosanoids have been designed to measure either new synthesis from endogenous arachidonic acid or the conversion of exogenous arachidonic acid, usually radiolabelled arachidonic acid. Several tissue preparations have been used, ranging from whole tissue or organ culture to subcellular enzyme preparations. Whatever the tissue preparation used, it should be emphasized that mechanical manipulation of tissue can stimulate the release of arachidonic acid and hence eicosanoid synthesis. When comparing the capacity of control and diseased tissue for eicosanoid biosynthesis, it is therefore important that all the tissues are handled in a uniform manner.

Organ culture
The synthesis of prostanoids by biopsies of human rectal mucosa has been studied using non-proliferative organ culture. The method, using colonic tissue, was described by Eastwood and Trier[16,17] and used by Sharon et al.[18] to demonstrate an increase in PGE$_2$ formation by rectal mucosa from patients with active ulcerative colitis. Biopsy samples of rectal mucosa, having an average weight of 10 mg, were placed on stainless-steel mesh over a culture dish well filled with culture medium. After an initial incubation of an hour the medium was replaced with fresh medium, presumably to remove any

prostanoid formed during tissue handling, and incubated for a further 23 hours. The levels of prostanoids in the medium were then measured, either directly or following lipid extraction, using specific RIA[18-20] or laminar flow bioassay[20]. In early experiments, the culture medium used contained foetal calf serum but in subsequent studies, in which thromboxane B_2 (TxB_2) was measured, the foetal calf serum was omitted since it interfered with the estimation of immuno-reactive TxB_2. As well as demonstrating an increase in prostanoid formation by inflamed colonic mucosa from IBD patients, this technique has been used to study the *in vitro* effect of drugs, such as sulphasalazine and prednisolone, on prostanoid synthesis by the cultured tissue[18-21]. These drugs were added directly to the incubation medium.

One of the major considerations when using organ culture is the viability of the tissue[17]. Each cell *in vivo* is within a few microns of the capillaries which supply nutrients and oxygen. In contrast, many cells *in vitro*, particularly those in the centre of the biopsy, may be several hundred microns from nutrient medium or surrounding oxygen and are therefore greatly dependent on diffusion into the tissue.

Tissue fragments
Fragments of human biopsy or rat colonic tissue have been used in short incubation procedures and therefore largely overcome the problems of cell viability. In drug studies, fragments (50–60 mg) of intestinal tissue were preincubated with drugs for 60 min at 4°C to allow drug penetration into the tissue before a subsequent incubation at 37°C. The prostanoids released into the medium were measured by RIA[22].

The capacity of fragments of rectal mucosal biopsy (20–48 mg) to synthesize eicosanoids has been determined using mechanical stimulation of the tissue. A vortex-mixing procedure was used to agitate the tissue. The 'generated' prostacyclin was measured immediately by bioassay, utilizing the potent anti-platelet aggregatory activity of prostacyclin to measure its concentration[23]. Using this method, inflamed tissue from patients with ulcerative colitis was found to have an increased capacity to generate prostacyclin compared with control tissue[24].

Homogenates
The whole-tissue preparations described so far have been used to measure eicosanoid synthesis from endogenous substrate. In studies in which exogenous arachidonic acid metabolism is used, usually [14C]arachidonic acid ([14C]AA), it is beneficial to homogenize the tissue to enable the exogenous substrate direct access to metabolizing enzymes. This method was originally used in IBD studies by Harris *et al.*[25] to determine 'prostaglandin synthetase activity' in biopsies of human rectal mucosa. In these studies, the tissue was homogenized for 'not greater than 15 seconds' in a buffer solution containing a number of cofactors, including glutathione and EDTA.

In our own studies[26], human colon was obtained at operation from patients undergoing resection for carcinomas of the colon. The mucosa was taken > 5 cm away from the tumour and was histologically normal. Colon from patients undergoing colectomy for ulcerative colitis was also used. The colonic

17

mucosa from these patients had the histological appearance of severe inflammation. None of the patients were receiving any drugs known to affect arachidonic acid metabolism.

At operation, mucosal tissue was stripped from the underlying muscle of the resected human colon and stored at $-70°C$. After storage (1 week to 1 month), the mucosal tissue was thawed and was homogenized in 50 mmol L^{-1} Tris buffer (pH 7.4), either manually using a 'Dual' ground glass homogenizer or mechanically using 15 × 1 sec strokes of an Ultra-Turax homogenizer, to give a 100 mg ml^{-1} final suspension.

Aliquots (1 ml) of homogenate were added to 1 ml of Tris buffer, either alone or containing the compounds under investigation, to give a final volume of 2 ml (50 mg ml^{-1} tissue homogenate). The addition of cofactors was avoided since they have been shown to alter the profile of arachidonic acid metabolites formed. The aliquots were preincubated for 20 min at 0°C before adding [^{14}C]AA (840 ng, 160 nCi) and incubating for a further 20 min in a shaking water bath at 37°C (Figure 2.2). Aliquots of boiled homogenate were also incubated with [^{14}C]AA (20 min) to assess any non-enzymic degradation which may occur during the experiments.

In all the experiments, tissue incubations with the cyclo-oxygenase inhibitor indomethacin[27] and the combined cyclo-oxygenase/lipoxygenase inhibitor

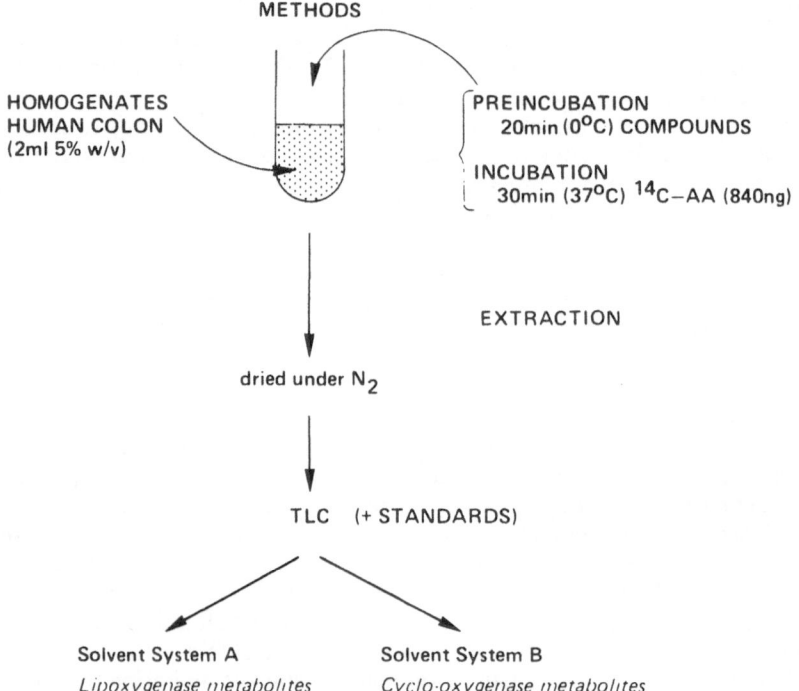

Figure 2.2 Method used to study [^{14}C]arachidonic acid metabolism by homogenates of human colonic mucosa. Solvent system A separates the lipoxygenase metabolites, while solvent system B separates the prostanoids

BW755C[28] were included in order to confirm the enzymic origin of the metabolites formed.

In these studies, the homogenates of human colonic mucosa formed the lipoxygenase products, 12- and 15-HETE, as well as forming cyclo-oxygenase metabolites from [14C]AA. Products co-migrating with 5-HETE and LTB$_4$ were also formed but their enzymic origin could not be confirmed as lipoxygenase because their synthesis was also inhibited by indomethacin[26].

In a subsequent study by Sharon and Stenson[29] in which human colonic mucosa was used, scrapings of fresh tissue were incubated with [14C]AA in a buffer containing glucose, calcium and the calcium ionophore, A23187. After 5 min, the tissue was placed on ice and immediately homogenized in a Polytron homogenizer[29]. Under these incubation conditions, products identified by HPLC as LTB$_4$ and 5-HETE were also formed by the colonic mucosa.

The formation of eicosanoids by homogenates of tissue may depend on whether the tissue is fresh or has been stored (frozen), or whether cofactors are added to the incubation media. Homogenization or freezing the tissue may lead to some damage of the enzymes and therefore possibly an underestimate of enzyme activity. However, homogenization is essential to allow [14C]AA adequate access to enzymes and this method of assessing arachidonic metabolite has several advantages as will be described below.

Cell culture

In an attempt to characterize the cell type responsible for the enhanced synthesis of prostanoids in inflammatory bowel disease, Zifroni et al.[30] have separated and isolated intestinal epithelial and mononuclear cells. The isolated cells were cultured for 18 h and prostanoid synthesis measured by RIA. When using such isolation cell techniques, it is of great importance to determine the purity of the isolated cells. Platelet contamination of isolated cell preparations has been common, and, even in preparations where platelets are a small proportion of the total number of cells, they could contribute substantially to the levels of thromboxane found in the cell cultures. As isolation techniques become more sophisticated and markers for different cell types are identified, studies on isolated cells could assume greater importance.

Subcellular preparations

Microsomal preparations of intestinal tissue have been used to assess cyclo-oxygenase activity[31]. This crude enzyme preparation can be used to evaluate the effect of drugs such as sulphasalazine, and to define the concentrations required to interact directly with the cyclo-oxygenase enzymes in the absence of other cell constituents.

Preparations of high-speed supernatant of intestinal and non-intestinal tissue have been used to measure the activity of the major prostaglandin metabolizing enzymes, prostaglandin-15-hydroxydehydrogenase (PGDH) and Δ^{13} reductase[32]. The activity of these enzymes in the supernatant is very low and the addition of the cofactor NAD is necessary to measure activity over short incubation periods. Using these preparations, an increase in PGDH activity was demonstrated in supernatants from inflamed colonic mucosa from IBD patients[33]. In addition, sulphasalazine was found to be a potent inhibitor of this enzyme[32,33].

Future studies with subcellular preparations may be important in studying the activity of lipoxygenase enzymes in intestinal tissue and could provide a useful model for drug evaluation studies.

In summary, a range of tissue preparations have been used to measure eicosanoid synthesis in IBD. These preparations vary from tissue microsomes to organ culture. Each preparation has its own advantages and can be used to assess eicosanoid synthesis. To some extent, the source of substrate is important when deciding which preparation to use and also the assay method employed to measure eicosanoids. All the preparations used have added greatly to the present understanding of the role of eicosanoids in IBD.

METHODS USED TO MEASURE EICOSANOIDS

Bioassay

The prostaglandins were originally discovered by bioassay. Although in recent years sophisticated physicochemical assay techniques have become more freely available, bioassay has contributed to several major advances in our knowledge of prostaglandins and, more recently, of the products of the lipoxygenase enzymes including the leukotrienes. Indeed, the first measurement of prostaglandins in IBD was determined using bioassay of lipid extracts from faeces. The extracts were bioassayed against standard PGE_2 using the rat stomach strip preparation[1]. In a later investigation, the medium from organ culture of rectal mucosa was extracted and the activity of products, co-migrating on TLC with PGE_2, bioassayed against authentic PGE_2 using superfused stomach strips from rat or hamster[29]. Bioassay techniques exploiting the platelet anti-aggregating activity of prostacyclin has also been employed to determine its formation from colonic tissue[24]. The use of bioassay techniques, however, requires a degree of expertise and is time-consuming. Bioassay also has limitations in the degree of selectivity and sensitivity in detecting low levels of eicosanoids. Many investigators have therefore preferred to use more direct methods of measuring eicosanoids.

Radioimmunoassay

Radioimmunoassay (RIA) is probably the most widely-used procedure to measure prostaglandins. Various antisera have been raised which are both highly sensitive and specific for individual prostaglandins, thromboxane B_2 and, more recently, for some of the leukotrienes[5]. The simplicity, sensitivity and reproducibility of the assay procedure enable the processing of many samples at relatively low running cost and make it ideal for routine eicosanoid assay.

Several investigators have used RIA to measure prostaglandin synthesis in IBD. Lipids extracts from the faeces of patients with ulcerative colitis[12], the incubation media from organ and cell culture[18-20], and the level of eicosanoids in dialysates[14,15] have all been measured using specific RIA. More recently,

Table 2.2 Assay methods used to identify and measure eicosanoid formation in human colonic mucosa

	Eicosanoids					
	Cyclo-oxygenase			Lipoxygenase		
Assay method	PGE_2	PGI_2 6-keto-$PGF_{1\alpha}$	TxA_2	12,15-HETE	5- HETE	LTB_4
Bioassay	1, 12, 20	24				34
RIA	12, 14, 15, 18, 20, 21, 22, 30	19, 21, 22, 30	19, 21, 30			15, 34
[^{14}C]AA-TLC	25, 26, 29, 35, 38	19, 26, 38	26, 38	26, 29, 35	26, 35	35
GC–MS/HPLC	37	37	37	26, 35, 37	15, 35	15, 34, 35

Identification and measurement of eicosanoid synthesis in human colonic mucosa by: bioassay; radioimmunoassay (RIA); conversion of [^{14}C]arachidonic acid and subsequent separation of metabolites by TLC ([^{14}C]AA-TLC); or by gas chromatography–mass spectrometry and high performance liquid chromatography (GC–MS/HPLC). Citations as in reference list

the formation of leukotriene C_4 and leukotriene B_4 by chopped human colon has also been determined by specific RIA[34]. In some of these investigations, extraction of eicosanoids was performed before RIA, while in others, they were measured directly. It is important to stress that appropriate tissue blanks and dilution should always be made, and standards curves used in each assay, for the immunoreactive activity to represent accurately the amount of eicosanoid present. Separation of metabolites by thin layer chromatography (TLC) or high performance liquid chromatography (HPLC) can be used as a further purification and identification step before RIA.

Although RIA is a highly specific assay method, only a single eicosanoid can be measured by each assay, and therefore multiple assays with different antisera are necessary if the profile of arachidonic acid metabolites are to be assessed.

Conversion of [^{14}C]AA: thin layer chromatography

The conversion of [^{14}C]AA by biopsy samples of colonic mucosa was first used by Harris *et al.*[13] to show that there was an increase in PGE_2 and $PGF_{2\alpha}$-like material in inflamed tissue from patients with ulcerative colitis. In these studies, following treatment of the patients with sulphasalazine, the formation of the eicosanoids from [^{14}C]AA returned to control levels.

In our studies, the biosynthesis of lipoxygenase and cyclo-oxygenase products from [^{14}C]AA was studied in homogenates of human colonic mucosa[26]. Using the procedure described in the previous section (Figure 2.2), homogenates of human colonic mucosa were incubated with [^{14}C]AA, and the metabolites formed were extracted and separated as described below.

Extraction

At the end of the incubation, the samples were acidified (pH 3.5) with citric acid (2.3 mol L^{-1}) and placed on ice. The lipids were extracted by adding diethyl ether (2 vol) and after mixing (1 min) and centrifugation (2000 g, 10 min), the pellet was extracted into a further 2 volumes of diethyl ether. The two extracts were combined and dried (50°C) under a steam of nitrogen.

TLC

The dry residues were redissolved in 75 µl of chloroform : methanol (2 : 1) and spotted onto multi-lane silica gel TLC plates (Whatman LK 5D). In each experiment, duplicate TLC plates were prepared and dried at room temperature (10 min).

Each TLC plate was developed using one of two different solvent systems.

(1) *Solvent system A*

Ether : hexane : acetic acid, 60 : 40 : 1 (v : v : v)

The system separates TxB$_2$ and prostaglandins (which remain together on the origin) from the mono- and dihydroxylipoxygenase products. The Raa values (chromatographic mobility of products with respect to arachidonic acid) were for leukotriene B$_4$: 0.15; 5-HETE: 0.44; HHT: 0.63; and 11-, 12-, 15-HETE (which run together): 0.75.

(2) *Solvent system B*

The organic phase of: ethylacetate : trimethyl pentane : H$_2$O : acetic acid, 110 : 50 : 100 : 20 (v : v : v : v)

The system facilitates the separation of the individual prostaglandins and TxB$_2$. The Raa values were: 6-keto-PGF$_{1\alpha}$: 0.29; PGF$_{2\alpha}$: TxB$_2$: 0.50; PGE$_2$: 0.59; PGD$_2$: 0.73.

Radioactive metabolites were located by autoradiography. The developed TLC plates were overlaid with photographic film (Kodak NS 2T) and sandwiched using a glass plate. After 3 days' contact, the film was developed and fixed using standard photographic reagents. Using the autoradiogram as a template, the radioactive bands were located on TLC plates by underlighting with an X-ray viewer. The extremities of each band were marked by scoring the silica gel of the TLC plate.

The individual silica gel zones corresponding to each radioactive band were wetted with distilled water and the silica gel scraped off, using a scalpel, into scintillation vials. After adding scintillant (5 ml), the radioactivity was determined by liquid scintillation counting. The dpm for each band was calculated and expressed as a percentage of the total dpm within the particular TLC lane. After subtraction of boiled tissue blanks, the data was calculated as the proportion of [^{14}C]AA converted to individual products and expressed as ng g^{-1} mucosal tissue.

Product identification

Products were identified by co-chromatography with authentic cold standards of PGD$_2$, PGE$_2$, TxB$_2$, PGF$_{2\alpha}$, 6-keto-PGF$_{1\alpha}$, 5-HETE, 15-HETE, 12-HETE and LTB$_4$. These standards (stored in ethanol at -20°C) were applied to spare lanes on the silica-gel plates. On completion of the chromatography, the standards were visualized colorimetrically by spraying the relevant lanes with an ethanolic solution of phosphomolybdic acid (10%) and heating (70°C).

In addition, the lipoxygenase metabolites formed on incubation of [14C]AA with rabbit peritoneal polymorphonuclear leukocytes and human washed platelets were regularly used as standards.

Products with the chromatographic mobility (in solvent system B) of PGE_2, $PGF_{2\alpha}$, PGD_2, TxB_2 and 6-keto-$PGF_{1\alpha}$ were formed from [14C]AA by homogenates of human colonic mucosa. The formation of these cyclo-oxygenase products was inhibited by BW755C and indomethacin (Figure 2.3).

The predominant lipoxygenase products characterized using solvent system A had a chromatographic mobility of 11-, 12-, 15-HETE. Smaller amounts of another metabolite, product II, were also formed. Whereas indomethacin failed to inhibit the formation of these products, BW755C inhibited their production thereby confirming their identity as lipoxygenase products (Figure 2.4).

In studies using inflamed mucosa from two patients with ulcerative colitis[26], there was an overall three-fold increase in metabolite formation compared

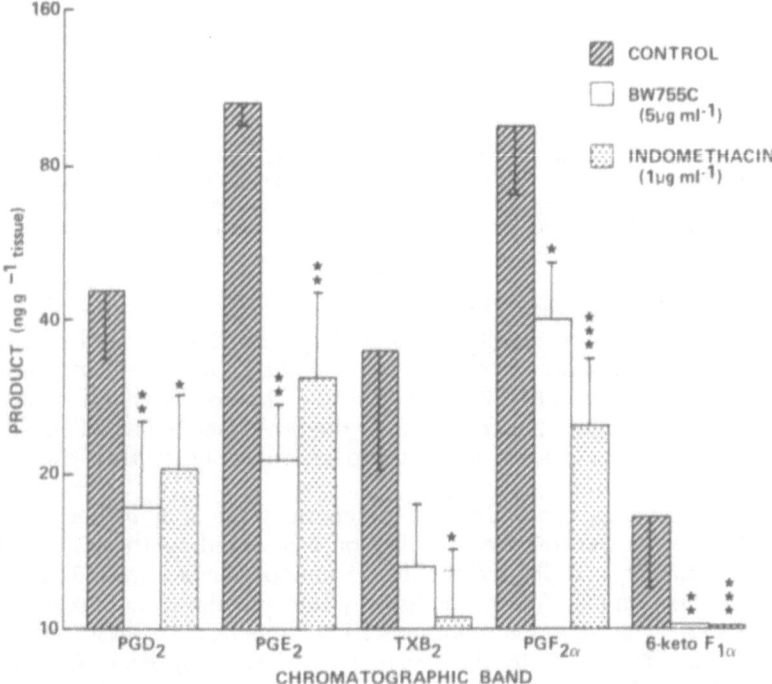

Figure 2.3 Cyclo-oxygenase products formed by homogenates of human colon mucosa from [14C]arachidonic acid and the inhibition of their formation by BW755C (5 μg ml^{-1}) and indomethacin (1 μg ml^{-1}). The metabolites were separated by TLC using solvent system B (see text). The results are the mean $\pm$ SEM of 5 experiments. *$p < 0.05$, **$p < 0.01$, ***$p < 0.001$. Data derived from Boughton-Smith, Hawkey and Whittle (reference 26)

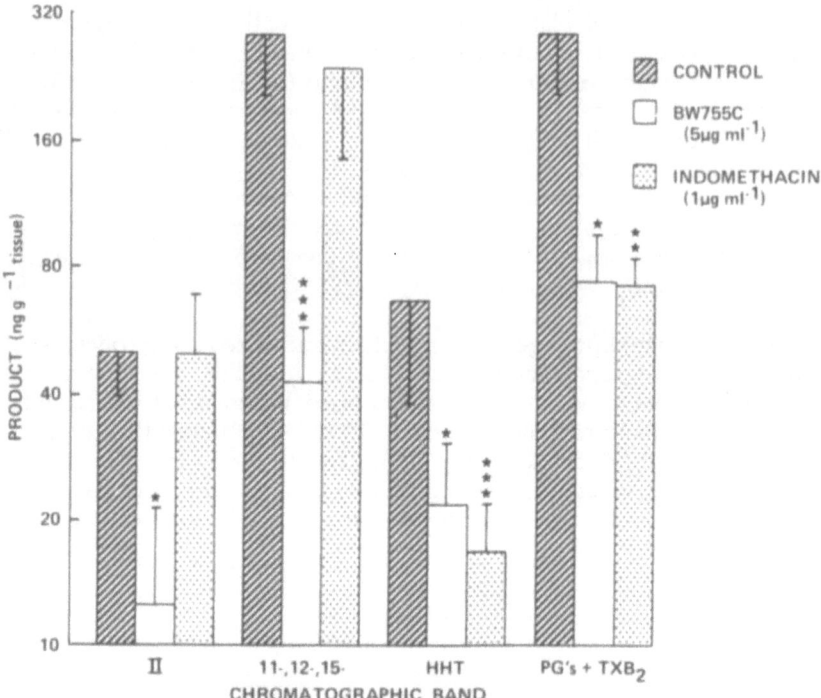

Figure 2.4 Lipoxygenase products formed by homogenates of human colonic mucosa from [^{14}C]arachidonic acid and the inhibition of their formation by BW755C (5 μg ml^{-1}) but not by indomethacin (1 μg ml^{-1}). The metabolites were separated by TLC using solvent system A (see text). The results are the mean $\pm$ SEM of 5 experiments. *$p < 0.05$, **$p < 0.01$, ***$p < 0.001$. Data derived from Boughton-Smith, Hawkey and Whittle (reference 26)

with control tissue (Figure 2.5). There was an increase in the formation of all the cyclo-oxygenase metabolites separated by TLC. There was also a marked increase in the formation of the products separated using solvent system A which correspond to 11-, 12-, 15-HETE and the combined PGs and TxB$_2$ band on the TLC plate. The formation of the other metabolites of arachidonic acid formed by the colonic mucosa and separated using this TLC system were also increased.

The methodology can be utilized to determine the *in vitro* effects of drugs used clinically in the treatment of IBD on eicosanoid synthesis. The effects of sulphasalazine and its metabolites, 5-amino-salicylic acid (5-ASA) and sulphapyridine on [^{14}C]AA metabolism by human colonic mucosa have been investigated[35]. An autoradiogram indicating the effects of these compounds is shown in Figure 2.6. In these experiments, sulphasalazine inhibited the formation of TxB$_2$. The inhibition was accompanied by a concentration-related enhancement of PGF$_{2\alpha}$ synthesis. At the higher concentration of sulphasalazine (1 mmol L^{-1}) there was a small inhibition of 6-keto-PGF$_{1\alpha}$ formation, but sulphasalazine had no effect on formation of the other major cyclo-oxygenase products. Sulphapyridine inhibited TxB$_2$ formation at the higher concentration

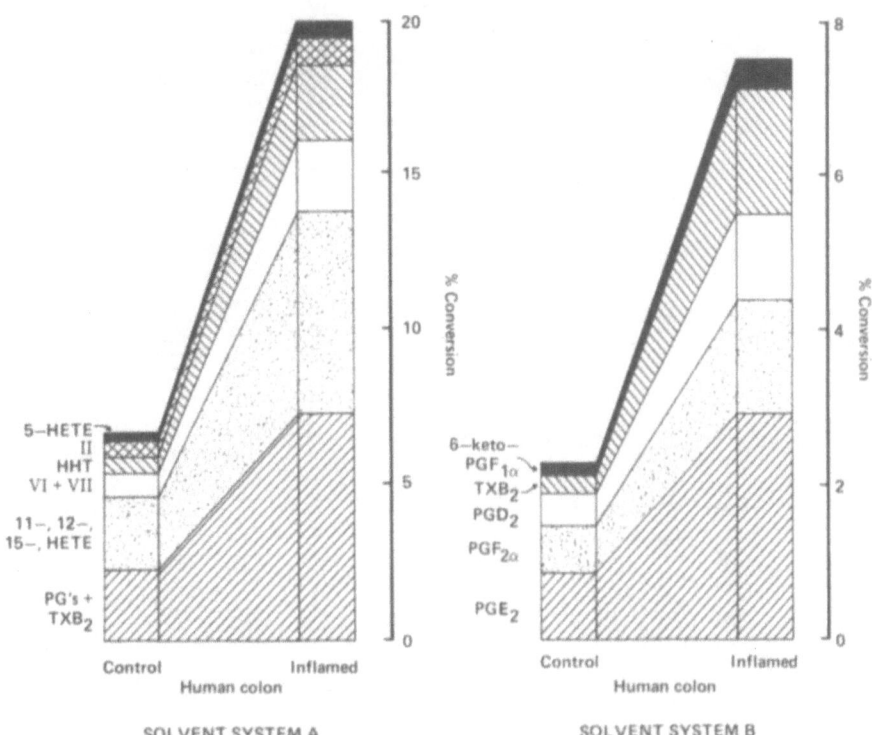

Figure 2.5 Schematic representation of the profile of [¹⁴C]arachidonic acid metabolites formed by homogenates of control human colonic mucosa and the increased formation by inflamed colonic mucosa from patients with ulcerative colitis. The overall conversion of [¹⁴C]arachidonic acid and the proportion of the individual products formed are shown, when separated by TLC using solvent system A and B

used ($1\,\mathrm{mmol\,L^{-1}}$) while, at this concentration, it enhanced PGE_2 formation. In contrast to both sulphasalazine and sulphyridine, 5-ASA ($1\,\mathrm{mmol\,L^{-1}}$) inhibited the formation of PGE_2, but had no effect on the other major arachidonate metabolites.

Assessment of the metabolic activity of human and animal tissue using [¹⁴C]AA conversion has the advantage of allowing the wide profile of arachidonic acid metabolites formed by these tissues to be revealed. If appropriate solvent systems are used, products of both the cyclo-oxygenase and lipoxygenase pathways of arachidonic acid can be separated by TLC. The identification of the [¹⁴C]AA metabolites depend on their chromatographic mobility compared with authentic standards. Since different metabolites may have the same mobility in a particular solvent system, wherever possible, a second solvent system should be used to confirm the identity of a particular metabolite. In addition, wherever possible, the enzymic origin of a metabolite should be confirmed using selective inhibitors of the different enzymes in the arachidonic acid cascade.

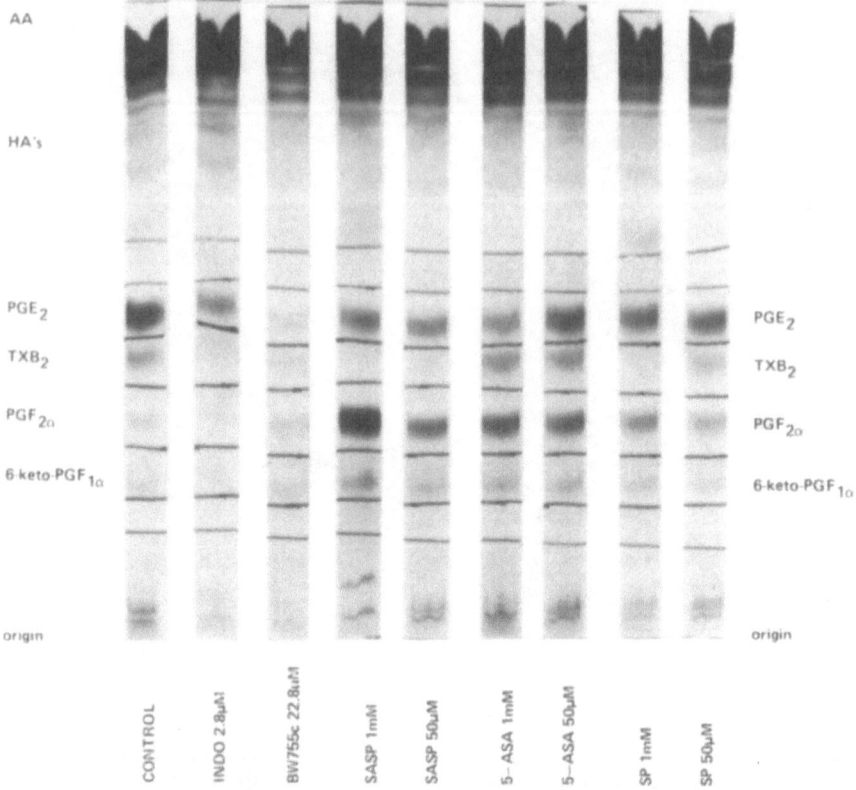

Figure 2.6 Autoradiogram of the prostanoids formed from [^{14}C]arachidonic acid by homogenates of human colonic mucosa and separated by TLC using solvent system B. The inhibition of TxB$_2$ formation by sulphasalazine (SASP) and sulphapyridine (SP) but not 5-aminosalicyclic acid (5-ASA) is shown. Also shown is the inhibition of metabolite formation by indomethacin (INDO) and BW755C. Data is derived from Hawkey, Boughton-Smith and Whittle (reference 35)

Conversion of [^{14}C]AA may not necessarily represent endogenous arachidonic metabolism. Indeed an increase in conversion of exogenous [^{14}C]AA may under some circumstances indicate a decrease in competition for enzymes by endogenous substrate. In addition, incubation conditions and tissue preparation can alter the profile of arachidonic acid metabolites formed. The conversion of [^{14}C]AA by homogenates of inflamed mucosa to 12- and 15-HETE in our study (6.4% of total conversion) was greater than reported by Sharon and Stenson[29] who used scrapings of inflamed colonic mucosa, incubated and homogenized in the presence of [^{14}C]AA and the calcium ionophore, A23187 (3.7% conversion). In contrast, the formation by homogenates of the product co-migrating with 5-HETE (0.59% conversion) was much less than that reported by Sharon and Stenson (3.0% conversion). These differences probably reflect the different incubation conditions used, particularly the use of the ionophore A23187. In the absence of A23187, the amount of 15-HETE synthesized by human polymorphonuclear leukocytes from added arachidonic acid is similar to or greater than the amount of 5-HETE formed[36]. However, if A23187 is present there is a 20-fold increase in the formation of 5-HETE with little change in 15-HETE synthesis. Thus, addition of ionophore can markedly affect the ratio of lipoxygenase metabolites formed from arachidonic acid *in vitro* and therefore is perhaps less likely to reflect the profile of products formed *in vivo*.

The separation of eicosanoids by TLC is both simple and rapid. However, not all the metabolites can be separated using this form of chromatography and more sophisticated chromatographic techniques are required to identify further the eicosanoids.

High pressure liquid chromatography and gas chromatography–mass spectrometry

In a study using GC–MS, Bennett *et al.*[37] identified a product corresponding to 12-HETE which was formed from endogenous arachidonic acid by normal human colonic mucosa and muscle. In addition, several cyclo-oxygenase metabolites were found to be present in these tissues. Gas chromatography coupled with mass spectrometry has become the most powerful analytical tool for qualitative and quantitative analysis of eicosanoids. However, the mandatory derivatization steps required for good chromatography are time consuming and the sophisticated instrumentation very expensive, which thus limit its availability to most investigators.

HPLC instrumentation is less expensive and allows the separation of arachidonic acid metabolites of very similar structure. In our own studies, we have used HPLC to separate the radio-labelled products comprising the 11-, 12-, 15-HETE TLC band, which ran together in most TLC systems[26].

In order to obtain sufficient radioactive material for resolution by HPLC, homogenates of inflamed or control colonic mucosa were incubated in bulk (250 mg in 5 ml) with [^{14}C]AA. The metabolites were extracted and resolved by TLC using solvent system A. The silica gel from the radioactive band corresponding to 11-, 12-, 15-HETE was scraped dry and crushed into a micro-column (a pasteur pipette plugged with glass wool). The column was eluted with methanol (20 ml) and the eluant filtered and dried under nitrogen.

The residue was redissolved in HPLC solvent (see below) before injection into a straight phase Zorbax sil column (Dupont 4.6 × 250 nm) which had been previously equilibrated at a flow rate of 3 ml min^{-1} with n-hexane : isopropyl alcohol : acetic acid (992 : 7 : 1, v : v : v) and standardized using authentic mono-HETE's (11-, 12- and 15-HETE). Elution of metabolites was monitored by U.V. absorbance (at 280 and 254 nm). Fractions, which were collected every 30 s, were decanted into scintillation vials, and, after adding scintillant (5 ml), radioactivity was measured by liquid scintillation counting.

Products were identified by coelution with authentic standards of 11-HETE, 12-HETE and 15-HETE. In addition, 15-HETE was added to each sample as an internal standard and in some experiments [^{3}H]12-HETE was also added as a further standard and to estimate procedural losses of radioactive metabolites.

Resolution by HPLC of a major product co-migrating on TLC with 11-, 12-, 15-HETE indicated that 12-HETE was the major identifiable mono-HETE formed by homogenates of uninflamed colon (Figure 2.7). A metabolite

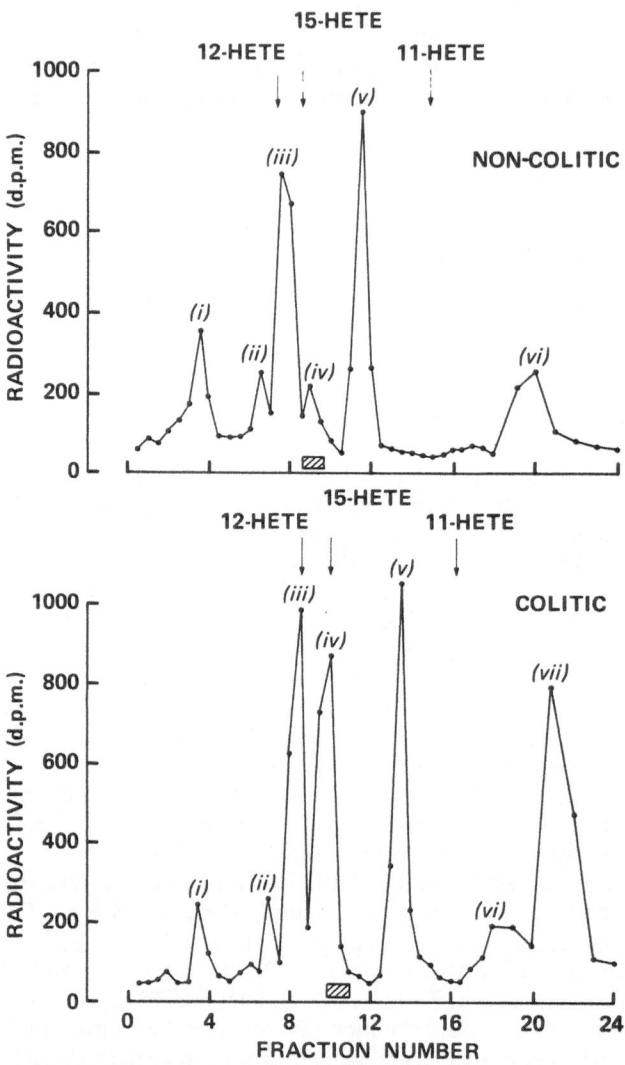

Figure 2.7 HPLC resolution of the products separated as the 11-, 12-, 15-HETE TLC band formed from [^{14}C]arachidonic acid by homogenates of inflamed colonic mucosa from patients with ulcerative colitis (colitic) or control uninflamed tissue (non-colitic). The position of the authentic 12-HETE, 15-HETE and 11-HETE are indicated by arrows. The hatched bar represents 15-HETE internal standards. Data is derived from Boughton-Smith, Hawkey and Whittle (reference 26)

co-migrating on HPLC with 12-HETE was also one of the major products formedfrom [^{14}C]AA by scrapings of human colonic mucosa stimulated with the calcium ionophore, A23187[29]. However, in another study using elaborate extraction procedures, the formation of HETE by human colonic mucosa could not be detected by TLC or gas–liquid chromatography[38].

Analysis by HPLC of the 11-, 12-, 15-HETE TLC band also revealed the novel finding that 15-HETE is formed by homogenates of human colonic mucosa (Figure 2.7). The formation of 15-HETE may reflect lipoxygenase activity derived from leukocytes which have infiltrated the mucosa, since, in addition to an increased synthesis of 15- and 12-HETE by inflamed colonic mucosa, the proportion of 15-HETE formed was greater. Furthermore, 15-HETE is the major mono-HETE formed in intact human polymorphonuclear leukocytes incubated with arachidonic acid[36] as well as in enriched human eosinophils[39].

Using TLC, HPLC and GC–MS, Sharon and Stenson demonstrated a considerable increase in the formation of LTB$_4$ by the inflamed colonic mucosa, both in the presence and absence of added arachidonic acid[29]. In addition, an increased formation of the sulphidopeptide-leukotrienes, LTC$_4$, LTD$_4$ and LTE$_4$, by inflamed human colon from patients with Crohn's disease was demonstrated using both specific RIA for LTC$_4$ and HPLC techniques[34].

LEUKOCYTE INFILTRATION IN INFLAMMATORY BOWEL DISEASE

Inflammatory cell infiltration into the intestinal mucosa is a characteristic of both ulcerative colitis and Crohn's disease. Since leukocytes are a major source of eicosanoids, especially for products of the lipoxygenase pathway, their presence in bowel tissue can have profound effects on the profile and amount of eicosanoids formed by inflamed tissue. Therefore, when investigating eicosanoid formation by inflamed tissue in IBD, it is important to determine the degree of cellular infiltration.

Histology

Histology has been used extensively to assess the presence of leukocytes in tissues. In detailed studies, serial sections of tissues are examined under light microscopy and cell numbers counted. This type of study is very time consuming and requires a great deal of expertise to identify individual cell types.

Myeloperoxidase

Inflammatory cell infiltration into the colon can also be assessed by measuring the activity of myeloperoxidase (MPO). This enzyme is a haemoprotein which catalyses the peroxidation of a wide variety of substrates and is involved in intracellular bacterial killing[40]. The enzyme is characteristically found in the azurophil granules of polymorphonuclear leukocytes, comprising up to 5% of the dry weight of the cell[41]. The activity of this enzyme has been used as a marker for polymorphonuclear leukocyte infiltration into a wide variety of tissues including human skin[42], rabbit eye[43], dog heart[44] and also in an acute model of intestinal inflammation in the rat[45] and in a chronic model of IBD in the rat[46].

In our studies[46], MPO was measured using a method similar to that described by Bradley *et al.*[42] (Figure 2.8). Segments of colon (stored at $-20°C$) were weighed and homogenized (Ultra-turax, 30 s) in 0.5% hexadecyltrimethyl-ammonium bromide (HTAB) in $50 \, mmol \, L^{-1}$ potassium phosphate buffer (pH 6.0) to give a $50 \, mg \, ml^{-1}$ w/v suspension. Aliquots (1 ml) of the suspension, pipetted into Eppendorf centrifuge tubes, were frozen (on cardice granules, $-20°C$) and thawed (immersion in warm water, $37°C$) three times. Following centrifugation ($10\,000\,g$, 2 min at $4°C$), aliquots of supernatant ($10 \, \mu l$) were mixed in a cuvette with 2.9 ml of $50 \, mmol \, L^{-1}$ phosphate buffer (pH 6.0) containing $0.167 \, mg \, ml^{-1}$ of O-dianisidine dihydrochloride and 0.0005% hydrogen peroxide, and the change in absorbance at 460 nm measured immediately (Beckman, spectrophotometer model 25). One unit of MPO activity was defined as that degrading one micromole of peroxidase

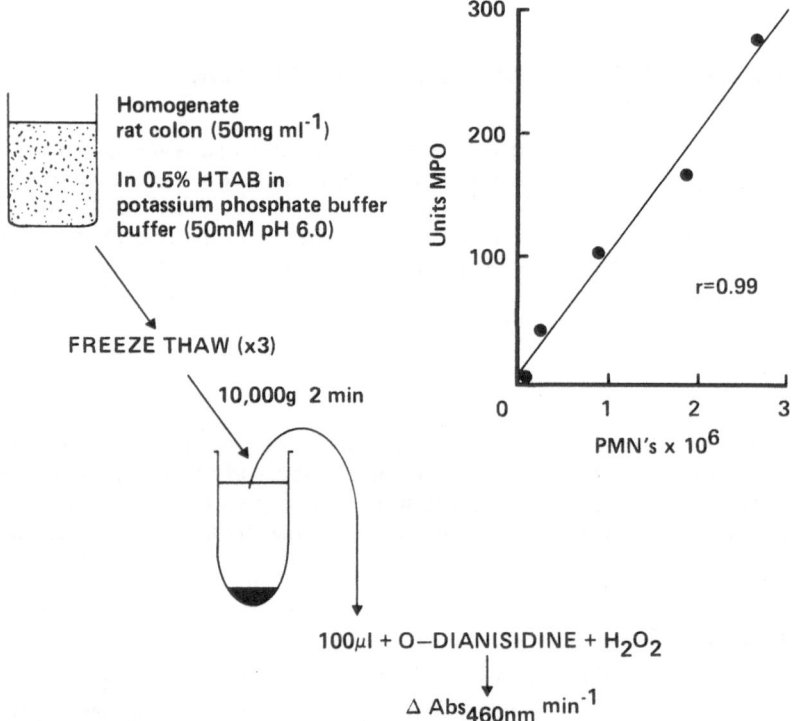

Figure 2.8 Method used to measure myeloperoxidase activity (MPO) in the rat colon, also showing the correlation between rat peritoneal polymorphonuclear leukocyte (PMN) concentration and MPO activity

per minute at 25°C. In control studies, the activity of MPO was directly correlated to the concentration of glycogen-elicited peritoneal PMN's (Figure 2.8). In addition, MPO activity was also directly correlated with the infiltration of leukocytes into the inflamed rat colon as assessed histologically.

Enzyme markers, such as MPO, provide a measurement of leukocyte infiltration without the prolonged and detailed histological studies involving serial sectioning of tissue, required for differential cell counting. As well as MPO, other enzyme markers have been used to assess inflammation in rectal biopsies from patients with IBD[47]. These include, 5-nucleotidase, a selective enzyme from lymphocytes[48], vitamin B_{12}-binding protein, which is exclusively located in the specific granules of neutrophils[49,50] and lysozyme, which is present in neutrophils[51] and mononuclear phagocytes[52]. Thus, assessment of inflammation using enzyme markers may give an insight into the inflammatory process within inflamed intestinal tissue and may also provide a means of measuring the activity of anti-inflammatory drugs in reducing leukocyte accumulation in inflamed tissue.

ANIMAL MODELS OF INFLAMMATORY BOWEL DISEASE

The need for a greater understanding of the aetiology of IBD and the search for more effective and novel therapy for the treatment of the disease, has led to the development of a variety of experimental animal models.

Spontaneous lesions

Several spontaneous colonic lesions have been observed in various species including rats, mice and in particular boxer dogs. Although some of the features of these spontaneous lesions are common to the human disease, none possesses the frequency of occurrence or is sufficiently similar in anatomical and histological appearance to human ulcerative colitis or Crohn's disease to serve as a convenient animal model[53]. A spontaneous colitis has recently been described in cotton-top tamarins, which is both chronic and responds to sulphasalazine treatment[54].

Vascular impairment

Mucosal ulceration of the dog colon can be produced by reduction of colonic blood flow induced either mechanically[55] or from muscular contractions which result from the administration of cholinergic agents[56]. The ulceration produced is directly related to the degree of ischaemia inflicted. Colonic lesions can be produced in rats and cats by exposure of the mucosa to chemical irritants such as acetic acid or ethanol. The lesions following topical damage, which heal slowly, are probably the result of impaired vascularization of the mucosa[57]. The lesions found in these models are similar to those seen in human ischaemic colitis which is a disease entity distinct from ulcerative colitis and Crohn's disease.

Bacterial infection

The similarities between ulcerative colitis and the colitis due to infection by specific pathogens led to investigations into bacterial induced colitis. Injection of dead *Escherichia coli* into the foot-pad of rats resulted in diarrhoea, bleeding and ulceration of the colonic mucosa[58]. Injection of *Escherichia coli* from patients with ulcerative colitis[59] or homologous colonic mucosa[60] into rabbits, induced colonic autoantibodies but failed to produce histological colitis. The induction of colitis by the injection of colonic extracts in other studies was found to be due to Salmonella contamination[61].

A colitis was produced in hamsters and guinea-pigs by the injection of antibiotics such as clindamycin and penicillin[62-64]. The colitis resulted from the release of specific toxins and could be reversed or prevented by administration of antibiotics against gram negative coliform bacteria. This animal model has many of the features of antibiotic-associated colitis in man, but as such does not provide a good model of non-specific IBD.

Hypersensitivity reactions

Various models of colitis have been developed by inducing Arthus, Schwartz, Auer and direct antigen—antibody hypersensitivity reactions in the colon[65]. Kirsner and colleagues originally described a model of colitis, induced by a modification of the Auer reaction, in which rabbits, sensitized to egg albumen, had dilute formalin instilled into the rectum followed by intravenous infusion of antigen[66]. Similarly, intravenous infusion of immune complexes (antigen—antibody complexes) to non-sensitized rabbits, after previous colonic instillation of dilute formalin, also produced a colitis[67]. The colitis induced by most of these immune complex-mediated reactions only lasted a few days, although a more chronic colitis could be induced by immunization with common enterobacterial antigen[68].

Carrageenin

A novel method for the development of large intestinal ulceration was described by Marcus and Watt[69,70]. A 5% aqueous solution of degraded carrageenin, derived from the red seaweed *Eucheuma spinosum*, was fed in the drinking water to guinea-pigs over a period of 20—45 days. By 30 days, all the animals had occult blood in the faeces and multiple ulcers in the caecum, colon and rectum. This ulceration of the bowel can also be induced in the rat, mouse[71], Rhesus monkey[72] and rabbit[73]. In contrast, others have failed to produce ulceration with carrageenin in the rat, hamster, squirrel, monkey or ferret[73]. The induction of the ulceration is totally dependent on the type and degree of degradation of the carrageenin[71,74].

In a small study, administration of sulphasalazine or prednisolone in the food failed to affect the mortality, occult blood or weight loss induced by 5% carrageenin in guinea-pigs[75]. In a study using 3% degraded carrageenin, a 'measure of protection' was observed following oral dosing with sulphasalazine, azathioprine or prednisolone[76]. In another study, sulphasalazine reduced the number of ulcers produced by 5% carrageenin, but a slow-release preparation of 5-ASA failed to have any effect[77].

The intestinal ulceration induced in guinea-pigs by carrageenin, unlike human IBD, is apparently dependent on anaerobic bacteria since it can be prevented by metronidazole and clindamycin and does not develop in germ-free rats[78,79].

Dinitrochlorobenzene

A model of colitis which is dependent on the development of cell-mediated immunity has been used by several investigators. The model, originally described by Rosenberg and Fischer[80], is based on the concept of contact dermatitis. The skin of guinea-pigs is painted with a solution of 1-chloro-2,4,-dinitrobenzene (DNCB) and seven days later a mixture of DNCB in an adherent dental paste (Orabase) is instilled intrarectally. After 24 h, histological examination of the colon reveals an allergic reaction consisting of oedema, vasodilatation and an intense perivascular accumulation of inflammatory cells, with some migration into the mucosa[81].

Sensitivity to DNCB can be transferred by inoculation of spleen and lymph node cells from sensitized animals to non-sensitized recipient guinea-pigs, but not by transfer of sensitized serum. The reaction is specific for the hapten used and can also be induced by primary sensitization of the intestine[81]. Similar cell-mediated immune models of IBD can be induced in miniature pigs[81] and in rabbits[82]. The immune nature of the DNCB colitis in guinea-pigs is not completely understood although both T-lymphocytes[83] and basophils[84,85] appear to be involved.

In our own studies we investigated the effect of the number of challenges and the challenge concentration of DNCB on previously sensitized guinea-pigs. The guinea-pigs (male, 280–440 g) were skin-sensitized by applying 50 μl of a 2.5% solution of DNCB, dissolved in ethanol, onto a previously shaved dorsal area (approximately 2 cm^2) for 3 consecutive days. After 10 days, the guinea-pigs were challenged with a mixture of DNCB in Orabase paste (Squibb & Sons Ltd) at concentrations which had no direct effect on the colon (0.25% and 1% DNCB), or with Orabase alone, for 3 consecutive days. A higher concentration of DNCB (5%) had a direct effect on the colon, even in non-sensitized animals, producing hyperaemia and rectal bleeding. The guinea-pigs were sacrificed after a further 24 h or groups of animals were killed 24 h after each challenge and assessed for inflammation of the distal colon. The degree and extent of small red areas of hyperaemia and vascular damage were used as a measure of inflammation, and each colon assigned a score in a blinded, randomized manner, depending on the severity of these parameters.

As shown in Figure 2.9, the inflammation score of the animals challenged with 1% DNCB was more consistent than the score of animals receiving 0.25% DNCB. In control guinea-pigs receiving 1% DNCB intrarectally after

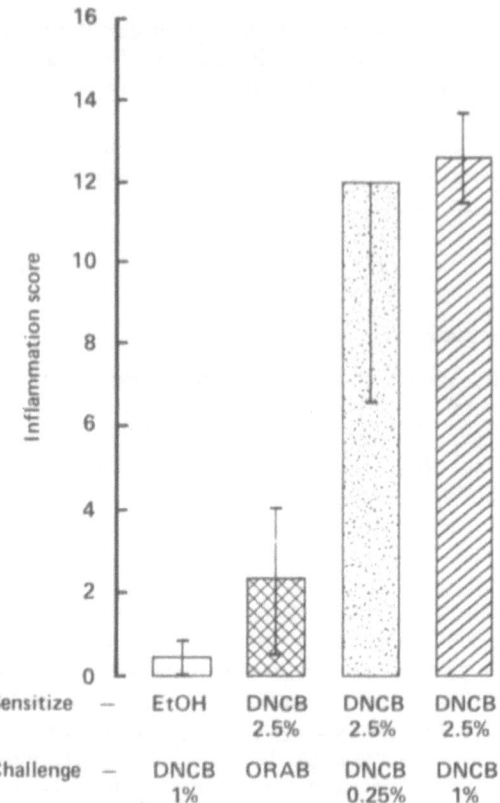

Figure 2.9 The effect of the intracolonic challenge concentration of DNCB on the production of colitis. Guinea-pigs were skin-sensitized with DNCB (2.5% in ethanol) or received ethanol alone (EtOH), and challenged with DNCB (0.25% or 1%) in Orabase or with Orabase alone (ORAB). The results, expressed as the inflammation score, are the mean $\pm$ SEM of 4–5 animals per group

application of ethanol to the skin, the inflammatory score was very low, with only one animal out of 5 showing gross signs of inflammation. A similar low inflammatory score was found in guinea-pigs challenged with Orabase vehicle after previous sensitization to DNCB.

The inflammation of the colon induced by DNCB (1%) was directly related to the number of intracolonic challenges to the previously sensitized guinea-pigs (Figure 2.10). There was a significant inflammation of the guinea-pig colon even after one challenge. In control animals (non-sensitized), the low level of inflammation increased slightly with the number of DNCB challenges.

Eicosanoid formation in models of inflammatory bowel disease

DNCB-induced colitis

Norris et al. originally reported that the level of PGE_2 was elevated in the inflamed colonic mucosa taken from guinea-pigs with DNCB colitis[86]. To

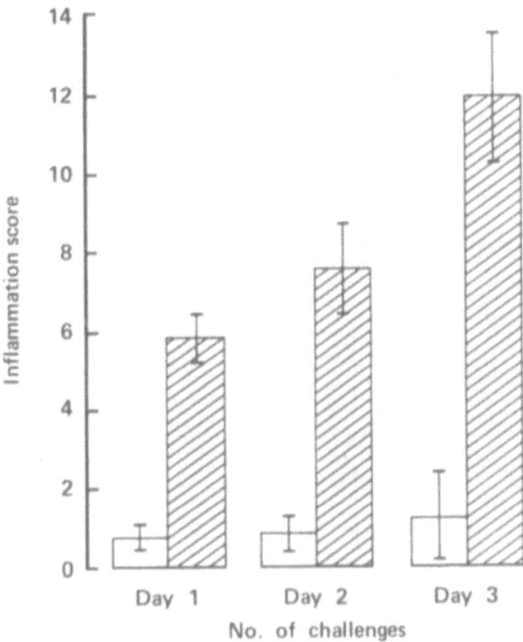

Figure 2.10 The effect of the number of intracolonic challenges with DNCB on the production of colitis (inflammatory score) in skin-sensitized (hatched columns) and non-sensitized (open columns) guinea-pigs. The results, expressed as the inflammation score, are the mean ± SEM of 5–8 animals per group

elucidate further the role of arachidonic acid metabolites in ulcerative colitis, we investigated the activities of both cyclo-oxygenase and lipoxygenase enzymes in inflamed colon taken from the DNCB guinea-pig model of colitis[87]. Arachidonic acid metabolism by guinea-pig colon was assessed as the conversion of [14C]AA, using the protocol shown in Figure 2.11.

Aliquots (1 ml) of homogenate were preincubated (15 min, 21°C) with enzyme inhibitor or Tris buffer (100 μl) before adding [14C]AA (0.25 μCi, 1.3 μg) and incubating for 30 min in a shaking water-bath (37°C).

The [14C]AA and its metabolites were extracted using a method similar to that described by Salmon et al.[88]. After adding acetone (2 ml, −20°C), the samples were vortexed and centrifuged (10 min, 2000 rpm). The supernatants were washed with hexane (2 ml). In the samples to be separated by TLC using solvent system A, the pH of the supernatants were first adjusted to pH 9.5–10, using 1 mol L^{-1} NaOH, before adding hexane (2 ml) to allow a more efficient extraction of the mono- and dihydroxy acid metabolites into the aqueous phase. This also resulted in a much greater extraction of unmetabolized [14C]AA into the aqueous phase and in the appearance of a TLC band co-migrating (solvent system A) with PGB_2, the dehydration product of PGE_2, formed in the alkaline extraction conditions.

The samples were then treated in an identical manner. Following vortexing (1 min) and centrifugation (10 min, 2000 rpm), the upper hexane layer was

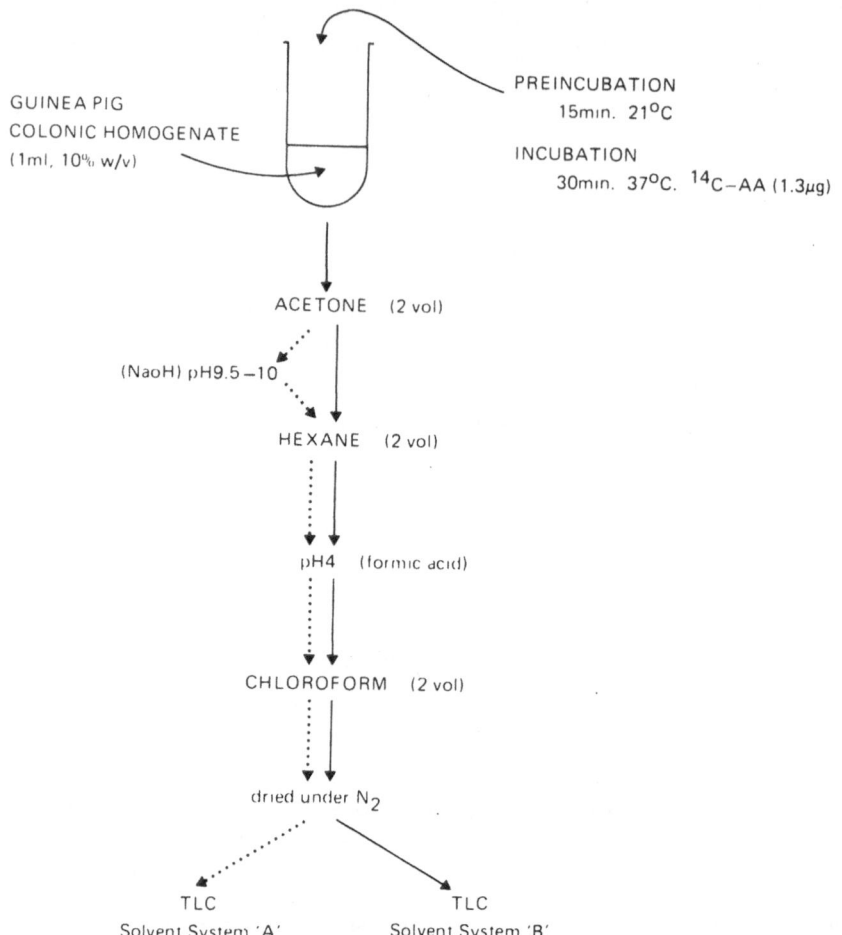

Figure 2.11 The incubation and extraction procedures used to study [^{14}C]arachidonic acid metabolism by homogenates of guinea-pig colon from the DNCB model of colitis. Following acetone extraction, the samples for subsequent TLC separation using solvent system A (dotted line) were alkalinized to increase the efficiency of extraction of lipoxygenase products

discarded and, after acidifying (pH 3.5) the remaining sample with formic acid, chloroform (2 ml) was added. After further vortexing and centrifugation (10 min, 2000 rpm), the lower chloroform layer was dried (50°C) under N$_2$.

In each experiment, duplicate TLC plates were prepared and developed, and the products quantitated using the two solvent systems described in detail already.

There was increased metabolism of [^{14}C]AA by homogenates of inflamed colon taken from guinea-pigs with colitis induced by DNCB[87]. The greatest increase in prostanoid formation was of PGE$_2$, while there were smaller increases in the formation of PGD$_2$, TxB$_2$, PGF$_{2\alpha}$ and 6-keto-PGF$_{1\alpha}$. In addition to prostanoids, there was also an increase in the formation by inflamed guinea-pig colon of [^{14}C]AA metabolites which co-migrated with HHT and 11-, 12-, 15-HETE. The enzymic origin of the TLC band corresponding to 11-, 12-, 15-HETE could not be confirmed as lipoxygenase, however, since its formation was inhibited by the cyclo-oxygenase inhibitor, indomethacin, as well as by the combined cyclo-oxygenase and lipoxygenase inhibitor, BW755C[87].

The formation from endogenous arachidonic acid of immunoreactive prostanoids was also increased in the inflamed colon taken from the guinea-pig model of colitis induced by DNCB[87]. The levels of PGE$_2$ formed by the homogenates of whole colon in our study were similar to those reported previously in the colonic mucosa alone[86] in a study using 0.25% DNCB to induce colitis in guinea-pigs. In that study blood-free segments of mucosal tissue were frozen in liquid nitrogen before subsequent homogenization[86]. The control level of immunoreactive PGE$_2$ formed by the colonic mucosa was also similar to our study using whole colon, as were the increases of PGE$_2$ formation in inflamed colonic mucosa. The formation of TxB$_2$ and 6-keto-PGF$_{1\alpha}$ was also increased in our study[87] on the inflamed guinea-pig colon, although, under the incubation conditions used, there was no change in immunoreactive LTB$_4$.

Eicosanoid formation in other models of IBD
An increase in PGE$_2$-like activity by microsomes and homogenates prepared from inflamed large bowel taken from a model of 'colitis' in carrageenin-fed guinea-pigs has also been reported[89], while supernatants of the same tissue were found to have a reduced capacity to metabolize PGF$_{2\alpha}$.

In another study[90], in which chopped colonic tissue from guinea-pigs sensitized to ovalbumin was challenged with antigen *in vitro*, there was a considerable release of immunoreactive LTC$_4$. An increase in prostanoid formation by vascular-perfused segments of inflamed colon, taken from DNCB and from immune complex-induced colitis in the rabbit, has recently been reported[91]. The perfused rabbit colons were prelabelled with [^{14}C]AA and the prostaglandins and thromboxane in the venous effluent identified by radiochromatography. Prostanoid formation was also measured by bioassay and immunoassay. The basal formation of PGE$_2$, TxB$_2$ and 6-keto-PGF$_{1\alpha}$ by inflamed tissue from both models of colitis was increased. Following bradykinin infusion, there was a further increase in prostanoid formation, particularly of TxB$_2$, which was accompanied by an increase in the vascular perfusion pressure. Angiotensin II also stimulated the formation of PGE$_2$ and 6-keto-PGF$_{1\alpha}$, but had little effect on TxB$_2$ synthesis by the rabbit colon[91].

In a model of colitis produced by instillation of acetic acid into the rat colon, there was also an increase in arachidonic acid metabolism[92]. Scrapings of inflamed colonic mucosa incubated with [^{14}C]AA in the presence and absence of calcium ionophore formed increased levels of radiolabelled metabolites, including LTB$_4$, the lipoxygenase-derived monohydroxy fatty acids as well as the cyclo-oxygenase products. The radiolabelled metabolites were separated by TLC and measured by liquid scintillation counting and unlabelled products were separated by HPLC and measured by UV absorbance[92].

A new model of inflammatory bowel disease

The rat is a species which has been widely used in the laboratory for studies into both gastrointestinal function and inflammation. The previously described methods of inducing experimental IBD in rats have not, however, provided a model which has both the chronicity and the pathological features of the disease.

Recently a new model of IBD was described in rats which is induced by the hapten, trinitrobenzene sulphonic acid (TNB)[93]. In this model, a single instillation of TNB into the rat colon produces a chronic ulceration and inflammation. The hapten is dissolved in ethanol and it is assumed that this acts as a 'barrier breaker', allowing the hapten access to the lamina propria which then induces the chronic inflammatory response. This model of IBD has many of the features of Crohn's disease. The damage produced includes open ulceration that persists for at least 5 weeks. The inflammation is transmural and produces a thickening of the bowel wall. Histopathological features include distorted crypt architecture, crypt atrophy, granulomata, giant cells, basal lymphoid aggregates and the presence of an inflammatory infiltrate.

As shown in Figure 2.12, the development of the chronic inflammation was investigated by measuring changes in arachidonic acid metabolism, and in the inflammatory cell infiltration into the colon, using both histological techniques and the activity of myeloperoxidase[46].

Inflammation of the colon was induced in female Wistar rats (200–250 g) by a single intracolonic administration of TNB. After anaesthetizing the rats with ether, the TNB solution (25 mg, dissolved in 0.25 ml of 30% ethanol) was administered into the colon via the anus using a rubber catheter (8 cm long, external diameter 2 mm). Groups of rats (3 or 4) were killed at various times (between 1 hour and 3 weeks) after TNB. The distal 6–8 cm of colon was removed, opened longitudinally and washed to remove luminal contents. The excised colon was pinned out flat on a wax block flooded with 0.9% saline. Small sections of colon were taken from two distinct areas from each colon and placed in storage fixative (glutaraldehyde 1% in 4% formaldehyde) for histology.

Coded histological sections were examined using light microscopy. Oedema, cellular infiltration and necrosis were assessed in a blind manner and each parameter given a score between 0–3 depending on the extent of the histological changes observed. A larger segment (> 50 mg) was immediately frozen ($-20°C$, cardice) for later estimation of MPO activity. A third segment (> 200 mg) was placed on ice for incubation with [^{14}C]AA. If gross colonic damage was apparent, the segments of tissue were taken from the areas involved; if not, segments were taken from a corresponding area of the colon. The metabolism of [^{14}C]AA to 11-, 12- and 15-HETE (HETE) and 6-keto-$PGF_{1\alpha}$, were used as indices of lipoxygenase and cyclo-oxygenase activity respectively.

There was an increase in HETE formation which reached a peak 24–36 h after TNB, but then fell to control levels 54 h after TNB administration. These changes in HETE were confirmed by separating the metabolites by TLC using two different solvent systems. The changes in 6-keto-$PGF_{1\alpha}$ formation were

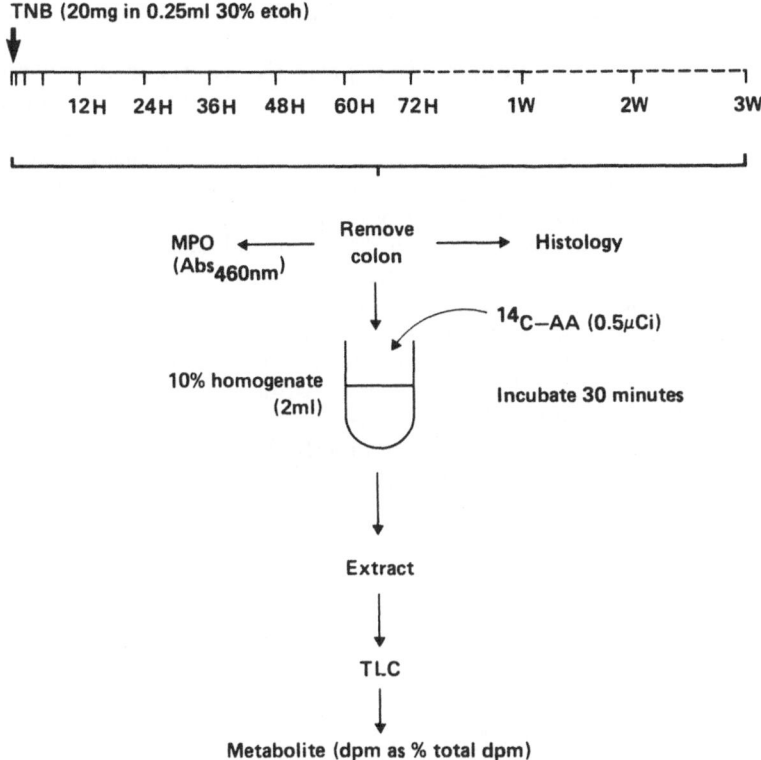

Figure 2.12 Experimental protocol used to study the inflammatory bowel disease induced in rats by intracolonic administration of TNB (20 mg in 0.25 ml of 30% ethanol). The metabolism of [14C]arachidonic acid by rat colon was measured at various times after TNB. In addition, leukocyte infiltration was assessed histologically and by measuring myeloperoxidase activity (MPO)

distinct from those of the lipoxygenase products. Following an initial significant fall, there was a gradual increase in 6-keto-$PGF_{1\alpha}$ which was maintained for up to 72 h after TNB. The formation of 6-keto-$PGF_{1\alpha}$ then returned to control levels after one week but subsequently fell below the level of the control 2 and 3 weeks after TNB[46].

Intestinal protection by prostaglandins

The well-documented ability of prostaglandins to protect the gastric mucosa from a variety of damaging agents[94-96] had led to studies on their protective activity in the intestine. Several prostaglandins and their analogues, particularly of the PGE_2 series, have been shown to protect the small intestine of animals from damage induced by indomethacin[97] or prednisolone[98], and the caecum from damage induced by the toxin *Clostridium difficile*[99]. Similarly, stable

39

prostacyclin analogues prevent indomethacin-induced lesions in the jejeunum and ileum[100].

In a recent study, we investigated the protective effects of 16,16-dimethyl PGE$_2$ in a model of acute damage of the rat colon induced by luminally-applied ethanol[101]. Twenty minutes after the intrarectal instillation of the prostaglandin analogue, 0.25 ml of 30% ethanol (v/v distilled water) was administered intrarectally. After a further 10 min, the colon was excised and the microscopically-visible damage was assessed. The damage was characterized as regions of extensive hyperaemia and haemorrhage. Histologically, the mucosal surface of the ethanol-treated colons was completely destroyed and there was extensive necrosis of the mucosal tissue. Disruption of mucosal cells was also assessed by measuring the intraluminal release *in vitro* of the cytoplasmic enzyme marker, lactate dehydrogenase, and the lysosomal enzyme, acid phosphatase. Pretreatment with the prostaglandin analogue reduced the ethanol-induced colonic damage, as assessed using all three of the parameters employed. Such methodology could also be utilized to assess the colonic damage in models of IBD and to demonstrate the effects of putative therapeutic agents.

SUMMARY

The methods described in this chapter to study eicosanoids have all helped to increase our understanding of their role in IBD. The biosynthesis of eicosanoids by intestinal tissue and their increased formation in IBD has been demonstrated by several investigators using a variety of tissue preparations, incubation conditions and analytical techniques. None of the methods used are ideal, all having their advantages and disadvantages, but overall these studies have enhanced our knowledge of the disease process. Most of the early studies were concerned with the measurement of prostanoid synthesis, while more recent investigations have included measurement of the products of the lipoxygenase pathways of arachidonic acid metabolism, including the biologically-active leukotrienes. These studies have largely satisfied the second and third criteria set down to identify and characterize a mediator of inflammation i.e. that the mediator is recoverable from the site of inflammation and is identified by appropriate pharmacological and physicochemical techniques. However, since inhibitors of cyclo-oxygenase have failed to be of clinical benefit in the treatment of ulcerative colitis, the products of this pathway of arachidonic acid metabolism, the prostaglandins and thromboxanes, do not fulfill the fourth criteria that inhibitors of the release of the mediator should reduce the inflammatory response proposed to be produced by it. The role of the products of the lipoxygenase pathway in inflammatory bowel disease clearly requires further investigation. In addition, the interaction of eicosanoids with other proposed mediators of inflammatory cell activity such as monokines and lymphokines will provide further valuable insight into their role in the disease. Some of the methods described in this chapter will aid in these investigations, while advances in our knowledge of these mediators and in technology will provide novel approaches for the study and understanding of the role of eicosanoid in the pathogenesis of inflammatory bowel disease.

REFERENCES

1. Gould, S.R. (1976). Assay of prostaglandin-like substances in faeces and their measurement in ulcerative colitis. *Prostaglandins*, **11**, 489–493
2. Flower, R.J. (1978). Steroidal anti-inflammatory drugs as inhibitors of phospholipase A$_2$. In Samuelsson, B. and Paoletti, R. (eds.) *Adv. Prostagl. Thrombox. Res.*, **3**, 105–112 (New York: Raven Press)
3. Higgs, G.A., Moncada, S. and Vane, J.R. (1984). Eicosanoids in inflammation. *Ann. Clin. Res.*, **16**, 287–299
4. Higgs, G.A., Palmer, R.M.J., Eakins, K.E. and Moncada, S. (1981). Arachidonic acid metabolism as a source of inflammatory mediators and its inhibition as a mechanism of action for anti-inflammatory drugs. *Mol. Aspects Med.*, **4**, 275–301
5. Salmon, J.A. and Flower, R.J. (1983). Prostaglandins and related compounds. In Gray, C.H. and James, V.H.T. (eds.) *Hormones in the Blood*, Vol. 5, pp. 138–165. (Academic Press)
6. Whittle, B.J.R. and Vane, J.R. (1983). Prostacyclin, thromboxanes, and prostaglandins – actions and roles in the gastrointestinal tract. In Jerzy-Glass, G.B. and Sherlock, P. (eds.) *Progress in Gastroenterology*, pp. 3–30. (New York: Grune and Stratton)
7. Rask-Madsen, J. and Bukhave, K. (1979). Prostaglandins and chronic diarrhoea: clinical aspects. *Scand. J. Gastroenterol.*, **14**, Suppl. 53, 73–78
8. Rachmilewitz, D. (1980). Prostaglandins and diarrhoea. *Dig. Dis. Sci.*, **25**, 897–899
9. Samuelsson, B., Borgeat, P., Hammarstrom, S. and Murphy, R.C. (1980). Leukotrienes: a new group of biologically active compounds. In Samuelsson, B., Ramwell, P. and Paoletti, R. (eds.) *Adv. Prostagl. Thrombox. Res.*, **6**, 1–18, (New York: Raven Press)
10. Samuelsson, B. (1983). Leukotrienes: mediators of immediate hypersensitivity reactions and inflammation. *Science*, **220**, 568–575
11. Rampton, D.S. and Hawkey, C.J. (1984). Prostaglandins and ulcerative colitis. *Gut*, **25**, 1399–1413
12. Gould, S.R., Brash, A.R., Conolly, M.E. and Lennard-Jones, J.E. (1981). Studies of prostaglandins and sulphasalazine in ulcerative colitis. *Prostagl. Med.*, **6**, 165–182
13. Harris, D.W., Swan, C.H.J. and Smith, P.R. (1978). Venous prostaglandin-like activity in diarrhoeal states. *Gut*, **19**, 1057–1058
14. Rampton D.S., Sladen G.E. and Youlten, L.J. (1980). Rectal mucosal prostaglandin E$_2$ release and its relation to disease activity, electrical potential difference, and treatment in ulcerative colitis. *Gut*, **21**, 591–596
15. Lauritsen, K., Laursen, L.S., Bukhave, K. and Rask-Madsen, J. (1985). Effects of topical 5-aminosalicylic acid (5-ASA) and prednisolone on prostaglandin (PG) E$_2$ and leukotriene (LT) B$_4$ levels determined by equilibrium *in vivo* dialysis of rectum in relapsing ulcerative colitis (UC). *Gastroenterology*, **88**, A1466
16. Eastwood, G.L. and Trier, J.R. (1973). Organ culture of human rectal mucosa. *Gastroenterology*, **64**, 375–382
17. Eastwood, G.L. and Trier, J.R. (1973). Epithelial cell renewal in cultured rectal biopsies in ulcerative colitis. *Gastroenterology*, **64**, 383–390
18. Sharon, P., Ligumsky, M., Rachmilewitz, D. and Zor, U. (1978). Role of prostaglandins in ulcerative colitis. Enhanced production during active disease and inhibition by sulfasalazine. *Gastroenterology*, **75**, 638–649
19. Ligumsky, M., Karmeli, F., Sharon, P., Zor, U, Cohen, F. and Rachmilewitz, D. (1981). Enhanced thromboxane A$_2$ and prostacyclin production by cultured rectal mucosa in ulcerative colitis and its inhibition by steroids and sulfasalazine. *Gastroenterology*, **81**, 444–449
20. Hawkey, C.J. and Truelove, S.C. (1981). Effect of prednisolone on prostaglandin synthesis by rectal mucosa in ulcerative colitis: investigation by laminar flow bioassay and radioimmunoassay. *Gut*, **22**, 190–193
21. Hawkey, C.J. and Truelove, S.C. (1983). Inhibition of prostaglandin synthetase in human rectal mucosa. *Gut*, **24**, 213–217

22. Hoult, J.R.S. and Page, J. (1981). 5-Aminosalicylic acid, a co-factor for colonic prostacyclin synthesis? *Lancet*, **1**, 255

23. Whittle, B.J.R. (1981). Temporal relationship between cyclo-oxygenase inhibition, measured as prostacyclin biosynthesis, and the gastrointestinal damage induced by indomethacin in rat. *Gastroenterology*, **80**, 94–98

24. Sinzinger, H., Silberbrauer, K. and Seyfried, H. (1979). Rectal mucosa prostacyclin formation in ulcerative colitis. *Lancet*, **1**, 444

25. Harris, D.W., Smith, P.R. and Swan, C.H.J. (1978). Determination of prostaglandin synthetase activity in rectal biopsy material and its significance in colonic disease. *Gut*, **19**, 875–877

26. Boughton-Smith, N.K., Hawkey, C.J. and Whittle, B.J.R. (1983). Biosynthesis of lipoxygenase and cyclo-oxygenase products of [^{14}C]-arachidonic acid by human colonic mucosa. *Gut*, **24**, 1176–1182

27. Vane, J.R. (1971). Inhibition of prostaglandin synthesis as a mechanism of action for the aspirin-like drugs. *Nature*, **231**, 232–235

28. Higgs, G.A., Flower, R.J. and Vane, J.R. (1979). A new approach to anti-inflammatory drugs. *Biochem. Pharmacol.*, **28**, 1959–1961

29. Sharon, P. and Stenson, W.F. (1984). Enhanced synthesis of leukotriene B$_4$ by colonic mucosa in inflammatory bowel disease. *Gastroenterology*, **86**, 453–460

30. Zifroni, A., Treves, A.J., Sachar, D.B. and Rachmilewitz, D. (1983). Prostanoid synthesis by cultured intestinal epithelial and mononuclear cells in inflammatory bowel disease. *Gut*, **24**, 659–664

31. Schlenker, T. and Peskar, B.M. (1981). Dual effect of sulphasalazine in colonic prostaglandin synthetase. *Lancet*, **1**, 815

32. Hoult, J.R.S. and Moore, P.K. (1978). Sulphasalazine is a potent inhibitor of prostaglandin 15-hydroxydehydrogenase: possible basis for therapeutic action in ulcerative colitis. *Br. J. Pharmacol.*, **64**, 6–8

33. Hillier, K., Mason, P.J., Pacheco, S. and Smith, C.L. (1982). Ulcerative colitis: effect of sulphasalazine, its metabolites and indomethacin on the ability of human colonic mucosa to metabolize prostaglandins *in vitro*. *Br. J. Pharmacol.*, **76**, 157–161

34. Peskar, B.M., Dreyling, K.W., Hope, U., Schaavschmidt, K., Goebell, H. and Peskar, B.A. (1985). Formation of sulfidopeptide-leukotrienes (SP-LT) in normal human colonic tissue, colonic carcinoma and Crohn's disease. *Gastroenterology*, **88**, A1537

35. Hawkey, C.J., Boughton-Smith, N.K. and Whittle, B.J.R. (1985). Modulation of human colonic arachidonic acid metabolism by sulfasalazine. *Dig. Dis. Sci.*, **30**, 1161–1165

36. Borgeat, P. and Samuelsson, B. (1979). Arachidonic acid metabolism in polymorphonuclear leukocytes: effect of ionophore A23187. *Proc. Natl. Acad. Sci.*, **76**, 2148–2152

37. Bennett, A., Hensby, C.N., Sanger, G.J. and Stamford, I.F. (1981). Metabolites of arachidonic acid formed by human gastrointestinal tissues and their actions on the muscle layers. *Br. J. Pharmacol.*, **74**, 435–444

38. Aly, A., Johansson, C., Slezak, P. and Green, K. (1984). Bioconversion of arachidonic acid in the human gastrointestinal tract. *Biochem. Med.*, **31**, 319–331

39. Turk, J., Maas, R.L., Brash, A.R., Jackson Roberts, L. and Oates, J.A. (1982). Arachidonic acid 15-lipoxygenase products from human eosinophils. *J. Biol. Chem.*, **257**, 7068–7076

40. Harkness, R.A. (1981). The characteristic cell of acute inflammation, the polymorphonuclear neutrophil leucocyte, and its biochemistry. *Molec. Aspects Med.*, **4**, 191–207

41. Schultz, J. and Kaminker, K. (1962). Myeloperoxidase of the leukocyte of normal blood content and localization. *Arch. Biochem. Biophys.*, **96**, 456–467

42. Bradley, P.P., Priebat, D.A., Christensen, R.D. and Rothstein, G. (1982). Measurement of cutaneous inflammation: estimation of neutrophil content with an enzyme marker. *J. Invest. Dermatol.*, **78**, 206–209

43. Williams, R.N. and Paterson, C.A. (1985). Anomalous effects of anti-inflammatory corticosteroids in endotoxin-induced ocular inflammation. *Eur. J. Pharmacol.*, **106**, 113–119

44. Mullane, K.M., Fraemer, R. and Smith, B. (1985). Myeloperoxidase activity as a quantitative assessment of neutrophil infiltration into ischaemic myocardium. *J. Pharmacol. Meth.*, **14**, 157–167

45. Krawisz, J.E., Sharon, P. and Stenson, W.F. (1984). Quantitative assay for acute intestinal inflammation based on myeloperoxidase activity. *Gastroenterology*, **87**, 1344–1350

46. Boughton-Smith, N.K., Wallace, J.L. and Whittle, B.J.R. (1985). Arachidonic acid meta-

bolism and leukocyte infiltration, as measured by myeloperoxidase activity in a model of IBD. *Gut*, **26**, A1148

47. O'Morain, C., Smethhurst, P., Levi, A.J. and Peters, T.J. (1983). Biochemical analysis of enzymic markers of inflammation in rectal biopsies from patients with ulcerative colitis and Crohn's disease. *J. Clin. Pathol.*, **36**, 1312–1316

48. Seymour, C.A. and Peters, T.J. (1977). Enzyme activities in human liver biopsies. Assay methods and activities of some lysosomal and membrane-bound enzyme in control tissue samples. *Clin. Sci. Mol. Med.*, **52**, 229–239

49. Kane, S.P. and Peters, T.J. (1975). Analytical subcellular fractionation of human granulo-cytes with reference to the localisation of vitamin B12 binding protein. *Clin. Sci. Mol. Med.*, **49**, 171–182

50. Rachmilewitz, D., Ligumsky, M., Rachmilewitz, B., Rachmilewitz, M., Tarcic, N. and Schlesinger, M. (1980). Transcobalomin II level in peripheral blood monocytes – a bio-chemical marker in inflammatory bowel disease. *Gastroenterology*, **78**, 43–46

51. Flemming, A. (1922). On a remarkable bacteriolytic element found in tissues and secretions. *Proc. Roy. Soc. B*, **93**, 306–312

52. Lippman, M.F. and Finch, S.C. (1972). A quantitative study of muramidase distribution in normal and nitrogen mustard treated rats. *Yale J. Biol. Med.*, **45**, 463–470

53. MacPherson, B. and Pfeiffer, C.J. (1976). Experimental colitis. *Digestion*, **14**, 424–452

54. Madara, J.L., Podolsky, D.K., King, N.W., Sehgal, P.K., Moore, R. and Winter, H.S. (1985). Characterization of spontaneous colitis in cotton-top tamarins (saguinus oedipus) and its response to sulfasalazine. *Gastroenterology*, **88**, 13–19

55. Marston, A., Marcuson, R.W., Chapman, M. and Arthur, J.E. (1969). Experimental study of devascularization of the colon. *Gut*, **10**, 121–130

56. Kirsner, J.B. (1961). Experimental 'colitis' with particular reference to hypersensitivity reactions in the colon. *Gastroenterology*, **40**, 307–312

57. Pfeiffer, C.J. (1985). Animal models of colitis. In Pfeiffer, C.J. (ed.) *Animal Models of Intestinal Disease*, pp. 148–155. (Florida: CRC Press)

58. Halpern, B., Zweibaum, A., Oriol Palou, R. and Morard, J.C. (1967). Experimental immune ulcerative colitis. In *Immunopathology. 5th Int. Symp. Mechanisms of Inflammation induced by Immune Reactions.* pp. 161–178. (New York: Grune and Stratton)

59. Cooke, E.M., Filipe, M.T. and Dawson, I.M.P. (1968). The production of colonic auto-antibodies in rabbits by immunization with *Escherichia coli. J. Pathol. Bacteriol.*, **96**, 125–130

60. Rabin, B.S. and Herrington, E. (1980). Antibody-mediated complement-dependent cyto-toxicity in immunologically induced experimental colon disease. *Int. Arch. Allergy Immun.*, **63**, 205–211

61. Kraft, S.C. and Kirsner, J.B. (1971). Immunological apparatus of the gut and inflammatory bowel disease. *Gastroenterology*, **60**, 922–951

62. Humphrey, C.D., Lushbaugh, W.B., Condon, C.W., Pittman, J.C. and Pittman, F.E. (1979). Light and electron microscopic studies of antibiotic associated colitis in the hamster. *Gut*, **20**, 6–15

63. Rehg, J.E. (1980). Cecal toxin(s) from guinea pigs with clindamycin-associated colitis, neutralized by clostridium sordellii antitoxin. *Infect. Immun.*, **27**, 387–390

64. Rothman, S.W. (1981). Presence of clostridium difficile toxin in guinea pigs with penicillin-associated colitis. *Med. Microbiol. Immunol.*, **169**, 187–196

65. Melnyk, C.S. (1980). Experimental enteritis and colitis. In Kirsner, J.B. and Shorter, R.G. (eds.) *Inflammatory Bowel Disease*. pp. 25–43 (Philadelphia: Lea and Febiger)

66. Kirsner, J.B., Elahlepp, J.G., Goldgraber, M.B., Ablaza, J. and Ford, H. (1959). Production of experimental ulcerative 'colitis' in rabbits. *Arch. Pathol.*, **68**, 392–408

67. Hodgson, H.J.F., Potter, B.J., Skinner, J. and Jewell, D.P. (1978). Immune-complex mediated colitis in rabbits. *Gut*, **19**, 225–232

68. Mee, A.S., McLaughlin, J.E., Hodgson, H.J.F. and Jewell, D.P. (1979). Chronic immune colitis in rabbits. *Gut*, **20**, 1–5

69. Marcus, R. and Watt, J. (1969). Seaweeds and ulcerative colitis in laboratory animals. *Lancet*, **2**, 489–490

70. Watt, J. and Marcus, R. (1971). Carrageenan-induced ulceration of the large intestine in the guinea pig. *Gut*, **12**, 164–171

71. Watt, J., McLean, C. and Marcus, R. (1979). Degradation of carrageenan for the experimental production of ulcers in the colon. *J. Pharm. Pharmacol.*, **31**, 645–646
72. Benitz, K.-F., Goldberg, L. and Coulston, F. (1973). Intestinal effects of carrageenans in the rhesus monkey. *Food Cosmet. Toxicol.*, **11**, 565–575
73. Grasso, P., Sharratt, M., Carpanini, F.M.B. and Gangolli, S.D. (1973). Studies on carrageenan and large-bowel ulceration in mammals. *Food Cosmet. Toxicol.*, **11**, 555–564
74. Norris, A.A., Lewis, A.J. and Zeitlin, I.J. (1981). Inability of degraded carrageenan fractions to induce inflammatory bowel ulceration in the guinea-pig. *J. Pharm. Pharmacol.*, **33**, 612–613
75. Boxenbaum, H.G. and Dairman, W. (1977). Evaluation of an animal model for the screening of compounds potentially useful in human ulcerative colitis: effect of salicylazosulfapyridine and prednisolone on carrageenan-induced ulceration of the large intestine of the guinea pig. *Drug Dev. Ind. Pharm.*, **3**, 121–130
76. Watt, J., Marcus, S.N. and Marcus, A.J. (1980). The comparative prophylactic effects of sulphasalazine, prednisolone and azathioprine in experimental colonic ulceration. *J. Pharm. Pharmacol.*, **32**, 873–874
77. Jensen, B.H., Andersen, J.O., Poulsen, S.S., Skov Olsen, P., Norby, S., Rasmussen, S., Hansen, H. and Hvidberg, E.F. (1984). The prophylactic effect of 5-aminosalicylic acid and salazosulphapyridine on degraded-carrageenan-induced colitis in guinea pigs. *Scand. J. Gastroenterol.*, **19**, 299–303
78. Onderdonk, A.B., Hermos, J.A., Dzink, J.L. and Bartlett, J.L. (1978). Protective effect of metronidazole in experimental ulcerative colitis. *Gastroenterology*, **74**, 521–526
79. Onderdonk, A.B. and Bartlett, J.G. (1979). Bacteriological studies of experimental ulcerative colitis. *Am. J. Clin. Nutr.*, **32**, 258–265
80. Rosenberg, E.W. and Fischer, R.W. (1964). DNCB allergy in the guinea pig colon. *Arch. Dermatol.*, **89**, 159–163
81. Bicks, R.O., Azar, M.M., Rosenberg, E.W., Dunham, W.G. and Luther, J. (1967). Delayed hypersensitivity reactions in the intestinal tract. I. Studies of 2,4-dinitrochlorobenzene-caused guinea pig and swine colon lesions. *Gastroenterology*, **53**, 422–436
82. Rabin, B.S. and Rogers, S.J. (1978). A cell-mediated immune model of inflammatory bowel disease in the rabbit. *Gastroenterology*, **75**, 29–33
83. Glick, M.E. and Falchuk, Z.M. (1981). Dinitrochlorobenzene-induced colitis in the guinea-pig: studies of colonic lamina propria lymphocytes. *Gut*, **22**, 120–125
84. Askenase, P.W., Boone, W.T. and Binder, H.J. (1978). Colonic basophil hypersensitivity. *J. Immunol.*, **120**, 198–201
85. Mitchell, E.B. and Askenase, P.W. (1982). Suppression of T cell-mediated cutaneous basophil hypersensitivity by serum from guinea-pigs immunized with mycobacterial adjuvant. *J. Exp. Med.*, **156**, 159–172
86. Norris, A.A., Lewis, A.J. and Zeitlin, I.J. (1982). Changes in colonic tissue levels of inflammatory mediators in a guinea-pig model of immune colitis. *Agents Actions*, **12**, 243–246
87. Boughton-Smith, N.K. and Whittle, B.J.R. (1985). Increased metabolism of arachidonic acid in an immune model of colitis in guinea-pigs. *Br. J. Pharmacol.*, **86**, 439–446
88. Salmon, J.A., Simmons, P.M. and Palmer, R.M.J. (1982). A radioimmunoassay for leukotriene B$_4$. *Prostaglandins*, **24**, 225–235
89. Hoult, J.R.S., Moore, P.K., Marcus, A.J. and Watt, J. (1979). On the effect of sulphasalazine on the prostaglandin system and the defective prostaglandin inactivation observed in experimental ulcerative colitis. *Agents Actions*, **4**, 232–244
90. Wolbling, R.H., Aehringhaus, U., Peskar, B.A., Morgenroth, K. and Peskar, B.M. (1983). Release of slow-reacting substance of anaphylaxis and leukotriene C$_4$-like immunoreactivity from guinea pig colonic tissue. *Prostaglandins*, **25**, 809–822
91. Zipser, R.D., Patterson, J.B., Kao, H.W., Hauser, C.J. and Lecke, R. (1985). Hypersensitive prostaglandin and thromboxane response to hormones in rabbit colitis. *Am. J. Physiol.*, **249**, G457–463
92. Sharon, P. and Stenson, W.F. (1985). Metabolism of arachidonic acid in acetic acid colitis in rats. Similarity to human inflammatory bowel disease. *Gastroenterology*, **88**, 55–63
93. Morris, G.P., Rebetro, L., Herridge, M.M., Szewczuk, M. and Depew, W. (1984). An animal model for chronic granulomatous inflammation of the stomach and colon. *Gastroenterology*, **86**, A1188

94. Robert, A. (1976). Antisecretory anti-ulcer, cytoprotective and diarrheogenic properties of prostaglandins. In Samuelsson, R. and Paoletti, R. (eds.) *Adv. Prostagl. Thrombox. Res.*, **2**, 507–520. (New York: Raven Press)

95. Miller, T.A. (1983). Protective effects of prostaglandins against gastric mucosal damage: current knowledge and proposed mechanism. *Am. J. Physiol.*, **254**, G601–623

96. Hawkey, C.J. and Rampton, D.S. (1985). Prostaglandins and the gastrointestinal mucosa: are they important in its function, disease, or treatment? *Gastroenterology*, **89**, 1162–1188

97. Robert, A. (1975). An intestinal disease produced experimentally by a prostaglandin deficiency. *Gastroenterology*, **69**, 1045–1047

98. Lancaster, C. and Robert, A. (1978). Intestinal lesions produced by prednisolone: Prevention (cytoprotection) by 16,16-dimethyl prostaglandin E_2. *Am. J. Physiol.*, **235**, E703–E708

99. Robert, A., Bundy, G.L., Field, S.O., Nezamis, J.E., Davis, J.P., Hanchar, A.J., Lancaster, C. and Ruwart, M.J. (1985). Prevention of colitis in hamsters by certain prostaglandins. *Prostaglandins*, **29**, 961–980

100. Whittle, B.R.J. and Boughton-Smith, N.K. (1979). 16-Phenoxy prostacyclin analogs – potent selective antiulcer compounds. In Vane, J.R. and Bergstrom, S. (eds.) *Prostacyclin*, pp. 159–170. (New York: Raven Press)

101. Wallace, J.L., Whittle, B.J.R. and Boughton-Smith, N.K. (1985). Prostaglandin protection of rat colonic mucosa from damage induced by ethanol. *Dig. Dis. Sci.*, **30**, 866–876

3
Clinical uses of prostaglandins in peptic ulcer disease

S. J. Konturek

INTRODUCTION

For several decades the clinical understanding and medical management of peptic ulcer disease have been focused on the control and neutralization of the major aggressive factor, i.e. gastric acid–pepsin secretion. The progress in this direction has been highlighted by the discoveries of powerful inhibitors of the parietal cell receptors such as H2-receptor antagonists (cimetidine and ranitidine), muscarinic receptor (M1 and M2) inhibitors (pirenzepine) and possible gastrin-receptor inhibitors (proglumide). Furthermore, the inhibitors of second messengers of the parietal cells (calcium ions and cyclic AMP), such as calcium-channel blockers and prostaglandins as well as proton pump inhibitors (omeprazole), have been added to the spectrum of acid suppressing therapeutic agents.

There is, however, no direct evidence that acid–pepsin secretion and its abnormalities play a crucial role in the pathogenesis of peptic ulceration and that the inhibition of acid secretion is a prerequisite of ulcer healing. Hence, there has been a shift of emphasis from studies of aggressive factors towards the more careful examination of defence mechanisms. It has been correctly pointed out that while a substantial number of individuals show gastric acid–pepsin hypersecretion only a few develop peptic ulcerations. Thus peptic ulcer may occur because of too little mucosal resistance rather than too much acid–pepsin secretion.

Among the mechanisms protecting the gastroduodenal mucosa against damage and ulcer formation, attention has been directed to the possible importance of

(1) Mucus–alkaline secretion that provides a continuous cover of the mucosa and the barrier between the epithelial cells and acid pepsin in the lumen;
(2) The hydrophobic mucosal barrier preventing the penetration of luminal acid into the mucosa;

(3) Rapid epithelial cell renewal for a quick recovery from the mucosal insults;
(4) Rich mucosal blood flow providing oxygen and necessary nutrients to increased cell resistance, and
(5) The presence in the mucosa of natural protective factors, particularly certain prostaglandins (PG).

Gastrointestinal mucosa, which is constantly exposed to a variety of irritants and damaging factors, including its own secretions (acid, pepsin, bile acids), spicy food, micro-organisms, nicotine, ethanol or drugs, is capable of maintaining its integrity due to the activation of the protective mechanisms. The mucosa is capable of generating substantial amounts of various metabolites of arachidonic acid, particularly E and I series PG, which have been implicated in the mucosal protective mechanisms and the mediation of the 'adaptation' of the stomach to a hostile environment and tissue repair. Acute deficiency of PG in the mucosa caused by the administration of noxious agents such as non-steroidal anti-inflammatory compounds (NOSAC) has been considered an important factor in the disruption of the gastric mucosal barrier, gastric bleeding and gross mucosal lesions. There is an increasing body of evidence that chronic deficiency of mucosal PG or the inadequate capacity of the mucosa to biosynthesize PG may be an important factor in the pathogenesis of chronic gastroduodenal ulcerations.

Following an understanding of mucosal protective mechanisms, several therapeutic agents which do not inhibit or neutralize gastric acid but which activate these mechanisms have been successfully used in peptic ulcer therapy. PG and their stable analogues are now recognized as standard gastroprotective compounds but they appear to increase the healing rate of gastroduodenal ulcerations only when larger, gastric inhibitor doses of these agents are used. Other agents such as carbenoxolone, colloidal bismuth subcitrate (De-Nol), basic aluminium sucrose octasulphate (sucralfate) and certain flavonoids (Solon) have been found to increase the mucosal PG biosynthesis and to have efficacy in the management of ulcer disease similar to that of agents acting via the anti-secretory mechanism.

This review discusses the involvement of prostaglandins and related compounds in the control of gastric functions, mucosal integrity and in the pathogenesis and treatment of peptic ulcer disease.

BIOCHEMISTRY OF EICOSANOIDS

PG are products of cellular metabolism of polyunsaturated 20-carbon fatty acids. Additional products of cellular metabolism of these acids, differing in structure from PG, include the thromboxanes (Tx) and leukotrienes (LT), which are functionally interrelated with PG. These compounds have been given the generic term eicosanoids (*eicosa* = twenty).

The common precursor of PG, Tx and LT are three naturally occurring eicosapolyenoic acids, including trienoic (dihomo-γ-linolenic acid), tetraenoic (arachidonic acid − AA) and pentaenoic acid. In man, AA is by far the most common and gives rise to dienoic PG. It is derived from dietary linoleic acid or is ingested as a constituent of meat. After absorption from the gut, it is esterified and is present ubiquitously in the body as the major component of the phospholipids of cell membranes or is found in ester linkage in other complex lipids[1].

Alteration of the content of essential fatty acids in the diet may be one of the routes for modulating PG biosynthesis in the body. The hydrolysis of esterified AA present in the phospholipid pool of cell membranes provides the first rate-controlling step in PG formation. The activity of the AA 'cascade' depends on the availability of free AA at the precursor storage site in membrane phospholipids. The formation of PG precursors from dietary linoleic or dihomo-γ-linolenic acids depends on the nutritional state and the presence of other dietary fatty acids that may compete with AA for the cyclo-oxygenase or lipoxygenase pathway. Linoleic acid is a classic essential fatty acid; it is transformed to longer-chain fatty acid derivatives such as dihomo-γ-linoleic acid (precursor of PG of series I). This metabolic transformation to longer-chain fatty acid derivatives occurs mainly in the liver. The balance between the levels of linoleic acid and dihomo-γ-linolenic acid in the diet modulates the relative rate of formation of longer-chain fatty acids derived from them. Various dietary regimes in humans may modulate the biosynthesis of PG and Tx[1,2]. A deficiency of essential fatty acids decreases the biosynthesis of PG, whereas dietary loading of these acids enhances PG production in the body. Patients on a rich diet in dihomo-γ-linolenic acid also show signs of increased production of PG of series I and reduced formation of Tx resulting in decreased platelet aggregation and a lower incidence of cardiovascular diseases. The most direct way of provoking dietary stimulation of PG synthesis would be to feed dihomo-γ-linolenic acid or AA, combined with a low fat diet to reduce competition from other unsaturated fatty acids. Consumption of large amounts of eicosapentaenoic acid (EPA), present in certain fish oils, increases the content of this acid in membrane phospholipids at the expense of AA. EPA competes with AA for cyclo-oxygenase or lipoxygenase and is converted to PGI_3 and less pro-aggregatory TxA_3. These changes in PG and Tx, caused by ingestion of large amounts of EPA, occur naturally in Greenland Eskimos. It has also been shown experimentally in man that, following ingestion of either cod liver oil or mackerel, a shift of prostanoid formation from the dienoic to the trienoic series occurred and PGI_3 and TxA_3 were generated[2,3]. It is uncertain whether the diet-induced modifications in prostanoid formation are limited only to the platelets and vascular wall or whether they also occur in other tissues, such as altering PG biosynthesis in the gastrointestinal tract of PG-deficient peptic ulcer patients.

BIOSYNTHESIS AND MEASUREMENT OF EICOSANOIDS IN THE GASTROINTESTINAL TRACT

In the gastrointestinal mucosa, as in other tissues, biosynthesis of eicosanoids depends primarily upon the release of free AA from the phospholipid stores in cell membranes by various acyl hydrolases, particularly phospholipases A_2 and C. A wide variety of divergent physical, chemical and hormonal factors appears to contribute to the activation of these enzymes, probably through release of cellular calcium ions and calmodulin[1]. The chain of events leading to the release of AA may be initiated by a variety of physical and neuro-hormonal factors. The major stimulus for PG synthesis in the gastrointestinal tract appears to be mechanical strain such as distention, contraction or deformation of the gut wall associated with perturbation of the membranes of mucosal cells. Other factors activating the synthesis of eicosanoids include vagal stimulation and neurotransmitters (acetylcholine)[4], hyperosmolar solutions[5], acidification[6] or alkalinization[7] of the mucosa, ethanol[8], bile salts[9] and emptying of the gastric content of the duodenum[10].

Gastroduodenal mucosa, like other tissues, is capable of synthesizing the whole range of products of AA metabolism via the cyclo-oxygenase or lipoxygenase pathway. The first product of cyclo-oxygenase is an unstable cyclic endoperoxide derivative, PGG_2, which may proceed, either spontaneously or by a peroxidase, to PGH_2. PGH_2 is the common intermediate for TxA_2, PGD_2, PGE_2, $PGF_{2\alpha}$ and PGI_2. An endoperoxide isomerase can convert PGH_2 to either PGE_2 or to its isomer PGD_2. The combined action of this isomerase and reductase yields $PGF_{2\alpha}$. There is also a 9-keto-reductase which catalyses the interconversion of PGE_2 to $PGF_{2\alpha}$. PGH_2 may be converted by prostacyclin synthetase to PGI_2, first discovered in vascular and gastric walls. PGI_2 is unstable in physiological conditions, particlarly at low pH, hydrolysing to a stable compound 6-keto-$PGF_{1\alpha}$. The other route for PGH_2 metabolism is to TxA_2, yet another unstable and highly active compound formed by an enzyme complex, thromboxane synthetase. TxA_2 is hydrolysed non-enzymatically to the hemiacetal oxane, TxB_2 (Figure 3.1).

In addition to PG of the E, F and I series and Tx, the metabolites of another pathway converting AA to hydroperoxides (HPETE and HETE) have been discovered[1,11,12]. The most important enzyme involved in peroxidization of AA in different positions is a 5-lipoxygenase giving rise to 5-HPETE and its degradation products 5-HETE and a 5,6-epoxide known as LTA_4. The latter may be transformed to LTB_4 by an epoxide hydrolase or LTC_4 by the action of glutathione-S-transferase. The sequential removal of peptides from LTC_4 yields LTD_4 and LTE_4. The final step is the formation of LTF_4 by the reincorporation of the glutamyl group into LTE_4.

Most of these products of AA metabolism via the cyclo-oxygenase or lipoxygenase pathways have been identified, though their measurement has sometimes given difficulty. Since the synthesis of eicosanoids is activated by tissue trauma and cell perturbation, any attempt to collect mucosal samples from the stomach or duodenum should alter this synthesis. Measurement of the 'actual' level of tissue PG is problematical because biopsy itself and tissue homogenization may change PG synthesis[13]. Particular problems arise in the interpretation of luminal release of PG, especially into the gastric lumen, because gastric mucosa has an extraordinarily high catabolic capacity[14] resulting in a much reduced luminal concentration of PG. Organ culture has been used by some investigators[15,16], but it is uncertain whether substrate release due to tissue degradation is not an artifactual stimulus for PG synthesis. Whittle[17] introduced the technique of measuring the capacity of a fresh tissue sample to generate PG by vortexing it under standard conditions. This results in maximal stimulation of biosynthesis and release of PG into a tissue medium

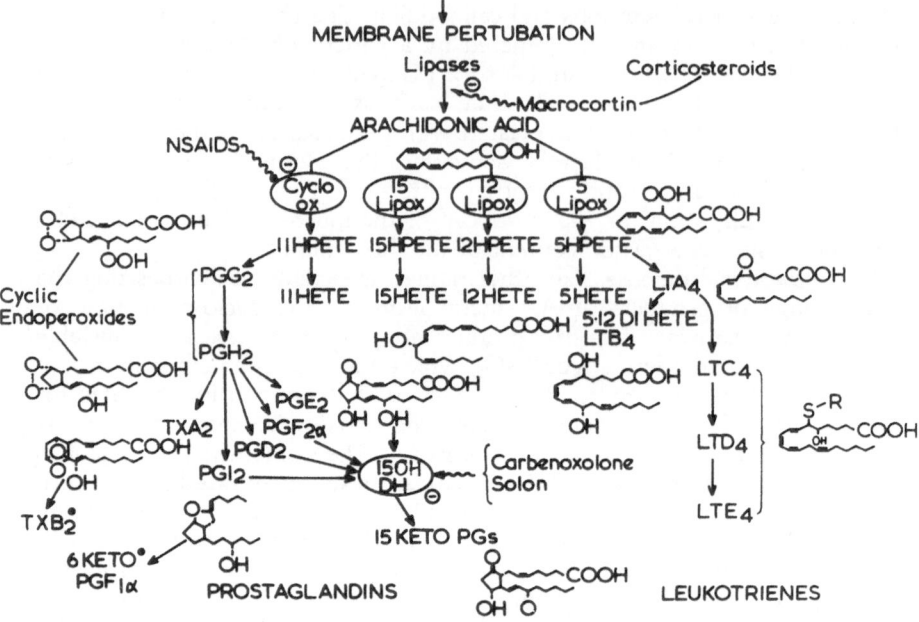

Figure 3.1 Main recognized pathways of arachidonic acid metabolism through cyclo-oxygenase and lipoxygenase. Corticosteroids inhibit phospholipase A_2 through the induction of synthesis of macrocortin. The inhibitor action of non-steroidal anti-inflammatory agents, carbenoxolone or Solon is indicated by arrows. Closed circles indicate stable products arising by non-enzymatic degradation. R = glutathione (LTC_4), cysteinylglycyl (LTD_4), cysteinyl (LTE_4)[133]

in which they can be conveniently determined either by bioassay[18] or specific radioimmunoassays[8,9]. This particular technique provides quite reliable and reproducible results but, unfortunately, does not determine the actual tissue level of eicosanoids. The relationship between the biosynthetic capacity and actual levels of tissue PG is uncertain.

In spite of these methodological problems, various studies have succeeded in identifying various metabolites of AA in the gastrointestinal mucosa, including PGE_2, PGI_2, $PGF_{2\alpha}$, TxB_2 and LT[13–15,19–22]. The precise cellular origin of mucosal eicosanoids is not certain, but probably macrophages, platelets, endothelial cells and the lamina propria are the main sites of PG synthesis, whereas surface epithelial cells are the sites of eicosanoid catabolism[23].

PG LEVELS IN PATIENTS WITH PEPTIC ULCER DISEASE

Using both bioassay and radioimmunoassay techniques, the main primary eicosanoid found in the mucosa[13,15,19–22,24–26] or detected in the gastric juice[13,19,27–30] was PGE_2. First, Bennett[13] and Cheung et al.[28] recognized that PGE-like activity is synthesized in the mucosa and released into the gastric juice. Then, Hinsdale et al.[29] reported that duodenal ulcer patients have lower concentrations of PGE in their plasma and basal gastric juice and that this may be an important aetiological factor in peptic ulcer disease. Baker et al.[27] demonstrated a positive correlation between the gastric outputs of immunoreactive PGE and PGF and gastric acid outputs stimulated by pentagastrin and insulin. It was suggested that mucosal PG may play a role in the physiological control of gastric acid secretion as local feedback inhibitors. Since plasma PG levels in duodenal ulcer patients were not lower than in healthy controls and no correlation was found between plasma PGE and gastric acid secretion, the possible importance of PG deficiency in the pathogenesis of peptic ulcer disease was refuted. Other workers studying duodenal ulcer patients also failed to confirm that PGE deficiency either in basal or insulin-stimulated[28] gastric juice but noted a disruption in the rhythms of basal PGE_2 and acid secretion[30].

Our studies[25] on the mucosal distribution of bioassayable PGE_2 revealed that the gastroduodenal mucosa is capable of generating large amounts of this eicosanoid, which were, however, not significantly correlated with the gastric acid secretory status or serum gastrin level under basal or histamine-stimulated conditions. Thus we failed to confirm the notion that mucosal PG are involved in the feedback control of gastric acid secretion in duodenal ulcer patients[27]. This does not exclude the possible role of PG in gastric secretory mechanisms, as recently it was shown that the blockade of PG cyclo-oxygenase by indomethacin in man increases gastric acid secretion[31] and oral PGE_2 inhibits gastric acid secretion[32].

There are conflicting reports on the PGE content of mucosa in gastric ulcer (GU) or duodenal ulcer (DU) patients. Schlegel et al.[24] reported that PGE and PGF levels in the mucosa of gastric ulcer patients were higher, presumably due to associated gastritis. In contrast, Wright et al.[33] found subnormal levels of mucosal PG even in the presence of gastritis. Only in the ulcer edge were the PGE_2 levels relatively higher than on the opposite side, probably due to increased inflammatory cell infiltration and tissue vascularity. It is noteworthy that ulcer healing in this study resulted in bringing the mucosal PG levels back to normal. The discovery that gastric mucosa even with active inflammation exhibits reduced PG synthesis is rather surprising, particularly as gastritis without peptic ulcer was reported to be accompanied by increased mucosal PGE levels. There may be local inhibitors of PG synthesis in the mucosa of GU patients[14].

In our study[34] including GU patients with normal histology of the fundic mucosa, the mucosal PGE_2 levels were also significantly lower than in healthy subjects. This study suggests that PG deficiency in the gastric mucosa may be a general abnormality in peptic ulcer disease, and not merely secondary to mucosal changes or the presence of ulcers (Figure 3.2).

In patients with DU, the direct and indirect methods of measuring mucosal eicosanoids have also given discordant results. Using bioassay technique, we[25] were the first to report that the major type of PG in the gastroduodenal mucosa was PGE_2, and though DU patients tended to generate smaller amounts of this PG, both in the gastric and duodenal mucosa, the difference from healthy subjects was not statistically significant. Later combined bioassay and radioimmunoassay studies[35,36] of the same biopsy mucosal samples from

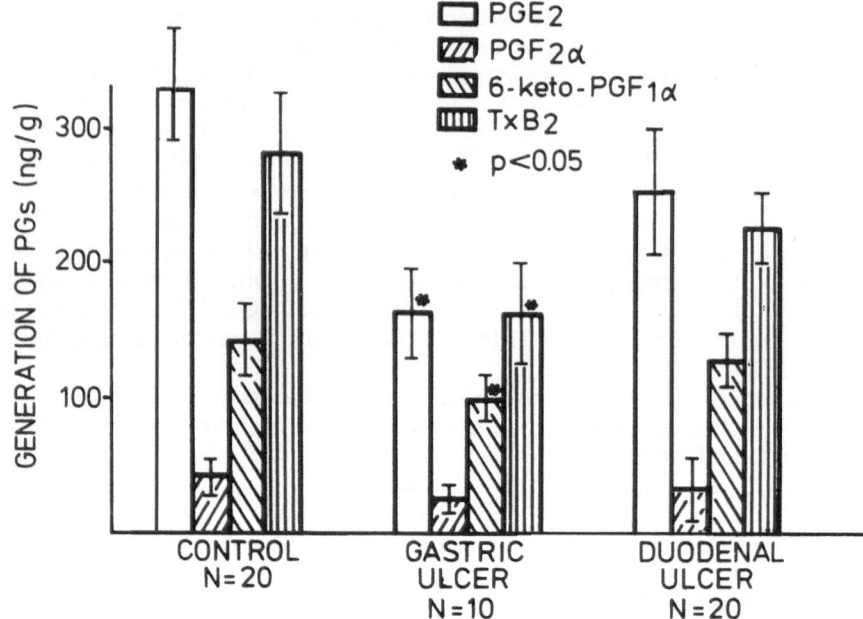

Figure 3.2 Generation of PGE_2, $PGF_{2\alpha}$, 6-keto-$PGF_{1\alpha}$, and TxB_2 by mucosal samples obtained by biopsy of the fundic portion of the stomach in healthy subjects, gastric ulcer and duodenal ulcer patients

healthy subjects and GU or DU patients confirmed that PGE_2 was the major eicosanoid. $PGF_{2\alpha}$ was detected in amounts less than 10% of PGE_2 levels, while PGI_2 (measured as stable metabolite 6-keto-$PGF_{1\alpha}$) and TxB_2 were found in quantities averaging, respectively, about 40% and 80% of PGE_2 amounts (Figure 3.2). PGE_2-like activity was also detected by RIA in the gastric juice in the basal state and following vagal stimulation (sham-feeding) or pentagastrin infusion ($2\,\mu g\,kg^{-1}\,h^{-1}$) (Figure 3.3). The generation of PGE_2, but not of PGI_2 or TxB_2, tended to decrease in DU patients both in gastric and duodenal mucosa, but this was not statistically significant[35].

Sharon et al.[16] reported that, in DU patients, cultured gastric mucosa (1.5 h) produced significantly less PGE_2, PGI_2 and TxB_2, while duodenal mucosa generated amounts of eicosanoids similar to those in normal subjects (Figure 3.4). It was suggested that the deficiency of mucosal PG formation may play an important role in the pathogenesis of DU. Since PG formed in the mucosa are considered to act locally, it is not clear how the deficiency of gastric PG might contribute to the pathogenesis of peptic ulcer in a duodenum whose mucosa retained the normal capacity for PG formation.

Recent studies have raised the possibility that the duodenal mucosa of DU patients may have a reduced capacity to generate PG of E and I series with subsequent disturbance in mucosal defence and repair mechanism. Hillier et al.[26] showed that the synthesis of PGI_2 and $PGF_{2\alpha}$, but not of PGE_2 or TxB_2, in duodenal mucosa taken both from the ulcer site and opposite this in the

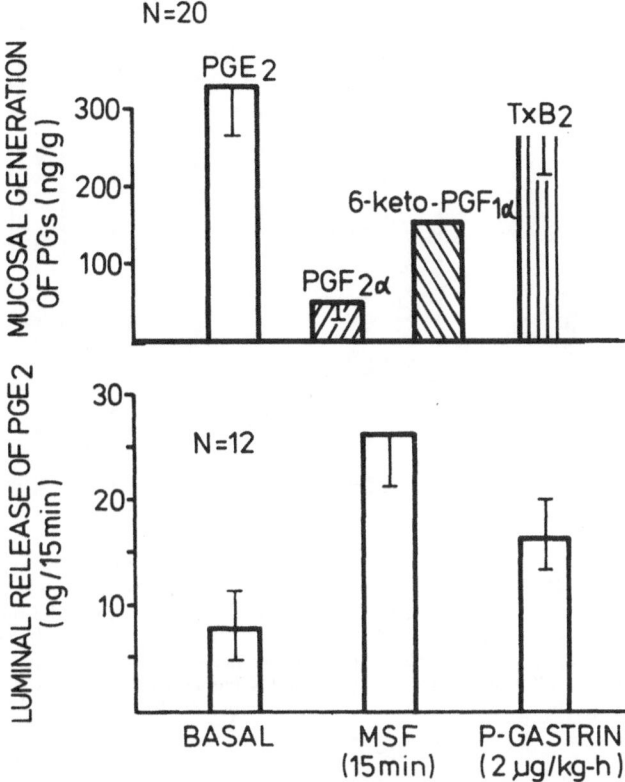

Figure 3.3 Mucosal generation of various PG and TxB_2 in fundic mucosa of healthy subjects (top) and luminal release of PGE_2-like immunoreactivity into the gastric lumen under basal conditions and following stimulation by modified sham-feeding (MSF) or pentagastrin $(2 \mu g \, kg^{-1} h^{-1})$ infusion. Reprinted from Konturek *et al.* (1983). 'The use of carprofen nonsteroidal anti-inflammatory agent in peptic ulcer disease', *Hepato-Gastroenterology*, **30**, 261–5 by permission of Georg Thieme Verlag, Stuttgart

same DU patients were significantly reduced as compared with normal mucosa (Figure 3.5). Arakawa *et al.*[37] reported that both PGE_2 and PGI_2 formation was greatly reduced in the duodenal mucosa of DU patients and that this might contribute to the decrease in the integrity of mucosa when exposed to endogenous acid. In another study[10], it was found that the duodenal mucosa of DU patients did not show any increase in PG formation after a meal. In normal subjects gastric emptying of an acidified meal into the duodenum (probably acting as 'mild irritant') was found to increase PG biosynthesis. In this study, however, the resting content of PG in the duodenal mucosa of ulcer patients was abnormally high, and in fact, fell postprandially.

Isenberg and his colleagues[38] showed that human duodenal mucosa secretes substantial amounts of bicarbonate and releases large quantities of PGE_2, particularly in response to topical acidification. Since the upper duodenum in DU patients was found to secrete significantly smaller amounts of both PGE_2

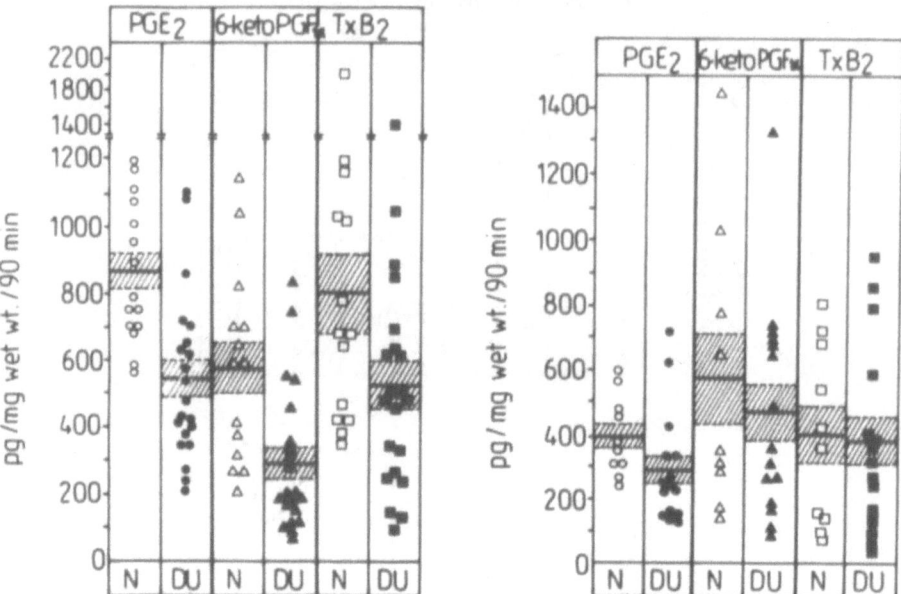

Figure 3.4 The release of PGE$_2$, 6-keto-PGF$_{1\alpha}$ and TxB$_2$ in the medium during 90 min of culturing the gastric mucosa (on the left) and the duodenal mucosa (on the right) of healthy subjects and duodenal ulcer patients[16]. Reprinted from 'Prostanoid synthesis by cultured gastric and duodenal mucosa: possible role in the pathogenesis of duodenal ulcer' by Sharon, P., Cohen, F., Zifroni, A., Karmeli, F., Ligumsky, M. and Rachmilewitz, D. from *Scandinavian Journal of Gastroenterology* by permission of Norwegian University Press (Universitetsforlaget AS), Oslo

and alkaline secretion in response to topical acidification[39], it is likely that the deficiency of duodenal PG may be the major factor in the pathogenesis of mucosal damage and ulcer formation.

ROLE OF PROSTAGLANDINS IN MUCOSAL INTEGRITY. EFFECTS OF DRUGS AFFECTING MUCOSAL PG BIOSYNTHESIS

Since PG are ubiquitous and cannot be eliminated from the body by the removal of their sources or by blocking their respective receptor sites, the results of suppression of their biosynthesis are of particular interest. As shown by Vane[40] and confirmed by others[51,52], the application of non-steroidal anti-inflammatory componds (NOSAC), such as aspirin or indomethacin, blocks PG biosynthesis by inhibition of cyclo-oxygenase activity. If the mucosal PG are implicated in the gastric protective mechanism, the suppression of their synthesis by NOSAC should result in mucosal damage. Indeed, clinical trials with NOSAC show that the most common side-effects of these agents in humans are various degrees of gastric mucosal damage including:

(1) Decrease in transmucosal potential difference[41];

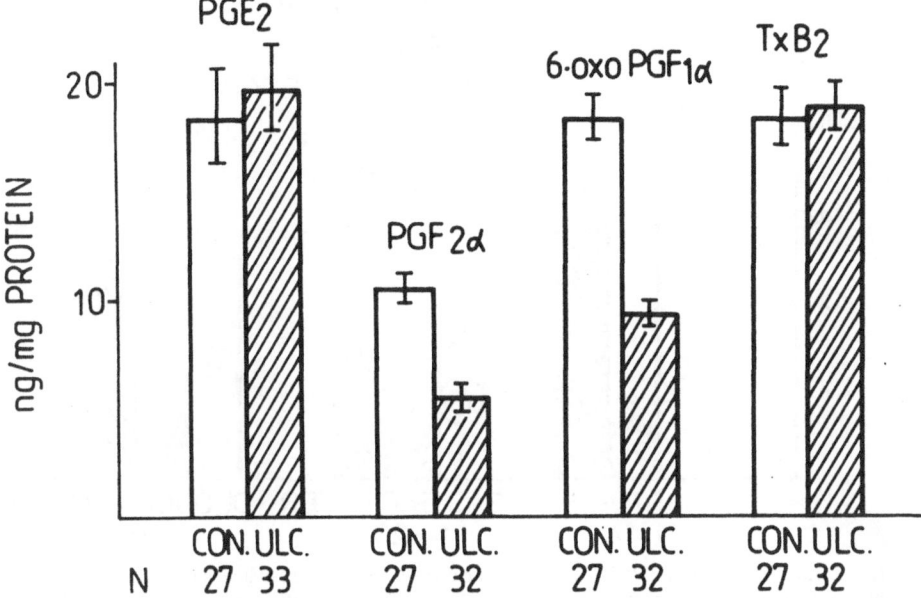

Figure 3.5 Biosynthesis of PGE_2, $PGF_{2\alpha}$, 6-keto-$PGF_{1\alpha}$ and TxB_2 by duodenal mucosa of normal subjects and duodenal ulcer patients[26]

(2) Increase in cell desquamation and DNA loss in the gastric lumen[25,34,35,41];
(3) Blood loss into the gastric lumen[41–45,47]; and
(4) The formation of mucosal lesions or frank acute ulcerations observed macroscopically[34–36,41,42,49,50].

These functional and morphological changes in the gastric mucosa were more advanced after the administration of NOSAC which have a strong inhibitory effect on PG biosynthesis (i.e. aspirin, indomethacin) than after agents with little (i.e. carprofen) or no such effect (i.e. paracetamol)[34,41,49,51] (Figure 3.6). They have been correlated with the reduction in mucosal PG generation and attributed at least in part to the suppression of PG biosynthesis. Patients with peptic ulcer in the stomach showing reduced mucosal PG generation were more sensitive to the deleterious effects of NOSAC than those with ulcer but without PG deficiency[34]. Animal studies showed that drugs with high gastric ulcerogenicity induced selective injury to the parietal, mucous, and microvascular cells coincident with depression in PGE_2 and PGI_2 levels, while drugs with low gastrotoxicity did not affect the mucosal cells and often did not reduce mucosal PG generation[46]. The presumption that NOSAC causes mucosal damage merely due to the reduction in mucosal PG biosynthesis has not been fully attested. Drugs may also inhibit the production of mucosal TxA_2[52] and this may help to offset the damage resulting from the suppression of PGE_2 and PGI_2. They may also divert arachidonate metabolism from cyclo-oxygenase to lipoxygenase products which may be deleterious to the mucosa. In addition to the sensitivity of mucosal cyclo-oxygenase or lipoxygenase to

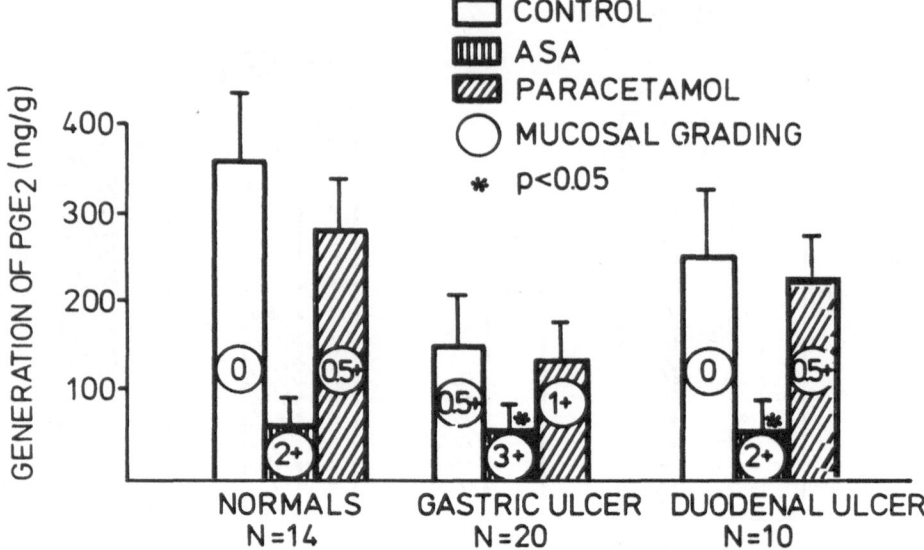

Figure 3.6   Generation of PGE_2 by the fundic mucosa of normal healthy subjects and patients with gastric or duodenal ulcers before and after administration of aspirin (2.5 g/d) or paracetamol (2.5 g/d). Numbers in circles indicate mucosal grading of the fundic mucosa according to Lanza *et al.*[49]. Reprinted with permission from Raven Press *Advances in Inflammation Research*, 'Actions of non-steroid anti-inflammatory compounds on gastric mucosal integrity and prostaglandin formation in healthy subjects and peptic ulcer patients', S.J. Konturek, Vol. 6 pp. 29–37, 1984

inhibition by NOSAC, other factors such as tissue penetration by drugs into the site of PG biosynthesis in the mucosa and the ability to produce free oxygen radicals, determine the deleterious effects of NOSAC on the gastric mucosa[13,53]. Furthermore, chronic administration of NOSAC such as aspirin results in some 'adaptation' of the mucosa[34,53] so that the acute mucosal lesions disappear in spite of continuation of the NOSAC therapy. Other agents such as steroids may affect the whole arachidonate 'cascade' but apparently it causes less mucosal damage than that observed after NOSAC.

The minimum level of tissue PG required to maintain structural integrity is uncertain, but studies in rats indicate that less than 10% of normal PG generation may be sufficient to maintain the mucosa intact[54]. Thus the reduction in mucosal PG and the resultant damage might not be closely coupled, but, in general, the results obtained with NOSAC administration in animals and man favour the conclusion that endogenous PG are implicated in the maintenance of mucosal integrity.

The role of PG in mucosal integrity is also supported by acute endoscopic studies showing that pretreatment with exogenous PGE_2 or stable analogues of PGE_1 or PGE_2 (abraprostil, misoprostol, enprostil, trimoprostil and rioprostil) reduced the gastric mucosal damage induced by aspirin[34,35,42,45,48] and by topical application of ethanol to the duodenal mucosa[55]. PGE and its analogues have also been reported to reduce the shedding of epithelial cells or DNA loss and microbleeding caused by aspirin[34,35,38,41,43–45,47] or ethanol[55,56] damage

to the duodenal mucosa. An exception may be mucosal injury caused by bile salts which appears to be resistant to the protective action of PG analogues[57].

PROSTAGLANDINS AND GASTRIC ACID SECRETION

Inhibition of gastric acid secretion has been the most extensively examined action of PG since it was first demonstrated in dogs in 1967 by Robert *et al.*[58]. The acid antisecretory action of intravenous PGA and PGE has been confirmed in humans[59–62]. When given orally to men, PGE_2 was reported to be without significant effect on gastric secretion, presumably due to its rapid degradation in contact with gastric mucosa[63]. Recently it has been reported, however, that large doses of PGE_2 administered orally may reduce stimulated acid secretion in humans[32,64].

Synthetic PG analogues, substituted in positions 15 or 16 to resist enzymatic degradation, are recognized as extremely potent inhibitors of gastric acid secretion in all species so far tested. They are active after both oral and parenteral administration[59]. They inhibit gastric acid secretion by such stimulants as vagal excitation[65,66], gastrin infusion[66,67] or a meal[66–69] (Figure 3.7).

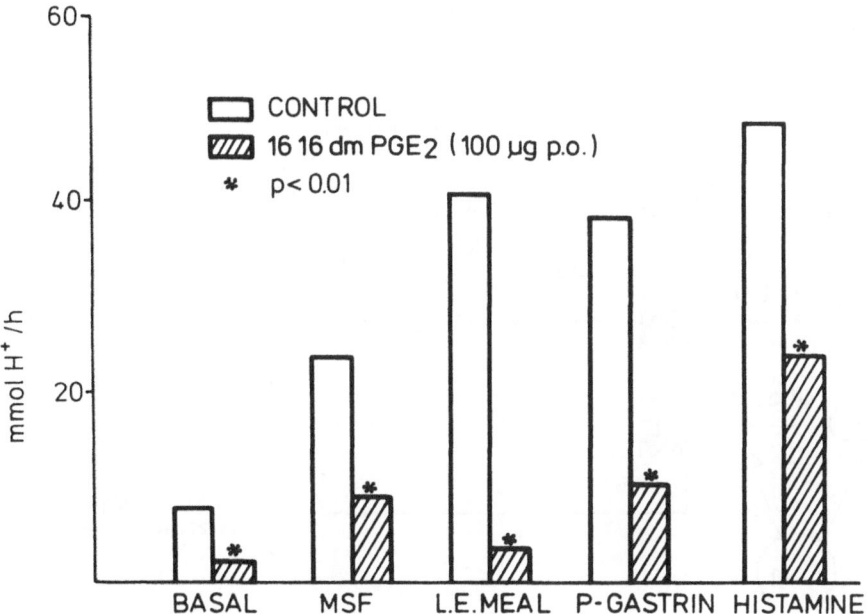

Figure 3.7 Effect of 16,16-dm PGE_2 given orally in a dose of 100 µg on basal gastric acid output and gastric secretion induced by vagal stimulation (modified sham-feeding), liver extract meal, pentagastrin ($2 \mu g\,kg^{-1}h^{-1}$) or histamine ($2.5 \mu g\,kg^{-1}h^{-1}$) infusion in 8 duodenal ulcer patients[66]

Two complementary mechanisms have been proposed to explain PG-induced inhibition: (1) direct suppression of the parietal cells probably via decreasing cyclic AMP production[70] (Figure 3.8), and (2) the reduction in gastrin release[67-69,71]. PG analogues appear to be particularly effective inhibitors when applied directly on the fundic mucosa. Experiments on animals[59] provide evidence that this may be due to their local action on the oxyntic glands. The suppression of gastrin release was also observed mainly after oral but not parenteral[72] administration of abraprostil[64,67,68] (Figure 3.9) and possibly enprostil[73,74], but not after misoprostol[75]. The failure of some PG to affect gastrin release might be attributed to the higher threshold dose of PG needed to affect G-cells compared with parietal cells[64].

Endogenous PG released locally in the antral mucosa have been suggested as mediators of the acid-induced suppression of gastrin release by vagal excitation and as contributors to somatostatin-induced suppression of gastrin release[76]. Recently it was reported[77] that pretreatment with indomethacin to block PG biosynthesis did not abolish the inhibitory action of somatostatin on gastric secretion. Thus PG do not appear to be required for the inhibition of gastric acid secretion by somatostatin in man.

Although there is little doubt that exogenous PG, particularly of the E series and their analogues can suppress all tested modes of gastric acid stimulation, the possible role of endogenously produced PG in the control

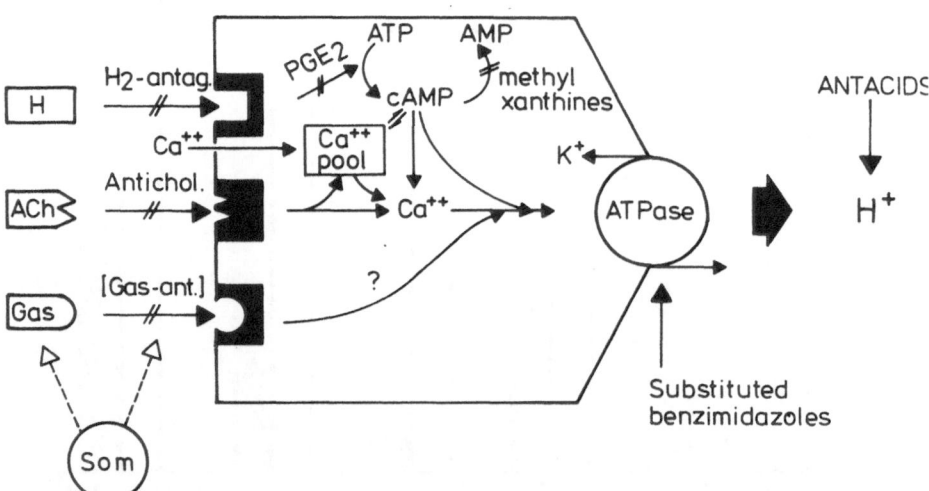

Figure 3.8 Schematic presentation of the parietal cell and the inhibition of its secretory activity by blocking the receptor sites (H2-receptor antagonists, anticholinergics, somatostatin), by acting on the formation of cyclic AMP (PGE$_2$), by suppressing the proton pump (substituted benzimidazoles) and by blocking the calcium channels

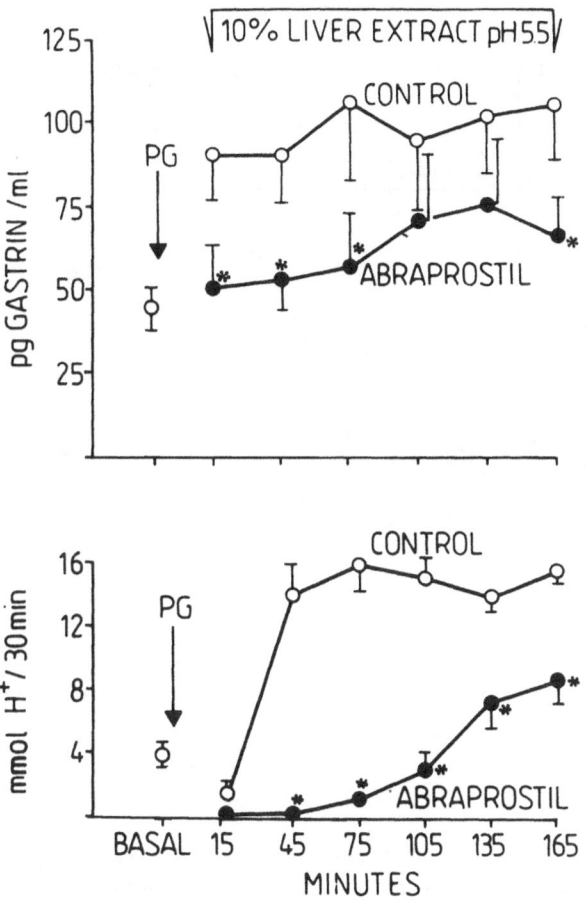

Figure 3.9 Effect of 15(R)15-methyl PGE$_2$ given orally in a dose of 2 µg/kg on peptone meal-induced gastric acid secretion and serum gastrin levels in healthy subjects[67]

of this secretion has not been elucidated. The disruption by aspirin of reciprocal circadian variations of released PGE$_2$ and acid outputs in the resting human stomach was not accompanied by significant changes in gastric acid secretion[78]. The blockade of PG biosynthesis by indomethacin or aspirin failed to affect basal and histamine[79] or vagally-stimulated gastric acid secretion[65] (Figure 3.10) though in some studies an increase in basal or histamine-provoked secretion was observed after indomethacin, presumably due to the inhibition of PG biosynthesis[67]. In another study, the increase in basal acid secretion after indomethacin was variable and not accompanied by significant changes in serum gastrin. Indomethacin failed to affect the postprandial gastric acid secretion or gastrin release[80].

The common feature of these studies is their short-term design. The effect of chronic treatment with blockers of PG synthesis does not appear to affect

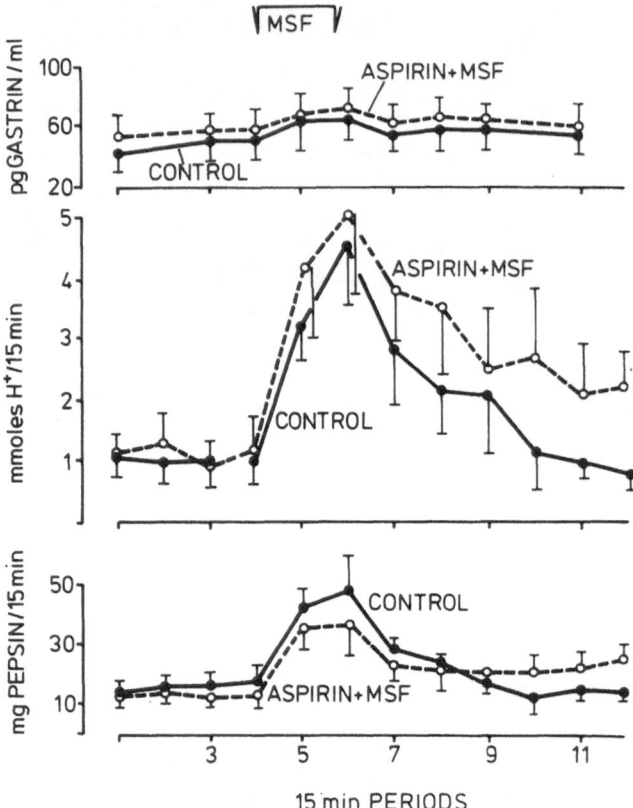

Figure 3.10 Effect of aspirin (given orally in a dose of 2.5 g that suppressed the gastric mucosal generation of PG by about 80%) on basal and vagally stimulated (modified sham-feeding) gastric acid and pepsin secretion in duodenal ulcer patients[65]

gastric acid secretion significantly in most patients with rheumatic diseases[34,64]. These studies indicate that endogenous PG play little if any role in the regulation of basal or postprandial gastric acid secretion or gastrin release. It is unknown whether the deficiency of the gastric mucosal PG such as occurs in some peptic ulcer patients contributes to the alteration in gastric acid secretion and whether the acute suppression of PG biosynthesis in ulcer patients by NOSAC affects gastric secretion to a similar extent in healthy subjects.

PROSTAGLANDINS AND GASTRODUODENAL MUCUS-ALKALINE SECRETION

Mucus is constantly secreted by the gastroduodenal mucosa and forms two phases, one is water insoluble and adheres to the mucosal surface, and the other is the product of the degradation and washing out of the adherent mucus gel[81]. Adherent mucus provides a stable 'unstirred' layer over the mucosal surface and plays an important role as the first line of mucosal defence against gastric acid and pepsin in the gastric juice. In humans, the thickness of adherent mucus gel averages 180 μm and consists of glycoprotein units in polymeric structure.

Both the thickness and the structure of mucus gel change in physiological conditions and in peptic ulcer disease. Topical application of PG stimulates rapid secretion of adherent mucus and this may enhance the protective capability of the mucous barrier by ensuring the continuity of mucus cover and providing a better layer for pH-gradient and better barrier between the epithelial cells and luminal pepsin[81]. Adherent gastric mucus gel in patients with peptic ulcer shows a decreased polymerization of glycoproteins resulting in a weaker structure and poorer quality of the mucus barrier in this disease[82]. The mucus layer in GU or DU patients tends to be thinner than in healthy subjects. Thus, both the quality and quantity of the adherent gastric mucus gel may be impaired in peptic ulcer disease but it may also result from the gastritis and increased mucosal cell shedding associated with that disease.

Although the existence of alkaline secretion by the gastroduodenal mucosa was recognized long ago, it received increased attention only in recent years, mainly because of its proposed role in mucosal protection against luminal acid and pepsin.

Studies in animals both *in vivo* and *in vitro* have revealed that mucosal bicarbonate secretion from gastric fundic and duodenal mucosa is an active, energy-dependent process than can be stimulated by various factors, particularly by exogenous PG, and inhibited by blockers of cyclo-oxygenase[84-87]. Topical acidification of the mucosa was found to cause strong stimulation of alkaline secretion, particularly from the duodenal mucosa, and an increase in PGE_2 release. Both these effects may be suppressed by inhibitors of cyclo-oxygenase[87].

Although the amounts of gastric alkaline secretion vary in different species from 2% to 10% of the maximal rate of acid secretion[83,85], this secretion is believed to be important because it contributes to the formation of the pH gradient within the mucus gel adherent to the gastric mucosa. Due to continuous bicarbonate secretion, mucus can sustain a significant pH gradient from the acid lumen to the almost neutral pH of the epithelial surface.

In humans, the measurements of alkaline secretion based on a two-component model of gastric secretion showed that basal bicarbonate secretion averaged 2.6 mmol/h which corresponds to about 50% of basal acid secretion[88]. Using more direct measurements based on recording the gastric content pH and pCO_2, and calculation by means of the Henderson–Hasselbach equation, it was found that mean basal bicarbonate secretion in healthy subjects averaged about 0.4 mmol/h[89]. In spite of the technical differences, it was confirmed that in humans, as in animals, gastric alkaline secretion increased after topical PG application[88,89] and cholinergic or vagal stimulation[88,90,91] but declined after administration of indomethacin or anticholinergics[80,90].

The importance of the mucus-alkaline system in gastric mucosal protection in humans is not clear because the pH gradient within the adherent mucus layer is dissipated at a low luminal pH (pH 1.8) which may occur physiologically in the stomach[92]. It is unknown whether patients with gastroduodenal ulcerations exhibit any significant changes in the gastric alkaline secretion. Cigarette smoking in DU patients was reported to reduce luminal release of PGE by the gastric mucosa[93] and this has been implicated in the impairment of mucosal integrity possibly due to the decrease in the mucus-alkaline secretion. The upper portion of the duodenum in DU patients was found to secrete significantly less bicarbonate and to release smaller quantities of PGE_2[39] than healthy subjects and this has been considered to be an important factor in the pathogenesis of duodenal ulceration. Studies in animals showed that exogenous PG and carbenoxolone increase the thickness of the mucus layer lying on the gastric mucosa[94] and stimulate alkaline secretion[84,85] but the protection of this mucosa by exogenous PG or mild irritants may be demonstrated in the absence of any acute changes in the gel mucus thickness[95].

Most animal experiments demonstrated that PG of the E series and their analogues prevent or reduce the gastric mucosal permeability to hydrogen ion or potential difference occurring after the exposure of gastric mucosa to various noxious agents[59]. In humans PGE analogues were also found to prevent a drop in the gastric mucosal barrier to hydrogen ion and in mucosal potential difference after topical administration of aspirin, indomethacin or bile salts[96,97]. The nature of this barrier and the possible contribution of PG in strengthening it is not clear but it may be related, at least in part, to the mucus-alkaline secretion[85]. Exogenous PG and gastroprotective agents may affect mucus permeability and adhesiveness by directly interacting with mucus components[99,100]. Topical application of agents that adhere to and reinforce the mucus barrier, such as sucralfate or colloidal bismuth (De-Nol), may provide an extra physical barrier. In addition, they may increase the hydrophobicity of the mucosa due to the accumulation of surfactant-like phospholipids[98]. All these effects contribute to strengthening the gastric mucus barrier and may have potential in peptic ulcer therapy.

PROSTAGLANDINS IN THE TREATMENT OF GASTRODUODENAL ULCERATION

The finding that PG in animals are gastroprotective against various noxious agents at doses low enough to be claimed non-antisecretory and physiological[59], raised the hope that these agents might be ideal drugs in the therapy of acute and chronic gastroduodenal ulcerations. Although the nature of PG-induced gastroprotection is not clear, in some way it is related to enhancement of the mucosal resistance to damage[101]. All the suggested mechanisms of cytoprotection, including an increase in mucus-alkaline secretion, mucosal vasodilation, strengthening of gastric mucosal barrier and stimulation of restitution of disrupted surface epithelium, might contribute to ulcer healing but there is no evidence that PG administered in cytoprotective or non-antisecretory doses significantly accelerate the healing rate of pre-existing ulcers in animals or in man. Ishibashi et al.[102] found in rats that while the PGE_2 analogue at non-antisecretory doses accelerated the healing of chronic acetic acid ulcers in the stomach, it had no effect on the healing of such ulcers in the duodenum. In another study, Ishihara and Okabe[103] also were unable to demonstrate any beneficial effect of oral 16,16-dimethyl-PGE_2 at a cytoprotective dose on the healing of chronic duodenal ulcers induced by mepirizole, a non-steroidal anti-inflammatory drug. It is worthwhile mentioning that PGE_2 analogues, in a dose range without effect on pre-existing chronic duodenal ulceration in rats, prevented the formation of acute gastric or duodenal lesions induced by necrotic agents. Thus the results obtained from experimental models indicate that the ulcer preventive and ulcer healing properties of PG may not be the same. The question arises as to what extent the gastroprotective effect of PG might contribute to their healing effect on chronic gastroduodenal ulceration in humans.

The suggestion that PG may be helpful in peptic ulcer therapy originates from an old observation in China where semen, which is rich in PG, was used as a remedy for gastric ulcerations[104]. Natural PGE_2 at a dose of 0.5 mg t.i.d. and 1 mg at night resulted in an increase in duodenal ulcer healing rate within 4 weeks' therapy to 83% as compared with 43% when using a placebo[105]. Since a dose of 1 mg of PGE failed to affect pentagastrin-induced gastric acid secretion in some of these patients, the acceleration in ulcer healing observed has been attributed to the cytoprotective effects of this PG. This may not be the case however, because other workers[32] have demonstrated that 1 mg of oral PG is inhibitory for certain forms of gastric acid secretion.

Wider placebo-controlled studies using abraprostil, misoprostol or enprostil (Figure 3.11) for 2–8 weeks revealed that all of these given orally approximately doubled the placebo healing rate of gastroduodenal ulcerations. Gibinski et al.[106], who performed the first larger double-blind clinical trial involving 177 patients, observed that in two weeks of treatment with abraprostil healing reached about 75% in the DU patients compared with 50% healed in a placebo group. In another study from the same centre carried out on 117 patients, the healing rate with abraprostil was about 72% and with placebo 50%[107].

Unlike DU patients, those with GU treated with abraprostil were healed to a similar extent (about 40%) to those on placebo, indicating that abroprostil was not effective, at least during 2 weeks' therapy, in healing GU. A multicentre study[108] conducted on 173 DU patients showed that abraprostil at 100 μg q.i.d. healed 37% compared with 12% healed on placebo. After 4 weeks' treatment the respective healing rates were 67% and 30% (Figure 3.12).

In all these studies abraprostil was administered in doses inhibiting gastric acid secretion, so it is not clear whether its ulcer healing action was simply due to gastric acid inhibition or to its protective properties. GU patients who exhibited some deficiency in mucosal PG did not respond favourably to PG therapy, indicating that 'replacement' treatment in these patients is not advantageous. The major side-effects were loose stools and diarrhoea observed in about 30% patients. The potent uterotonic effect excluded the administration of this agent in women of child-bearing age.

Misoprostol, a synthetic agent structurally related to PGE_1 and a potent gastric inhibitory and gastroprotective agent in animals[109] has recently been launched as the first PG for peptic ulcer therapy. A multicentre double-blind

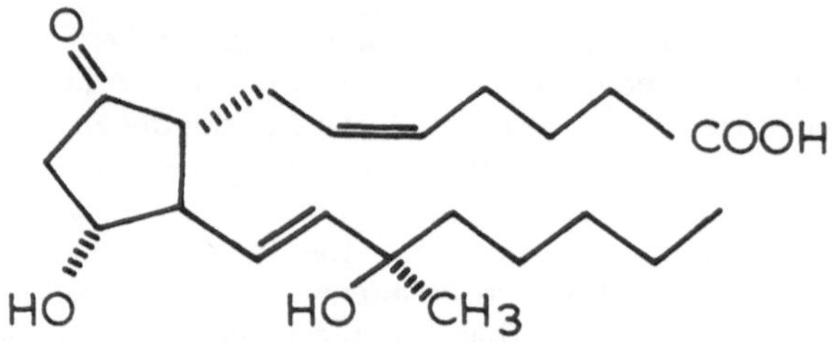

ABRAPROSTIL

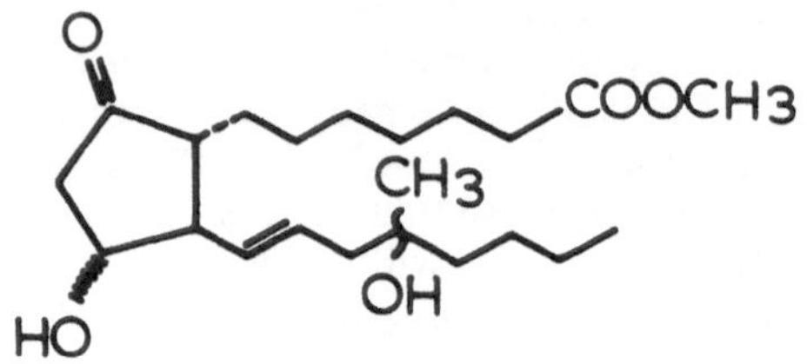

MISOPROSTOL (SC-29333)

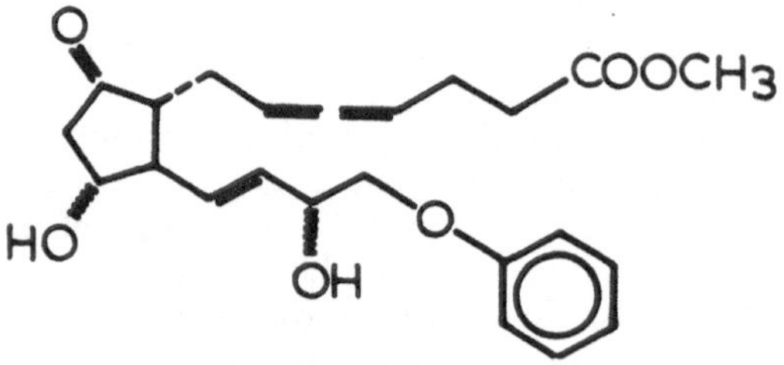

ENPROSTIL

Figure 3.11 The structure of three PG methyl analogues presently used in the treatment of peptic ulcer disease

controlled trial[110] involving 308 DU patients showed that during 4 weeks' treatment with misoprostol at 50 μg q.i.d. the healing rate was about 51% and that at 200 μg q.i.d about 77% as compared with 46% healed on placebo, so that, as in abraprostil trials, the smaller cytoprotective dose of misoprostol was ineffective (Figure 3.13). This provides evidence that cytoprotection does not play any significant role in the ulcer-healing effect of this drug. There was a greater percentage of healed ulcers among non-smokers than smokers, whereas those with a history of alcohol usage were more likely to heal their ulcers by misoprostol.

Misoprostol was effective in healing GU but required longer treatment. In a trial[111] performed on 299 GU patients the healing rate with misoprostol (100 μg q.i.d. for 8 weeks) was 62% compared to 45% in a placebo group (Figure 3.14). A lower dose (25 μg q.i.d. for 8 weeks) was ineffective in the healing of GU. Misoprostol was somewhat better tolerated than abraprostil;

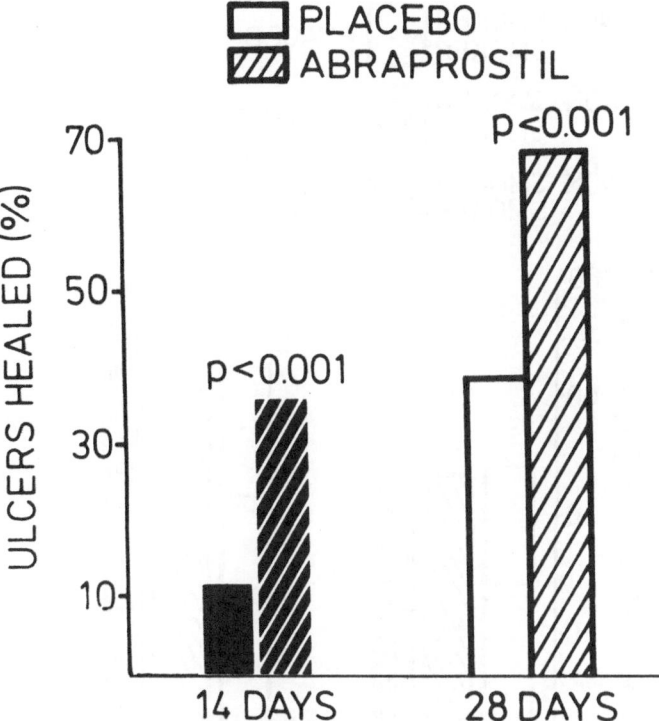

Figure 3.12 Percentage of duodenal ulcers completely healed after 2 and 4 week's therapy with abraprostil given orally at 100 μg q.i.d.[108]. Reprinted with permission from 'Effect of 15(R)15-methyl prostaglandin E$_2$ (Abraprostil) on the healing of duodenal ulcer', by Vantrappen et al., Gastroenterology, **83**, 357–363. Copyright 1982 by the American Gastroenterological Association

the diarrhoea was moderate and occurred only in 13% of patients but the uterotonicity remained a problem.

Enprostil, another PGE analogue that has also been studied extensively and recently launched on the market as an anti-ulcer agent, seems to exhibit a longer inhibitory action on gastric secretion, and, unlike misoprostol, tends to decrease gastrin release. Recent clinical trials[112,113] showed that enprostil administered during 4 weeks at 70 and 35 μg b.i.d. in DU patients increased the healing rate to 77% and 51% respectively as compared with 46% on placebo. The same regimen in 128 GU patients did not affect the healing rate at 2 and 4 weeks' treatment, but at 6 weeks the healing rate was 82% as compared with 39% on placebo.

In general, in spite of theoretical benefits, exogenous PG and their stable analogues so far tested in various clinical trials do not seem to be superior in ulcer healing or ulcer prevention to the conventional anti-ulcer drugs, such as cimetidine, ranitidine or pirenzepine, available at present. The major adverse reactions limiting their clinical use are the diarrhoeagenic and uterotonic effects. The ulcer recurrence rate upon the withdrawal of PG therapy does

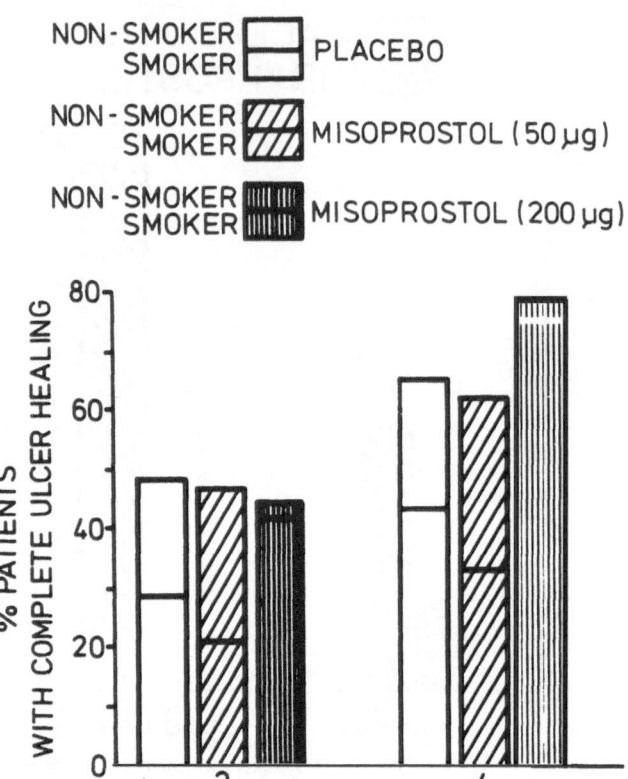

Figure 3.13 Percentage of DU patients (smokers and non-smokers) with complete ulcer healing after 2 and 4 week's treatment with misoprostol given orally at a dose of 50 and 200 μg q.i.d.[110]. Reprinted with permission from Brand *et al.* (1985) *Digestive Diseases and Sciences*, **30**, 147S–158S (Plenum Publishing Corporation)

not seem to be lower than after conventional anti-ulcer treatment. There is no evidence that cytoprotective properties contribute to the ulcer healing action of exogenous PG.

ROLE OF PG IN ULCER TREATMENT WITH DRUGS ACTING BY A MECHANISM OTHER THAN INHIBITION OF GASTRIC SECRETION

Following an appreciation of cytoprotective mechanisms, a family of therapeutic agents which enhances these factors has been developed for the treatment of peptic ulcerations. Besides PG, gastroprotective agents are carbenoxolone, basic aluminium sucrose octasulphate (sucralfate), colloidal bismuth subcitrate (De-Nol) and certain flavonoids (Solon).

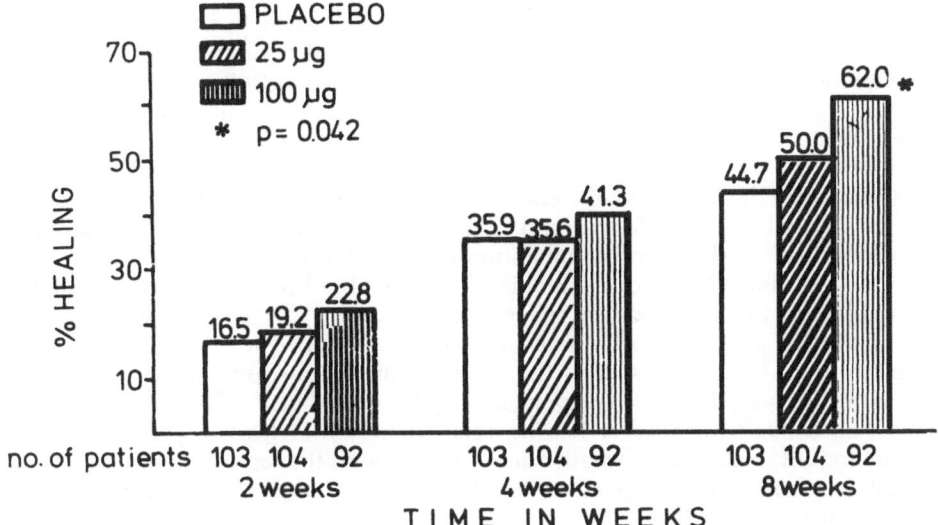

Figure 3.14 Percentage of GU patients with complete ulcer healing after 2, 4 and 8 weeks of treatment with misoprostol[111]. Reprinted with permission from Agrawal *et al.* (1985) *Digestive Diseases and Sciences*, **30**, 164S–170S (Plenum Publishing Corporation)

Natural liquorice root extracts or similar synthetic compounds (carbenoxolone, deglycyrrhizinized liquorice) have been used for many years in the treatment of gastroduodenal ulcerations though they do not affect gastric acid secretion[114,115]. They are known to stimulate gastric mucus secretion, stabilize the cell membranes and stimulate epithelial renewal[116]. These effects are probably mediated by an increase in mucosal PG due to the inhibition of their deactivation (see Figure 3.1) or the inhibition of the synthesis of thromboxanes and leukotrienes[117,118]. Because of aldosterone-like action, this drug, found to be cytoprotective in animals[119] and as effective as cimetidine in healing of gastric ulcers[114], has been practically abandoned.

Sucralfate was found to be clinically effective in healing gastric and duodenal ulcers[115,120], in preventing the recurrence of peptic ulcers[121] and preventing stress ulcerations in critically ill patients[122]. The postulated mechanisms of the therapeutic action of sucralfate include formation of a protective barrier consisting of stable complexes of the drug with proteins on the ulcerated mucosa, deactivation of pepsin, binding of pepsin and bile acids, and strengthening of the gastric mucosal barrier[120]. Sucralfate is gastroprotective in animals against various noxious agents[123–125] acting at least in part by stimulating the biosynthesis of endogenous PG. The latter effect also applies to human gastric mucosa[126] and may explain the therapeutic and prophylactic efficacy of this drug.

Bismuth-containing compounds were used for a long time in the treatment of gastrointestinal disorders but have been abandoned because of neurotoxicity. Colloidal bismuth subcitrate (De-Nol) at recommended doses is apparently without toxic side-effects and highly effective in peptic ulcer therapy[115,120]. It exhibits various properties not shown by other bismuth-containing salts, including the formation of a protective coat on the ulcer base due to chelating with the proteinaceous material, the inhibition of peptic activity, the stimulation of mucus-alkaline secretion and antibacterial activity[120]. Some of these effects are related to the stimulation of PG biosynthesis due to 'mild' irritation of the mucosa by De-Nol crystals precipitating at lower pH in the mucus layer adherent to the surface of the epithelial cells[125,127]. De-Nol only has a limited capacity to buffer gastric acid, and so its gastroprotective effects in laboratory animals are unrelated to the inhibition of gastric acid secretion[125].

The healing efficacy of De-Nol in GU or DU has been compared with that of placebo or cimetidine in several clinical trials[115,120]. De-Nol was found superior to placebo in all studies and comparable to cimetidine[120,128,129]. An interesting finding was that the relapse rate seems retarded after prior treatment with De-Nol as compared with cimetidine[129]. These favourable effects of De-Nol on ulcer healing seem to result, at least in part, from its binding of epidermal growth factor (EGF) and the accumulation of this mitogenic peptide in the ulcer area to promote tissue repair and ulcer re-epithelialization.

Solon is a synthetic flavonoid derived from sophoradin, an extract of the root of a Chinese medical plant. In experimental animals it is highly gastroprotective against various noxious agents acting in part by increasing PG generation in the gastric mucosa and decreasing PG deactivation in a similar manner to carbenoxolone[130]. It does not affect gastric acid secretion but increases the healing rate of gastroduodenal ulcerations. This suggests that its major mechanism of action is an increase in mucosal resistance resulting from increased PG generation. Solon is widely used in Japan in the therapy of gastroduodenal ulceration in man[131,132].

REFERENCES

1. Moncada, S., Flower, R.J. and Vane, J.R. (1985). Prostaglandins, prostacyclin, thromboxane A_2 and leukotrienes. In Goodman Gilman, A., Goodman, L.S., Rall, T.W. and Murad, F. (eds.) *The Pharmacological Basis of Therapeutics*, pp. 660–673. (New York: MacMillan Publ. Co.)
2. Willis, A.L. (1981). Nutritional and pharmacological factors in eicosanoid biology. *Nutr. Rev.*, **39**, 289–301
3. Fischer, S. and Weber, P.C. (1984). Prostaglandin I_3 formed *in vivo* in man after dietary eicosapentaenoic acid. *Nature*, **307**, 165–171
4. Coceani F., Pace-Asciak, C., Volta, F. and Wolfe, L.S. (1967). Effect of nerve stimulation on prostaglandin formation and release from the rat stomach. *Am. J. Physiol.*, **213**, 1056–1064
5. Knapp, H.R., Oelz, O., Sweetman, B.J. and Oates, J.A. (1979). Synthesis and metabolism of prostaglandins E_2, F_2 and D_2 by the rat gastrointestinal tract. Stimulation by a hypertonic and environment *in vitro*. *Prostaglandins*, **15**, 751–757
6. Konturek, S.J., Bilski, J., Tasler, J. and Laskiewicz, J. (1984). Gastroduodenal alkaline response to acid and taurocholate in conscious dogs. *Am. J. Physiol.*, **247**, G149–G154
7. Robert, A., Nezamis, J.E., Lancaster, C., Davis, J.P., Field, S.O. and Hanchar, A.J. (1983). Mild irritants prevent gastric necrosis through 'adaptive cytoprotection' mediated by prostaglandins. *Am. J. Physiol.*, **245**, G113–G121
8. Konturek, S.J., Piastucki, I., Brzozowski, T. and Redecki, T. (1982). Role of locally generated prostaglandins in adaptive gastric cytoprotection. *Dig. Dis. Sci.*, **27**, 967–971

9. Konturek, S.J., Brzozowski, T., Piastucki, I., Radecki, T. and Dembinska-Kiec, A. (1983). Role of prostaglandin and thromboxane biosynthesis in gastric necrosis produced by taurocholate and ethanol. *Dig. Dis. Sci.*, **28**, 154–160

10. Ahlquist, D.A., Dozois, R.R., Zinsmeister, A.R. and Malagelada, J.R. (1983). Duodenal prostaglandin synthesis and acid load in health and duodenal ulcer disease. *Gastroenterology,* **85**, 522–529

11. Bray, M.A. (1983). The pharmacology and pathophysiology of leukotriene B_4. *Br. Med. Bull.*, **39**, 249–254

12. Samuelsson, B. (1983). Leukotrienes: mediators of immediate hypersensitivity reaction and inflammation. *Science*, **220**, 568–575

13. Bennett, A. (1985). Prostanoids in human gastric mucosa. *Gastroenterol. Clin. Biol.*, **9**, 30–32

14. Saeed, S.A., Drew, M., Denning-Kendall, P.A., McDonald-Gibson, W. and Collier, H.O. (1981). Inhibitors and stimulants of prostaglandin cyclo-oxygenase in stomach extracts. *Biochem. Soc. Trans.*, **9**, 92–93

15. Ligumsky, M., Sharon, P., Karmeli, F. and Rachmilewitz, D. (1979). Prostaglandins and the pathogenesis of duodenal ulcer: no correlation with the gastric mucosal PGE_2 content. *Isr. J. Med. Sci.*, **15**, 171–174

16. Sharon, P., Cohen, F., Zifroni, A., Karmeli, F., Ligumsky, M. and Rachmilewitz, D. (1983). Prostanoid synthesis by cultured gastric and duodenal mucosa: possible role in the pathogenesis of duodenal ulcer. *Scand. J. Gastroenterol.*, **18**, 1045–1049

17. Whittle, B.J.R. (1978). Potential endogenous inhibitor of prostaglandin synthetase in plasma, failure to inhibit cyclo-oxygenase in platelets and the gastric mucosa. *J. Pharm. Pharmacol.*, **30**, 467–468

18. Vane, J.R. (1964). The use of isolated organs for detecting active substances in the circulating blood. *Br. J. Pharmacol. Chemother.*, **23**, 360–373

19. Bennett, A., Hensby, C.N., Sanger, G.J. and Stamford, I.F. (1981). Metabolites of arachidonic acid formed by human gastrointestinal tissue and their action on the muscle layers. *Br. J. Pharmacol.*, **74**, 435–444

20. Peskar, B.M., Seyberth, H.W. and Peskar, B.A. (1980). Synthesis and metabolism of prostaglandins by human gastric mucosa. *Adv. Prostagl. Thromboxane Res.*, **8**, 1511–1514

21. Green, K., Aly, A. and Johansson, C. (1981). Measurements of prostaglandin biosynthesis in gastrointestinal tract: biochemical and technical problems. *Prostaglandins*, **21** (Suppl.), 1–8

22. Aly, A., Johansson, C., Slezak, P. and Green, K. (1984). Bioconversion of arachidonic acid in the human gastrointestinal tract. *Biochem. Med.*, **31**, 319–331

23. Smith, G.S., Warhurst, G. and Turnberg, L.A. (1982). Synthesis and degradation of prostaglandin E_2 in the epithelial and subepithelial layers of the rat intestine. *Biochem. Biophys. Acta,* **713**, 684–687

24. Schlegel, W., Wenk, K., Dollinger, H.C. and Raptis, S. (1977). Concentrations of prostaglandin A, E and F-like substances in gastric mucosa of normal subjects and of patients with various gastric diseases. *Clin. Sci. Mol. Med.*, **52**, 255–258

25. Konturek, S.J., Obtulowicz, W., Sito, E., Oleksy, J., Wilkon, S. and Dembinska-Kiec, A. (1981). Distribution of prostaglandins in gastric and duodenal mucosa of healthy subjects and duodenal ulcer patients. *Gut*, **22**, 283–289

26. Hillier, K., Smith, C.L., Jewell, R., Arthur, M.J.P. and Ross, G. (1985). Duodenal mucosa synthesis of prostaglandins in duodenal ulcer disease. *Gut*, **26**, 237–240

27. Baker, R., Jaffe, B.M. and Venables, C.W. (1979). Endogenous prostaglandins in peptic ulcer disease. *Gut*, **20**, 394–399

28. Cheung, L.Y., Jubiz, W. and Moore, J.G. (1976). Gastric prostaglandin E output during basal and stimulated acid secretion in normal subjets and patients with duodenal ulcer. *J. Surg. Res.*, **20**, 369–372

29. Hinsdale, J.G., Engel, J.J. and Wilson, D.E. (1974). Prostaglandin E in peptic ulcer disease. *Prostaglandins*, **6**, 459–500

30. Tonnesen, M.G., Jubiz, W., Moore, J.G. and Frailey, J. (1974). Circadian variation of prostaglandin E (PGE) production in human gastric juice. *Am. J. Dig. Dis.*, **19**, 644–648

31. Levine, R.A. and Schwartzel, E.H. (1984). Effect of indomethacin on basal and histamine-stimulated human gastric acid secretion. *Gut*, **25**, 718–722

32. Reele, S.B. and Rohan, D. (1984). Oral antisecretory activity of prostaglandin E_2 in man. *Dig. Dis. Sci.*, **29**, 390–393
33. Wright, J.P., Young, G.O., Klaff, L.J., Weers, L.A., Price, S.K. and Marks, I.N. (1982). Gastric mucosal prostaglandin E levels in patients with gastric ulcer disease and carcinoma. *Gastroenterology*, **82**, 263–267
34. Konturek, S.J. (1984). Actions of non-steroidal anti-inflammatory compounds on gastric mucosal integrity and prostaglandin formation in healthy subjects and peptic ulcer patients. *Adv. Inflamm. Res.*, **6**, 29–37
35. Konturek, S.J., Obtulowicz. N. and Oleksy, J. (1984). Generation of prostaglandins in gastric mucosa of patients with peptic ulcer disease; effect of non-steroidal anti-inflammatory compounds. *Scand. J. Gastroenterol.*, **19** (Suppl. 101), 75–77
36. Konturek, S.J., Kwiecien, N., Obtulowicz, W., Zmuda, A., Polanski, M., Kopp, B., Sito, E. and Oleksy, J. (1983). The use of carprofen, a non-steroidal anti-inflammatory agent in peptic ulcer disease. *Hepato-Gastroenterology*, **30**, 261–265
37. Arakawa, T., Kobayashi, K. and Nakamura, H. (1985). Endogenous prostaglandin E_2 and prostacyclin in duodenal ulcer disease. *Gastroenterology*, **88**, 1308
38. Aly, A., Selling, J.A., Hogan, D.L., Isenberg, J.I., Koss, M.A. and Johansson, C. (1985). Gastric and duodenal prostaglandin E_2 (PGE_2) in humans; effect of luminal acidification and indomethacin. *Gastroenterology*, **88**, 1305
39. Isenberg, J.I., Hogan, D.L., Selling, J.A. and Koss, M.A. (1985). Duodenal bicarbonate secretion in normal subjects and duodenal ulcer patients. *Dig. Dis. Sci.*, **30**, 381
40. Vane, J.R. (1971). Inhibition of prostaglandin synthesis as a mechanism of action for aspirin-like drugs. *Nature*, **231**, 232–235
41. Konturek, S.J., Kwiecien, N., Obtulowicz, W., Dembinska-Kiec, A., Polanski, M., Kopp, B., Sito, E. and Oleksy, J. (1982). Effect of carprofen and indomethacin on gastric function, mucosal integrity and generation of prostaglandin in man. *Hepato-Gastroenterology*, **29**, 267–270
42. Cohen, M.M., McCready, D., Clark, L. and Sevelius, H. (1985). Protection against aspirin-induced antral and duodenal damage with enprostil. A double blind endoscopic study. *Gastroenterology*, **88**, 382–386
43. Hunt, J.N. and Franz, J.D. (1981). Effect of prostaglandin E_2 on gastric mucosal bleeding caused by aspirin. *Dig. Dis. Sci.*, **26**, 301–305
44. Johansson, C., Kolberg, B., Nordeman, R., Samuelsson, K. and Bergstrom, S. (1979). Protective effects of prostaglandin E_2 in the gastrointestinal tract during indomethacin treatment of rheumatic diseases. *Gastroenterology*, **78**, 479–493
45. Konturek, S.J., Kwiecien, N., Obtulowicz, W., Polanski, M., Kopp, B. and Oleksy, J. (1983). Comparison of prostaglandin E_2 and ranitidine in prevention of gastric bleeding by aspirin in man. *Gut*, **24**, 89–93
46. Rainsford, K.D. (1985). Anti-inflammatory drugs and the gastrointestinal mucosa. *Gastroenterol. Clin. Biol.*, **9**, 30–32
47. Hunt, J.N., Smith, C.L., Jiang, C.L. and Kessler, L. (1983). Effect of synthetic prostaglandin E analogue on aspirin-induced gastric bleeding and secretion. *Dig. Dis. Sci.*, **28**, 897–902
48. Gilbert, D.A., Surowicz, C.M., Silverstein, F.E., Weinberg, C.R., Saunders, D.R., Feld, A.D., Sanford, R.L., Bergman, D. and Washington, P. (1984). Prevention of acute aspirin-induced gastric mucosal injury by 15-R-methyl prostaglandin E_2; an endoscopic study. *Gastroenterology*, **86**, 339–345
49. Lanza, F.L., Royer, G.L., Nelson, R.S., Chen, T.T., Seckman, C.E. and Rack, M.F. (1979). Effect of ibuprofen, indomethacin, aspirin, naproxen and placebo on the gastric mucosa of normal volunteers. A gastroscopic and photographic study. *Dig. Dis. Sci.*, **24**, 823–828
50. Silvoso, G.R., Ivey, K.R. and Butt, J.H. (1979). Incidence of gastric lesions in patients with rheumatic diseases on chronic aspirin therapy. *Ann. Intern. Med.*, **91**, 517–520
51. Peskar, B.M., Weiler, H. and Meyer, Ch. (1984). Inhibition of prostaglandin production in the gastrointestinal tract by anti-inflammatory drugs. *Adv. Inflamm. Res.*, **6**, 39–50
52. Whittle, B.J.R., Kauffman, G.L. and Moncada, S. (1981). Vasoconstriction with thromboxane A_2 induces ulcers in the gastric mucosa. *Nature*, **292**, 472–474
53. Rainsford, K.D. (1984). Mechanisms of gastrointestinal ulcerations by non-steroidal anti-inflammatory/analgesic drugs. *Adv. Inflamm. Res.*, **6**, 51–64

54. Ligumsky, M., Golanska, E.M., Hansen, D.G. and Kauffman, G.L. (1983). Aspirin can inhibit gastric mucosal cyclo-oxygenase without causing lesions in rats. *Gastroenterology*, **84**, 756–761

55. Tarnawski, A., Stachura, J., Ivey, J., Mach, T., Bogdal, J. and Klimczyk, B. (1981). Ethanol-induced duodenal lesions in man. Protective effects of prostaglandin. *Prostaglandins*, **21** (Suppl.) 147–153

56. Rupin, H., Person, B., Robert, A. and Domschke, W. (1981). Gastric cytoprotection in man by PGE$_2$. *Scand. J. Gastroenterol.*, **16**, 647–652

57. Fimmel, C.J., Muller-Lissner, S.A. and Blum, A.L. (1984). Bile salt-induced acute gastric mucosal damage in man; time course and effect of misoprostol, a PGE$_1$ analogue. *Scand. J. Gastroenterol.*, **19** (Suppl. 92), 184–187

58. Robert, A., Nezamis, J.E. and Phillips, J.P. (1967). Inhibition of gastric secretion by prostaglandins. *Am. J. Dig. Dis.*, **12**, 1073–1076

59. Robert, A. (1981). Prostaglandins and the gastrointestinal tract. In Johnson, L.R. (ed.) *Physiology of the Gastrointestinal Tract*, pp. 1407–1434. (New York: Raven Press)

60. Wilson, D.E., Phillipos, C. and Levine, R.A. (1971). Inhibition of gastric secretion in man by prostaglandin A. *Gastroenterology*, **61**, 201–206

61. Classen, M., Koch, H., Bickhardt, J. and Demling, L. (1971). The effect of prostaglandin E$_1$ on the pentagastrin-stimulated gastric secretion in man. *Digestion*, **4**, 333–344

62. Newman, A., Prado, P., De Moraes-Filho, J., Phillippakos, D. and Misiewicz, J.J. (1975). The effect of intravenous infusion of prostaglandin E$_2$ and F$_{2\alpha}$ on human gastric function. *Gut*, **16**, 272–276

63. Karim, S.M., Carter, D.C., Bhana, D. and Ganesan, P.A. (1973). Effect of orally administered prostaglandin E$_2$ and its 15-methyl analogues on gastric secretion. *Brit. Med. J.*, **1**, 143–146

64. Johansson, C. and Bergstrom, S. (1982). Prostaglandins and protection of the gastroduodenal mucosa. *Scand. J. Gastroenterol.*, **17** (Suppl. 77), 21–46

65. Konturek, S.J., Kwiecien, N., Obtulowicz, W. and Oleksy, J. (1983). Prostaglandins and vagal stimulation of gastric secretion in duodenal ulcer patients. *Scand. J. Gastroenterol.*, **18**, 43–47

66. Konturek, S.J. (1983). Pharmacological control of gastric acid secretion in peptic ulcer. *Mt. Sinai J. Med.*, **50**, 457–463

67. Konturek, S.J., Kwiecien, N., Swierczek, J., Oleksy, J., Sito, E. and Robert, A. (1976). Comparison of methylated prostaglandin E$_2$ analogues given orally in the inhibition of gastric responses to pentagastrin and peptone meal in man. *Gastroenterology*, **70**, 683–687

68. Peterson, W., Fieldman, M., Taylor, I. and Bremer, M. (1979). The effect of 15(R)-methyl prostaglandin E$_2$ on meal-stimulated gastric acid secretion, serum gastrin and pancreatic polypeptide in duodenal ulcer patients. *Dig. Dis. Sci.*, **24**, 381–384

69. Tytgat, G.N.J. and Huibreg, T.S.E. (1981). The effect of 15(R)-methyl prostaglandin E$_2$ on basal and meal-stimulated gastrin in duodenal ulcer patients. *Prostaglandins*, **21** (Suppl.), 53–56

70. Soll, A.H. (1980). Specific inhibition by prostaglandins E$_2$ and I$_2$ of histamine-stimulated [^{14}C]aminopyrine accumulation and cyclic adenosine monophosphate generation by isolated canine parietal cells. *J. Clin. Invest.*, **65**, 1222–1229

71. Ippoliti, A.F., Isenberg, J.I., Maxwell, V. and Walsh, J.H. (1976). The effect of 16,16-dimethyl prostaglandin E$_2$ on meal-stimulated gastric acid secretion and serum gastrin in duodenal ulcer patients. *Gastroenterology*, **70**, 488–491

72. Konturek, S.J., Oleksy, J., Bieranat, J., Sito, E. and Kwiecien, N. (1976). Effect of synthetic 15-methyl analog of PGE$_2$ on gastric acid and serum gastrin response to peptone meal, gastrin and histamine in duodenal ulcer patients. *Am. J. Dig. Dis.*, **21**, 291–300

73. Davis, G.R., Santa Ana, G.A., Morawski, S.G. and Fordtran, J.S. (1982). Effect of synthetic PGE$_2$ on food-stimulated gastric acid secretion. *Clin. Pharmacol. Ther.*, **31**, 215–220

74. Mahachai, V., Walker, K., Sevelius, H. and Thompson, A.B.R. (1984). Enprostil, a dehydro-prostaglandin E$_2$ has potent antisecretory and antigastrin properties in patients with duodenal ulcer disease. *Gastroenterology*, **86**, 1171

75. Steiner, J.A. (1985). Misoprostol clinical pharmacology. *Dig. Dis. Sci.*, **30** (Suppl.), 136S–141S

76. Befritis, R., Samuelsson, K. and Johansson, C. (1984). Gastric acid inhibition by antral

acidification mediated by endogenous prostaglandins. *Scand. J. Gastroenterol.*, **19**, 899–904

77. Mogard, M.H., Maxwell, V., Kovacs, T., Deventer, G.V., Elashoff, J.D., Yamada, T., Kaufmann, G.L. and Walsh, J.H. (1985). Somatostatin inhibits gastric acid secretion after gastric mucosal prostaglandin synthesis inhibition by indomethacin in man. *Gut*, **26**, 1189–1191

78. Child, C., Jubiz, W. and Moore, J.G. (1976). Effects of aspirin on gastric prostaglandin E (PGE) and acid output in normal subjects. *Gut*, **17**, 54–57

79. Winship, D.H. and Bernhard, G.C. (1970). Basal and histamine-stimulated human gastric acid secretion; lack of effect of indomethacin in therapeutic doses. *Gastroenterology*, **58**, 762–765

80. Feldman, M. and Colturi, T.J. (1984). Effect of indomethacin on gastric acid and bicarbonate secretion in humans. *Gastroenterology*, **87**, 1339–1343

81. Allen, A. and Leonard, A. (1985). Mucus structure. *Gastroenterol. Clin. Biol.*, **9**, 9–12

82. Allen, A., Ward, R.H., Cunlifee, W.J., Hutton, D.A., Pearson, J.P. and Venables, C.W. (1985). Changes in adherent mucus gel and pepsinolysis in peptic ulcer patients. *Dig. Dis. Sci.*, **30**, 365

83. Flemstrom, G. (1981). Gastric secretion of bicarbonates. In Johnson, L.R. (ed.) *Physiology of the Gastrointestinal Tract*, pp. 603–616. (New York: Raven Press)

84. Flemstrom, G. and Garner, A. (1982). Gastroduodenal HCO_3 transport. Characteristics and proposed role in acidity regulation and mucosal protection. *Am. J. Physiol.*, **242**, G183–G193

85. Garner, A., Flemstrom, G. and Allen, A. (1983). Gastroduodenal alkaline and mucus secretions. *Scand. J. Gastoenterol.*, **18** (Suppl. 87), 25–41

86. Flemstrom, G. and Turnberg, L.A. (1984). Gastroduodenal defence mechanism. *Clin. Gastroenterol.*, **13**, 327–353

87. Konturek, S.J., Bilski, J., Tasler, J. and Bielanski, W. (1986). Role of endogenous prostaglandins in duodenal alkaline response to luminal hydrochloric acid or arachidonic acid. *Digestion* (In press)

88. Feldman, M. (1983). Gastric bicarbonate secretion in humans. Effect of pentagastrin, bethanechol and 11,16,16-trimethyl prostaglandin E_2. *J. Clin. Invest.*, **72**, 295–303

89. Forsell, H. and Olbe, L. (1985). Continuous computerized determination of gastric bicarbonate secretion in man. *Scand. J. Gastroenterol.*, **20**, 767–774

90. Foresell, H., Stenquist, B. and Olbe, L. (1985). Vagal stimulation of human gastric bicarbonate secretion. *Gastroenterology*, **89**, 581–586

91. Feldman, M. (1985). Gastric H^+ and HCO_3^- secretion in response to sham-feeding in humans. *Am. J. Physiol.*, **248**, G188–G191

92. Bahari, H.M.M., Ross, I.N. and Turnberg, L.A. (1982). Demonstration of a pH-gradient across the mucus layer on the surface of human gastric mucosa *in vitro*. *Gut*, **23**, 513–516

93. McCready, D.R., Clark, L. and Cohen, M.M. (1985). Cigarette smoking reduces human gastric luminal prostaglandin E_2. *Gut*, **26**, 1192–1196

94. Bickel, M. and Kaufmann, G.L. (1981). Gastric gel mucus thickness; effect of distension, 16,16-dimethyl prostaglandin E_2 and carbenoxolone. *Gastroenterology*, **80**, 770–775

95. Robert, A., Bottcher, K. and Kaufmann, G.L. (1984). Lack of correlation between mucus gel thickness and gastric cytoprotection. *Gastroenterology*, **86**, 670–674

96. Cohen, M.M. and Pottett, J.M. (1976). Prostaglandin E_2 prevents aspirin and indomethacin damage to human gastric mucosa. *Surg. Forum.*, **27**, 400–401

97. Muller, P., Fisher, N., Dammann, H.G., Kather, H. and Simon, B. (1981). Simultaneous addition of 16,16-dimethyl PGE_2 prevents aspirin and bile salt damage to human gastric mucosa. *Z. Gastroenterol.*, **19**, 373–376

98. Lichtenberger, L.M., Graziani, L.A., Dial, E.J., Butler, B.D. and Hills, B.A. (1983). Role of surface active phospholipids in gastric cytoprotection. *Science*, **219**, 1327–1329

99. Slomiany, A., Takagi, A., Szymanska-Kosmala, M. and Slomiany, B.L. (1985). Prostaglandin protection against ethanol injury as reflected by biosynthesis, structure and secretion of mucus glycoprotein. *Gastroenterology*, **88**, 1591

100. Slomiany, B.L., Murty, V.L.N., Laszewicz, W., Piasek, A. and Slomiany, A. (1985). Effect of sucralfate on the viscosity and retardation of hydrogen ion diffusion by gastric mucus. *Gastroenterology*, **88**, 1591

101. Miller, T. (1983). Protective effects of prostaglandins against gastric mucosal damage; current knowledge and proposed mechanisms. *Am. J. Physiol.*, **245**, G601–G623

102. Ishibashi, A., Kasuya, Y., Takeuchi, K. and Okabe, S. (1979). Effects of 15(S)15-methyl PGE$_2$ methyl ester on healing of chronic gastric and duodenal ulcers in rats. *Jpn. J. Pharmacol.*, **29**, 807–810

103. Ishihara, Y. and Okabe, S. (1983). Effects of antiulcer agents on healing of mepirizole-induced duodenal ulcers in rats. *Digestion*, **27**, 29–35

104. Fung, W.P., Karim, S.M.M. and Tye, S.Y. (1974). Effect of 15(R)15-methyl prostaglandin E$_2$ methyl ester on healing of gastric ulcers. *Lancet*, **2**, 10–12

105. Kolberg, B., Slezak, P. and Johansson, C. (1982). The effect of prostaglandin E$_2$ on duodenal ulcer healing. *Prostaglandins*, **24**, 527–536

106. Gibinski, K., Rybicka, J., Mikos, E. and Nowak, A. (1977). Double-blind clinical trial on gastroduodenal ulcer healing with prostaglandin E$_2$ analogues. *Gut*, **18**, 636–639

107. Rybicka, J. and Gibinski, K. (1978). Methyl-prostaglandin E$_2$ analogues for healing of gastroduodenal ulcers. *Scand. J. Gastroenterol.*, **13**, 155–159

108. Van Trappen, G., Janssens, J., Popiela, T., Kulig, J., Tytgat, G.N., Huibregtse, K., Lambert, R., Pauchard, J.P. and Robert, A. (1982). Effect of 15(R)15-methyl prostaglandin E$_2$ (Abraprostil) on the healing of duodenal ulcer. *Gastroenterology*, **83**, 357–363

109. Bauer, R.F. (1985). Misoprostol preclinical pharmacology. *Dig. Dis. Sci.*, **30**, 118S–125S

110. Brand, D.L., Raufail, W.M., Thomson, A.B.R. and Tapper, E.J. (1985). Misoprostol, a synthetic PGE$_1$ analog in the treatment of duodenal ulcer. A multicenter double-blind study. *Dig. Dis. Sci.*, **30**, 147S–158S

111. Agrawal, N.M., Saffouri, B., Kruss, D.M., Callison, D.A. and Dajani, E.Z. (1985). Healing of benign gastric ulcer. *Dig. Dis. Sci.*, **30**, 164S–170S

112. Archambault, A.P., Halvorsen, L., Lee, S.P., MacLaurin, V.P., Sutherland, L.R., Sevelius, H. and Thomson, A.B.R. (1984). Efficacy and safety of enprostil, a synthetic prostaglandin, and placebo in patients with duodenal ulcer. *Am. J. Gastroenterol.*, **79**, 828–832

113. Bynum, L. (1985). Efficacy of enprostil vs placebo in gastric ulcer. Presented at the *Symposium on Protective and Therapeutic Effects of Gastrointestinal Prostaglandins*, November 12–14, Toronto, Canada

114. Morgan, A.G., McAdam, W.A. and Pascoo, C. (1982). Comparison between cimetidine and Caved-S in the treatment of gastric ulcerations and subsequent maintenance therapy. *Gut*, **23**, 545–551

115. Misiewicz, J.J. (1984). Medical management of peptic ulcer. *Postgrad. Med. J.*, **60**, 751–760

116. Van Huis, G.A. and Kramer, M.F. (1981). Effect of carbenoxolone on the synthesis of glycoprotein and DNA in rat gastric epithelial cells. *Gut*, **22**, 782–787

117. Peskar, B.M. (1980). Effect of carbenoxolone on prostaglandin synthesizing and metabolizing enzymes and correlation with gastric mucosal carbenoxolone concentrations. *Scand. J. Gastroenterol.*, **15** (Suppl.), 109–114

118. Peskar, B.M., Dreyling, K.M. and Peskar, B.A. (1985). Inhibition of sulfido-peptide–leukotriene (SP–LT) formation by carbenoxolone. *Gastroenterology*, **88**, 1538

119. Derelenko, M.J. and Long, J.F. (1981). Carbenoxolone sodium protects gastric mucosa against ethanol-induced necrosis. *Proc. Soc. Exp. Biol. Med.*, **166**, 394–397

120. Tytgat, G.N., Hameeteman, W. and Van Olften, G.H. (1984). Sucralfate, bismuth compounds, substituted benzimidazoles, trimipramine and pirenzepine in the short- and long-term treatment of duodenal ulcer. *Clin. Gastroenterol.*, **13**, 543–568

121. Marks, I.N., Lucke, W. and Wright, J.P. (1981). Ulcer healing and relapse rates after initial treatment with cimetidine and sucralfate. *J. Clin. Gastroenterol.*, **3** (Suppl. 2), 163–165

122. Borrego, E., Margolis, I. and Bank, S. (1984). A comparison between sucralfate and antiacids in the prevention of stress ulcers in critically ill patients. *Gastroenterology*, **86**, 10–32

123. Hollander, D., Tarnawski, A., Krause, W.J. and Gergely, H. (1985). Protective effect of sucralfate against alcohol-induced gastric mucosal injury in the rat. Macroscopic, histologic, ultrastructural and functional time sequence analysis. *Gastroenterology*, **88**, 366–374

124. Tarnawski, A. (1985). Prevention and treatment of gastrointestinal mucosal injury with cytoprotective agents. *Med. J. Aust.*, **142**, 513 517

125. Konturek, S.J., Radecki, T. and Piastucki, I. (1986). Gastroprotection by sucralfate and colloidal bismuth (De-Nol). Role of endogenous prostaglandins. *Gut* (In press)
126. Konturek, S.J., Kwiecien, N., Obtulowicz, W., Kopp, B. and Oleksy, J. (1986). Double-blind controlled study on the effect of sucralfate on gastric prostaglandin formation and microbleeding in normal and aspirin-treated humans. *Gut* (In press)
127. Lee, S.P. (1982). A potential mechanism of action of colloidal bismuth subcitrate; diffusion barrier to hydrochloric acid. *Scand. J. Gastroenterol.*, **17** (Suppl. 80), 17–21
128. Brodgen, R.N., Pinder, R.M. and Sawyer, P.R. (1976). Tripotassium dicitratobismuthate; a report of its pharmacological properties and therapeutic efficacy in peptic ulcer. *Drugs,* **12**, 401–411
129. Vantrappen, G., Schuurnans, P., Rutgents, P. and Janssens, J. (1982). A comparative study of colloidal bismuth subcitrate and cimetidine on the healing and recurrence of duodenal ulcer. *Scand. J. Gastroenterol.*, **17** (Suppl. 80), 23–30
130. Kyogoku, K., Hatayma, K., Yokomori, S., Saziki, R., Nakane, S., Sasajima, M., Sawada, J., Ohzeki, M. and Tanaka, I. (1979). Anti-ulcer effect of isoprenyl flavonoids. Synthesis and anti-ulcer activity of new chalone related to sophoradain. *Chem. Pharm. Bull.*, **27**, 2943–2945
131. Gomi, K., Kwayama, H., Abe, M., Okada, S., Tanaka, S. and Tanaka, Y. (1982). Clinical evaluation of SU-88 on peptic ulcer. *Jpn. Pharmacol. Therap.*, **10**, 1–5
132. Konturek, S.J., Radecki, T., Brzozowski, T. and Muramatsu, M. (1986). Antiulcer and gastroprotective effects of Solon, a synthetic flavonoid derivative of sofaradine. Role of endogenous prostaglandins. *Eur. J. Pharmacol.* (In press)
133. Hawkey, C.J. and Rampton, D.S. (1985). Prostaglandins and the gastrointestinal mucosa: Are they important in its function, disease, or treatment? *Gastroenterology,* **89**, 1162–1188

4
Animal models for studying the role of eicosanoids in peptic ulcer disease

S. Szabo and C. H. Cho

INTRODUCTION

Animal models of gastric and duodenal ulcer are important for the study of the pathogenesis of these disorders and testing of new antiulcer agents. Thus, these models should be as similar as possible to the human disease, and should be easy to produce, reproducible and economic to allow a continuous replication in various laboratories.

It is self evident, yet not always appreciated, that the preulcerogenic biochemical changes can be studied only in animal models. Human subjects do not present themselves for clinical investigation prior to the development of ulceration, and, in the biopsy material obtained from patients, the primary pathogenetic changes may be lost or cannot be distinguished from the secondary response to injury. Furthermore, especially in the pluricausal duodenal ulceration, alterations in other organs (e.g. brain, adrenals, pancreas) can be studied only in animal models of ulcer disease.

Prostanoids, especially prostaglandins (PG), are some of the endogenous chemicals beside sulfhydryls (SH) which have a role both as endogenous mediators or modulators of ulcer disease and as exogenously administered pharmacologic agents[1-3]. The involvement of PG in gastric ulceration has been suspected from data on the association of the use of aspirin-like drugs, which inhibit PG production, and the development of acute haemorrhagic gastric erosions or chronic ulcers both in humans and animals[2-4]. Supplementation with natural PGs, or their synthetic analogues, has been shown to prevent the formation of acute gastric lesions[4-5]. Administration of substances which increase synthesis in the stomach produces similar effects[6].

Recently, leukotriene (LT) metabolites of arachidonic acid, formed by the action of lipoxygenase, have also been shown to be involved in gastric lesion formation in rats. Namely, a gastrotoxic concentration of ethanol releases LT from gastric mucosa[7] and inhibitors of LT synthesis prevent ethanol-induced

75

gastric erosions[8,9]. Furthermore, intra-arterial infusion of LTC_4 or LTD_4 produces vascular damage which can develop into haemorrhagic erosions after intragastric administration of a low concentration of HCl or ethanol[9,10].

The involvement of PG in duodenal ulceration seems to be indicated but is not clear at the present stage. The experimental ulcers induced by the weak duodenal ulcerogen, acrylonitrile, may, at least in part, be due to inhibition of the protective PG synthesis[11]. Such a possibility is also implied for cysteamine-induced duodenal ulceration in rats[12]. Indeed, exogenously administered PG accelerates healing of duodenal ulcers in humans in some studies[4,5]. The duodenal PG synthesis in response to acid load is decreased in duodenal ulcer patients[13]. Thus, measurement of eicosanoid generation in gastric and duodenal mucosae represents a new biochemical approach in the elucidation of the pathogenesis of ulcer disease in the gastrointestinal tract.

This chapter reviews the animal models of gastric lesions and duodenal ulcer. The models discussed have been tested in several laboratories and can be used for biochemical, functional or morphological studies to gain insight into the pathogenesis of ulceration, as well as for pharmacological experiments to test new antiulcer agents.

Ulcer disease is defined as gastric and duodenal ulcers, which start as superficial and localized or multifocal mucosal necrosis, usually accompanied by haemorrhage, not extending beyond the muscularis mucosae (i.e. erosions), and often progress to a deep mucosal defect, reaching the muscularis propria (i.e. ulcer), which is resistant to healing. The pathogenesis and natural history of these lesions are poorly understood: hence the designation 'peptic ulcer' inappropriately overemphasizes one pathogenetic factor (i.e. pepsin) in the course of this multifactorial process[14,15]. A recently devised mechanistic classification of antiulcer agents (i.e. compounds which prevent the formation and/or accelerate the healing of existing lesions) has been suggested, using as a definition the specific biochemical process or target for the compound under consideration. This is applicable if the mechanism of action of the compound is understood or suggested, e.g. antisecretory agents which decrease acid or pepsin secretion, prosecretory agents which enhance bicarbonate or mucus secretion, etc.[16] (Table 4.1). If the mechanism of action of antiulcer agents is unknown, morphological terms according to the structural

Table 4.1 Mechanistic classification of antiulcer agents

Mechanism of action clarified[a] (defined by biochemical process or target)	Unknown mechanism(s) of action[b] (defined in morphological terms by structural target)
Antisecretory agents (HCl, pepsin)	'Cytoprotective' compounds
Prosecretory agents (HCO_3^-, mucus)	Organoprotective agents (e.g. for gastroprotection, enteroprotection)
Antioxidants (free radical scavengers)	
Oxidizing agents (mild stimulants, metals)	

Modified from Szabo and Bynum, (1988). *Scand. J. Gastroenterol.* (In press)
[a] It refers to at least one or a major mechanism so far detected.
[b] Although the biochemical mechanism is not known and may be multifactorial it probably does not include decrease in gastric acidity
(antisecretory and 'cytoprotective' doses of certain agents may, however, overlap in certain species, e.g. man vs. rat).

target may be used, such as 'cytoprotective' or organoprotective (e.g. gastroprotective, enteroprotective) agents[16]. These compounds usually prevent the induction of acute gastric mucosal lesions (e.g. haemorrhagic erosion): hence, the animal models of these lesions are reviewed in a separate category. This is followed by an overview of acute and chronic ulcer in the stomach and duodenum in small rodents.

ACUTE GASTRIC MUCOSAL INJURY

These animal models refer to chemically induced and rapidly developing diffuse surface epithelial injury in the gastric mucosa, as revealed by light and electron microscopy[17-19] and macroscopic histochemistry[20]. The grossly evident common end result of these lesions, which also develop rapidly, are multiple haemorrhagic erosions which can be graded, by measuring length or by surface planimetry[21]. The lesions are usually induced by the intragastric (i.g.) administration of chemicals (e.g. concentrated ethanol, NaOH,HCl) which induce mucosal injury in fasted rats without an obvious role for the presence of endogenous gastric HCl. These models have been used recently to study the role of endogenous prostanoids in the pathogenesis of lesions, and to test new cytoprotective agents.

The first suggestion that PG might protect the gastric mucosa from damage was made in 1975[22]. It was shown that 15-methyl PGE_2 could prevent the damage to the gastric mucosal barrier induced by either indomethacin or aspirin. Robert et al., in 1979, showed that pretreatment with various PG protected against acute haemorrhagic erosions caused by i.g. administration of noxious agents, such as concentrated ethanol, HCl, NaOH, hypertonic NaCl or boiling water[23]. This cytoprotective effect of PG is independent of their influence on gastric acid secretion[23]. Among the damaging agents, ethanol is probably the most widely used gastrotoxic agent in man, HCl is the naturally occurring gastric acid, and NaOH, like the other two chemicals, causes gastric erosions even in the presence of high gastric pH (low concentration of endogenous HCl). These animal models have been widely used to test the cytoprotective action of drugs.

Production of lesions

Young, adult, fasted rats of either sex and any strain are suitable. Oral (i.g.) administration of 50–100% ethanol, $0.2 \, mol \, L^{-1}$ NaOH or $0.6 \, mol \, L^{-1}$ HCl is performed by gastric intubation of 1 ml (for 100–200 g rats) using either rubber catheters (Rusch No. 8) or metallic tubes. The animals are usually killed one hour after the administration of damaging agent[23], although grossly evident haemorrhagic erosions develop dose-dependently and can be detected as early as one minute after ethanol exposure[21,24]. The gross appearance and speed of development of lesions induced by NaOH or HCl are similar to those produced by 100% ethanol[23,25].

The lesions appear mostly in the gastric corpus as elongated bands, 2–10 mm long and 1–3 mm wide parallel to the long axis of the stomach. The ethanol lesions are usually red, while the injury caused by NaOH or HCl appears brown or black. No gross lesion develops in the forestomach (non-secreting part covered with a squamous epithelium). The antrum is usually spared although microscopic lesions are frequently detected.

Histologically, the lesions consist of diffuse and superficial epithelial necrosis in the glandular stomach and the dead tissue is usually desquamated in one hour, with some evidence of repair by restitution[17,26]. Focally, the necrosis is deep and extends through two–thirds of the mucosa, occasionally involving the entire mucosal thickness. These erosions are accompanied by varying degrees of haemorrhage, mucosal and submuscosal oedema and congestion.

Evaluation of lesions

The lesions may be evaluated in the opened stomach semiquantitively by using a grade (e.g. scale 0–3) or quantitatively by planimetry of the stereomicroscopic image of haemorrhagic areas[21]. Since the lesions are usually uniform in width and depth, some investigators measure only the length of haemorrhagic erosions. This is also acceptable, unlike counting the lesions which provides misleading information, since the length of erosions is highly variable.

Indirect assessment of mucosal lesions is also possible by measuring the amount of blood loss into the gastric lumen, either as ^{51}Cr-labelled red blood cells[4] or as concentration of haemoglobin[27]. Biochemical measurement of released enzyme has also been used as the end-point of evaluation[28]. The most comprehensive evaluation of lesions may be obtained by light microscopic examination and morphometry of standardized sections of the stomach[17,18,26]. Histological evaluation may provide descriptive and quantitative assessment of both diffuse surface epithelial lesions and deep haemorrhagic erosions. On the other hand, this is time-consuming and is based only on certain sections of the stomach.

An optimal method of combining the quantitative assessment of diffuse surface cell injury is to use quantitative macroscopic histochemistry[20]. The freshly opened stomach is incubated in coloured substrates of dehydrogenases and lack of or differential staining of gastric surface coupled with planimetry provides a rapid and quantitative assessment of non-haemorrhagic diffuse epithelial damage. Stereomicroscopy and planimetry of haemorrhagic erosions before the incubation of the stomach quantitate the haemorrhagic component of lesions[20,21]. Cytoprotective agents usually decrease the haemorrhagic component but not the diffuse superficial epithelial lesions[17–21, 24].

Pathogenesis

The mechanism of acute gastric mucosal injury caused by concentrated solutions of ethanol, HCl or NaOH is poorly understood despite the considerable research efforts during the last decade. The initial cell injury in the surface epithelium is probably due to direct chemical toxicity. The high osmolality of alcohol and other solutions does not seem to be rate-limiting, since hypertonic solutions equi-osmolal to ethanol did not cause gastric erosions[24]. Solubility is not a major factor either, since both the lipid-soluble ethanol and aqueous HCl and NaOH produce quantitatively and qualitatively similar mucosal lesions in the stomach.

After initial injury to the surface epithelium, where the ethanol-induced lesions are the most investigated[29], the rate-limiting step seems to be the extent of vascular injury in subepithelial capillaries and venules[24, 30]. The early endothelial damage is accompanied by a slowing down of the microcirculation and increase in vascular permeability[24, 31]. The resultant intravascular haemo-concentration further decreases blood flow, resulting in circulatory standstill, as measured by laser-Doppler velocimetry in the early stage[31] or hydrogen gas clearance in the late phase of mucosal injury[32], and as visualized in histological sections[24, 33, 34]. Thus, in addition to the direct toxicity of the chemicals, vascular and hypoxic factors also contribute to the development of deep mucosal necrosis[35, 36] (Figure 4.1).

It appears that, in the pathogenesis of acute gastric mucosal injury induced by ethanol, HCl or NaOH, it does not matter which chemical is causing the superficial epithelial damage. The common rate-limiting step seems to be the vascular injury, which is produced either directly by the gastrotoxic exogenous chemicals or indirectly (e.g. by the release of LT from mast cells, macrophages, etc.) (Figures 4.1 and 4.2). It is important, from a pathogenetic point of view, that the gastric mucosal microvasculature represents a recently recognized target of interaction of damaging and protective agents[34–36]. New prostanoids or non-PG gastroprotective agents may thus be designed to directly or indirectly, prevent or minimize the vascular damage in the stomach. Namely, if the vascular injury is reduced or eliminated[24,30], blood flow is maintained[31,32] and restitution of surface epithelium[26] will lead to rapid repair of the gastric mucosa.

Pharmacology

It is well documented by now that the gastric erosions caused by ethanol, NaOH or HCl are prevented by PG in non-antisecretory doses in the rat[22,23,37,38]. This separation of cytoprotection and antisecretory doses of PG seems to be typical only for the rodent models of acute gastric mucosal

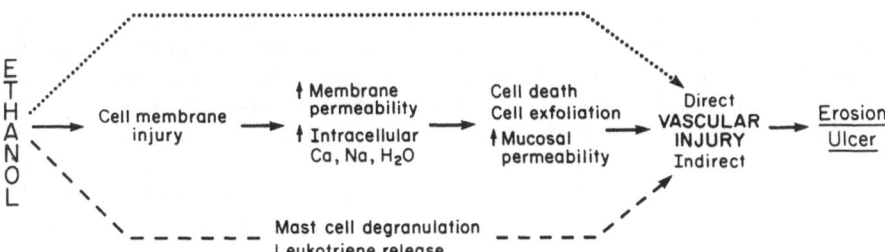

Figure 4.1 Pathogenesis of ethanol-induced gastric mucosal injury. (Modified and reprinted with permission from Szabo, S. (1987). *Scand J Gastroenterol.*, **22** Suppl. 127, 21–28)

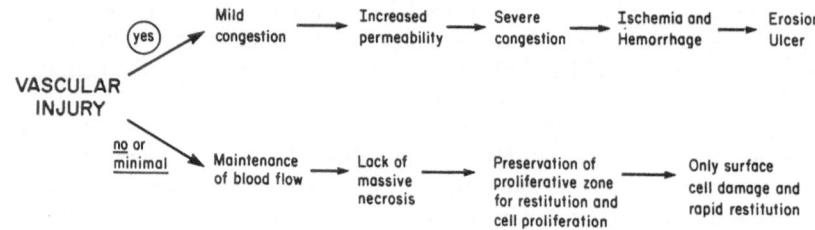

Figure 4.2 Importance of vascular injury in gastric mucosal injury and protection. (Reprinted with permission as in Figure 4.1)

injury, since, in humans, the PG doses for the two actions overlap[4,5,39]. More recently, direct or indirect inhibition of LT production was shown to decrease the acute gastric mucosal injury caused by ethanol, HCl or NaOH[7–10,40]. The animal models of acute gastric mucosal injury thus represent sensitive assays to detect new prostanoids, which may be relevant as endogenous modulators, or exogenously administered new pharmacological agents for amelioration of the acute gastric lesions.

ACUTE GASTRIC ULCERS

These animal models are used to study the pathogenesis of acute gastric ulceration and to detect new antiulcer agents which act mainly by inhibiting gastric acid secretion.

Aspirin, indomethacin

Aspirin and indomethacin are the oldest and probably most widely used non-steroidal anti-inflammatory drugs (NSAIDs). Since these drugs often cause gastrointestinal side-effects in patients (especially in those with rheumatoid arthritis requiring large daily doses of NSAIDs)[40], they are the most widely investigated NSAIDs inducing gastric ulcers in animals.

Induction of ulcers
In fasted rats, a single dose of aspirin or indomethacin produces exclusively gastric ulcers[41,42]. Daily subcutaneous (s.c.) injections of indomethacin (10 mg kg^{-1}) in rats induces multiple ulcers in the jejunum and ileum[43,44]. In the hamster, large doses of indomethacin (200 mg kg^{-1}) injected s.c. daily for five days, induce single antral or prepyloric acute and subacute ulcer[73].

The severity of aspirin-induced gastric ulcers is time- and dose-dependent[21]. Gastric erosions started to appear when the dose of acidified aspirin was increased from 20 to 50 mg kg^{-1} i.g., and the severity of lesions was slightly enhanced by the dose of 100 mg kg^{-1}. The haemorrhagic lesions appeared within 6–30 min, depending on the dose, and were maximal at 1 h after aspirin administration. The severity of lesions can be aggravated by HCl, either given with or shortly after aspirin ingestion[21,42].

The best method of obtaining reproducible ulcers with aspirin in fasted, young adult rats of either sex is to prepare a 1% solution of methyl cellulose (Sigma catalogue No. M–0512) with $0.2 \, mol \, L^{-1}$ HCl, and to prepare suspensions of aspirin $(100 \, mg \, ml^{-1})$[21]. This provides the optimal volume when given i.g. by rubber stomach tube (Rusch No. 8) at $100 \, mg \, kg^{-1}$. The animals are killed one hour after aspirin. For pharmacological experiments, rats may be pretreated with the test drug 30 min before aspirin.

Indomethacin-induced gastric erosions and ulcers develop more slowly than those caused by aspirin. After either i.g. or s.c. administration of indomethacin $(200-400 \, mg \, kg^{-1})$ in fasted rats, the animals are usually killed after 4 h.

Evaluation of ulcers
The semiquantitative and quantitative evaluation of these erosions and ulcers should meet the same criteria as those described for ethanol (see above). The only difference is that, since the NSAID-induced acute ulcers are usually of uniform size (e.g. about 1–2 mm in diameter), a lesion count is also an accepted method of evaluation[21].

Pathogenesis
The mechanism of aspirin- or indomethacin-induced gastric ulceration is more complex than the pathogenesis of ethanol-induced acute mucosal injury (Fig 4.3). Here, solubility of aspirin is important, since even the non-soluble crystals may cause physical damage to the gastric mucosa[4,36]. Since the pKa of aspirin is 3.5, the degree of ionization of salicylates decreases with low pH and it is the non-ionized, lipid-soluble form which most readily penetrates the gastric mucosa. In mice, Hingeson and Ito[45] reported that within 8 minutes after oesophageal intubation of aspirin, up to 80% of gastric surface epithelial cells exhibited morphological damage. Either following or parallel with epithelial necrosis, endothelial damage, like that seen following ethanol administration,

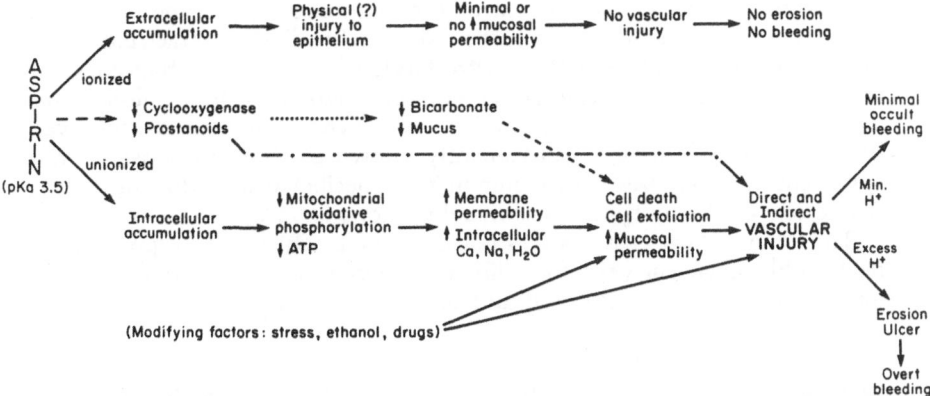

Figure 4.3 Pathogenesis of aspirin-induced acute gastric ulceration. (Modified and reprinted with permission as in Figure 4.1)

is the rate-limiting step in the pathogenesis leading to erosion and ulcer (Figures 4.2 and 4.3)[36]. The contributory role of inhibited PG synthesis and decreased mucus secretion should also be considered (Figure 4.3), although recent studies revealed no correlation between PG levels in gastric mucosa and ulcer development[46,47].

Aspirin may induce ulcers following either oral or parenteral administration[48,49]. Several experiments have indicated that intravenous (i.v.) aspirin produces primarily antral erosion in rats and cats[50,51]. Intrarectal or s.c. administration of salicylate was less severe than the oral route[52,53]. Intravenous infusion of aspirin over a 3 h period produced discrete antral lesions in rats when the stomach was perfused with HCl[53].

Pharmacology
Aspirin- or indomethacin-induced gastric erosions and acute ulcers are usually prevented or decreased by antisecretory agents in experimental animals. There is less agreement, however, about whether the aspirin-induced lesion can be diminished by non-antisecretory (cytoprotective) doses of cimetidine[42,50]. The sensitivity of indomethacin-induced gastric and intestinal lesions may also differ[43,44]. Nevertheless, these models of acute gastric ulcers represent good assays to test for new antiulcerogenic agents.

Stress

Stress is the non-specific response of the body to any demand[54]. It was Selye[54] who recognized, in 1936, that similar gastrointestinal erosions and ulcers develop in rats after exposure to various physical or chemical damaging agents: "if the organism is severely damaged by acute non-specific nocuous agents such as exposure to cold, surgical injury, production of spinal shock (transcision of the cord), excessive muscular exercise, or intoxication with sublethal doses of diverse drugs (adrenaline, atropine, morphine, formaldehyde, etc.) a typical syndrome appears, the symptoms of which are independent of the nature of the damaging agent or the pharmacological type of the drug employed and ... one observes acute erosions in the digestive tract, particularly in the stomach". Before 1936, gastroduodenal ulcers were thought to be specific responses to specific aggression, e.g. burn or Curling ulcers, brain-damage associated or Cushing ulcer[55,56]. The "syndrome produced by diverse nocuous agents"[54] became subsequently known as stress response or stress syndrome. It thus represents a common (non-specific) neuroendocrine pathway where one of the morphological manifestations is gastric ulcer.

The agent which causes stress is the stressor, which can be physical (e.g. heat, cold), chemical (e.g. formalin, epinephrine, atropine), biological (e.g. infectious agents) or psychological (e.g. emotional distress)[55,56].

Induction of ulcers
Over the years, various investigators have used, singly or in combination, various stressors, attempting to design an 'original' method to produce 'stress ulcers' in animals. For example, restraint plus cold[57] or water immersion[58]

appear to be synergistic in the production of gastric ulcers in the rat. Brodie and Hanson[59] reported a high incidence of ulceration by restraint alone in the rat, mouse and guinea pig, but not in the rabbit and monkey. Immobilization during the active phase of their daily cycle induced a high incidence of gastric erosions, but restraint during the inactive phase did not.

Restraint in animals can be accomplished by a variety of means, such as wrapping the animal in wire, immobilizing with a plaster of paris bandage, placing the animal in a small cage or a perforated metal tube, forcing the animal to stand on an electrified grid or run on an exercise wheel. All of these procedures have the same purpose, i.e. to restrict the animals from voluntary movements. It appears that the tighter the restraint, the more severe the stress and the higher the incidence of gastric lesions produced.

One of the most reproducible methods of inducing gastric erosions and ulcers in rats of either sex is immobilization on a restraining board and exposure to 4°C for 1–2 h. This procedure results in a similar number of gastric lesions as identical restraint at room temperature for 17 h[54]. Fasting is not a prerequisite, although it may aggravate the ulcers in certain strains of rats.

Evaluation of lesions
The gastric damage produced by the various stressors is essentially similar. The stomach shows multiple acute erosions and superficial ulcers, usually filled with blood. The lesions are punctuate or elongated and are localized in the acid producing part of the glandular stomach. Since the lesions are indistinguishable from ulcers induced by aspirin, the same evaluation criteria should be applied (see above). The NSAID-induced gastropathy is often classified as a stress ulcer, and, in this review, is separated only because of its distinct pharmacological properties (e.g. anti-inflammatory action, inhibition of PG synthesis) and clinical significance.

Pathogenesis
The mechanism of gastric ulceration during stress is not clarified and often controversial — more than 50 years after its original description. Extensive discussion of the pathogenesis and frequently contradictory data is beyond the scope of this review of animal models. The interested reader is referred to the multiplicity of contemporary reviews on the subject[54,56,60]. It is important to emphasize the strong central nervous system component in the pathogenesis of stress-induced acute gastric ulcers and some widely accepted pathogenetic factors, e.g. the presence of some gastric acid (not necessarily in great excess), occurrence of microcirculatory impairment, hypoxia, and probably decreased mucus and bicarbonate production. If these factors are eliminated, the superficial acute gastric ulcer rapidly heals.

Pharmacology
Stress-induced acute gastric erosions and ulcers are prevented by antacids, antisecretory agents and gastroprotective agents, such as sucralfate. The doses of PG needed to prevent the formation of stress-induced gastric ulcers are, however, larger than those needed to decrease ethanol-produced gastric

mucosal lesions[61]. It is also noted that sulphasalazine, an inhibitor of lipoxygenase and prostaglandin 15- hydroxydehydrogenase[62], protects against stress-induced gastric lesions in rats[63,64]. Thus, it is possible that various eicosanoids are involved in stress ulceration. The ready availability of these animal models could thus stimulate extensive new research into the pathogenesis and pharmacology of stress-induced gastric ulcers.

Other models

Acute gastric ulcers can also be induced by injecting high doses of endogenous monoamines, e.g. histamine in the guinea pig[65], or by stimulation of peripheral nerves[66], or of the brain[67,68]. These models are interesting because the gastric lesions may be caused by an imbalance of certain endogenous substances, in addition to the non-specific stress responses.

A special note of caution is also in order. Pylorus ligation in rats is often used to induce gastric ulcers (Shay ulcers). These lesions develop in the non-secretory forestomach which is lined by stratified squamous epithelium which has no counterpart in the human stomach. Since the procedure itself (i.e., pyloric ligation) is a drastic intervention, this animal model should be used neither for pathogenetic nor for pharmacological studies.

CHRONIC GASTRIC ULCERS

Most experimental acute erosions and ulcers in the stomach, induced by either NSAIDs or stress, heal rapidly (e.g. in a few hours or days) without scar formation. These lesions do not re-ulcerate spontaneously, the occurrence of which is a major and enigmatic feature of ulcer disease in man.

Acetic acid

This method, although artificial, represents one of the few reproducible models of chronic gastric ulcer.

Production and evaluation of ulcers
This method calls for injection in rats of 0.05 ml of 1–30% acetic acid into the submucosal layer through the serosa of the anterior wall of the glandular stomach. The site of injection is readily recognized by the localized swelling and blanching of the serosa at the injection site. A modified method consists of topical application of 0.06 ml of 100% acetic acid into the mold over the serosa and allowing it to remain for 60 s[69–71].

These methods produce a unified size of ulcer, which is quite useful for the assessment of the healing effect of different drugs. A defined acetic acid ulcer can be detected within three days after application and it can be maintained for at least 50 days. The amount of food present in the stomach can affect the ulcerogenic potential of acetic acid, i.e. a stomach distended with food produces more mucosal haemorrhage than the empty organ.

The single chronic ulcer can be easily quantitated by measuring the diameter of the ulcer crater in millimetres. With this model, histological evaluation is essential to assess the degree of necrosis, inflammation, epithelial regeneration and proliferation of fibrous connective tissue. Standard semiquantitative and morphometric methods should be used at the light microscopy level.

Pathogenesis and pharmacology
Cell injury and tissue necrosis in the muscle and serosa of the stomach are caused by the caustic nature of concentrated acetic acid, although this acid may hold some qualitative features not apparent in other caustic chemicals[71]. Thus, the epithelial necrosis is secondary to the destruction of underlying muscle and connective tissue stroma. This feature is at variance with the pathogenesis of human ulcer and other animal models where the pathogenetic factors originate from the gastroduodenal lumen and/or microcirculation.

This model can be used mainly to study ulcer healing and its modulation by eicosanoids or other drugs and growth factors. The model is thus applicable more to pharmacological than pathogenetic investigations.

Indomethacin

Indomethacin produces acute gastric erosions and ulcers in the fasted rat, small intestinal ulcers in the fed rat and solitary antral ulcers in the fed hamster. These techniques can be modified to obtain subacute and chronic gastric ulcers.

Induction of ulcers
Sprague–Dawley rats are fed chow pellets for 1 h after a 24 h fast. Indomethacin ($10-50 \, mg \, kg^{-1}$, s.c.) injected 30 min after the 1 h refeeding produces ulcers in the gastric antrum primarily along the lesser curvature and also in the small intestine[72]. These antral ulcers reach a maximum size in 6–10 h, penetrate the muscularis mucosae within 3 d and do not diminish in size for at least 7 d.

With indomethacin, the hamster model provides the advantage of inducing only antral ulcers, without lesions in the gastric corpus or intestines[73,74]. Con Olson or Syrian hamsters of either sex maintained on normal laboratory diet, should be injected s.c. with indomethacin, $200 \, mg \, kg^{-1}$, once daily for up to five days[73]. This dose produces 100% incidence of single perforated antral ulcers with 80% mortality (Figure 4.4). Decreasing the dose or number of injections results in a smaller incidence of non-perforated yet severe and solitary antral ulcers with low mortality so that animals may be maintained for a long time to study the healing process. A single s.c. injection of $50 \, mg \, kg^{-1}$ of indomethacin, for example, induces 3–5 ulcers per stomach in 5–8 h, while the same dose given twice daily for two days results in perforated antral ulcers[74].

Evaluation of ulcers
Following indomethacin, special attention should be given to whether the ulcers are localized in the stomach (as in the hamster) or in the intestines as

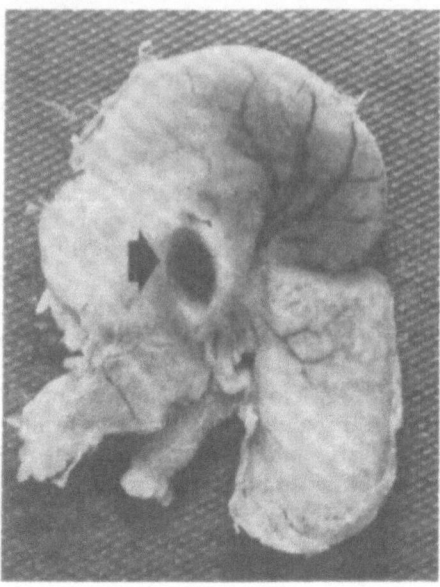

Figure 4.4 Indomethacin-induced subacute ulcer (arrow) which may develop into the chronic stage in the hamster. Indomethacin was injected at 200 mg kg^{-1} s.c. twice daily for five days and survivors were killed on the sixth day. (Reprinted with permission from Szabo *et al.* (1971). *Kisérletes Orvostudomány*, **23**, 316–320)

well (as in the rat). The acute ulcers are usually multiple and similar in size, implying that counting the ulcers provides a quantitative assessment. Subacute and chronic ulcers may vary greatly in size: hence diameter measurement is essential. Histological evaluation is also a sine qua non, as described for the acetic acid chronic ulcers (see above).

Pathogenesis
The mechanism of indomethacin-induced chronic gastric ulceration has not been extensively investigated. The pathogenesis of the antral ulcer in the rat does not involve an increase in acid secretion but little acid is needed for production of this ulcer[75]. In the hamster, the ulcer formation coincides with increased gastric acid secretion which may reach 295% that of controls[74]. The food content affects the formation of ulcers in the stomach. The nutritional component of food prevents the corpus lesions and the solid component of food (whether nutritive or not) plays an essential role in the formation of antral and intestinal lesions[76].

Pharmacology
The formation of the antral ulcer is prevented by PG or adrenalectomy, but not affected by cimetidine, atropine and/or vagotomy[72]. The development of subacute and chronic antral ulcers in the hamster is prevented by antisecretory agents, such as cimetidine, methscopolamine bromide, omeprazole or 16,16-dimethyl PGE$_2$[74]. PG, at non-antisecretory doses, also prevented the indome-

thacin-induced acute antral ulcers in the hamster[74], but the effect of cytoprotective PGs was not examined in the chronic model. Pretreatment with the hepatic microsomal enzyme inducer, spironolactone, on the other hand, significantly decreased the severity of subacute and chronic antral ulcers in the hamster, presumably because of enhanced metabolism of indomethacin[73].

Chronic antral ulcers, produced by indomethacin in the hamster and in the re-fed rat closely mimic human gastric ulcers with regard to location and histological pathogenesis. This experimental ulcer model thus seems to be especially useful for studies of the aetiology, pathogenesis and therapy of gastric ulcer disease.

Other models

Several methods exist to study the healing stage only of gastric ulceration. For example, mucosal wounds may be created by thermal injury at the fundic and pyloric area[77] which has much fragility and is the site of chronic gastric ulcer development[78]. The ulcer is sharply defined by the sixth day, with necrotic material present on the ulcer base. The ulcer area gradually diminishes in size from the third week.

A localized single wound may also be induced by external puncture of the rat stomach by a large needle and the healing process studied following this mechanical trauma[79]. The duration of ulceration induced by these methods is short and may not be long enough to assess the efficacy of drugs on ulcer healing.

ACUTE AND CHRONIC DUODENAL ULCERS

The ratio of gastric and duodenal ulcers has varied during the last century. Until the beginning of this century, gastric ulcer was prevalent, but, since then, duodenal ulcers have become 2–10 times more frequent. The frequency depends on geographical location, and, in certain countries, such as Japan and Chile, gastric ulcer is still more prevalent[2,14]. Despite the decline in the incidence of duodenal ulcer during the last decade, it still outnumbers those with gastric ulcer[3,5,14,80].

Despite the need for animal models of duodenal ulcer, until recently, only a few models were available in comparison with the plethora of experimental procedures for gastric ulcers. Pantothenic acid deficiency induces duodenal ulcer in a few weeks in about 60% of certain strains of rats[81–83]. Because of these technical and time restrictions, this animals model has not been widely used. It was, nevertheless, established that ulcer-susceptible strains of rats demonstrate increased gastric secretion and that the adrenal cortex is necessary for ulcer induction[83,84].

The subsequent models of duodenal ulcer may be divided into two groups (Table 4.3). Models (e.g. those produced by secretagogues) reproduce the multiple, irregular duodenal ulcers seen in patients with Zollinger–Ellison syndrome and pronounced gastric hypersecretion. The solitary or kissing duodenal ulcers induced by cysteamine, propionitrile, mepirizole and MPTP

Table 4.2 Models of mucosal injury, acute and chronic ulcer in the stomach

Damaging agent	Dose	Animal	Type of lesion		Suitable for pathogenetic study	Parmacological assay
			Acute	Chronic		
Ethanol, 50–100%	1 ml, i.g.	Rat	Erosion	—	yes	Cytoprotective agents
NaOH, 0.2 N	1 ml, i.g.	Rat	Erosion	—	yes	Cytoprotective agents
HCl, 0.5–0.6 N	1 ml. i.g.	Rat	Erosion	—	yes	Cytoprotective agents
Aspirin (acidified with 0.2 N HCL)	50–100 mg kg^{-1}, i.g.	Rat, mouse	Erosion ulcer	—	yes	Antiulcer, antisecretory (? cytoprotective) agents
Indomethacin (fasting + refeeding)	10–50 mg kg^{-1} i.g. or s.c.	Rat	Erosion ulcer	—	yes	Antiulcer, antisecretory (? cytoprotective) agents
Indomethacin	200 mg kg^{-1} s.c. × 2/day for 3–5 days	Hamster	Erosion ulcer	Ulcer	yes	Antiulcer, antisecretory agents
Stress	Restraint + cold	Rat	Erosion ulcer	—	yes	Antiulcer, antisecretory agents
Acetic acid	Local or topical application of acetic acid–(see text)	Rat, cat	Ulcer	Ulcer	no	Antiulcer agents

Table 4.3 Duodenal ulcerogens in rodents

Duodenal ulcerogens	Gastric secretion	Model for human disease	Suitable for pathogenetic study	Pharmacologic modulation Induction	Healing
Pantothenic acid deficiency	Decreased, then increased	Duodenitis(?) with ulcer	yes	+	±
Secretagogues (e.g. histamine, carbachol, pentagastrin)	Increased	Zollinger–Ellison and similar syndromes	yes	+	+
Acetic acid	?	?	no	–	+
Propionitrile	Increased/ no change	Non-specific acute duodenal ulcer(s)	?	+	±
Cysteamine	Increased/ no change	Non-specific acute and chronic 'peptic' duodenal ulcer(s)	yes	+	+
Mepirizole	Increased/ decreased	Acute stress and chronic duodenal ulcers	yes	+	+
MPTP	Decreased	Acute stress ulcer(s)	yes	+	±

89

represent models of stress-induced or non-specific duodenal ulcers. With local application of acetic acid, single or multiple duodenal ulcers may be produced.

Secretagogues

Hydrochloric acid seems to be necessary for duodenal ulceration, although less than half of duodenal ulcer patients are actually hypersecretors. Experimental duodenal ulcers may thus be induced in rats and guinea pigs by secretagogues, such as histamine, cholinergic drugs and pentagastrin[85,86]. The ulcers produced by these methods are selective for the duodenum; they are multiple and extend to the distal duodenum as in Zollinger–Ellison syndrome or other human hypersecretory states.

Induction and evaluation of ulcers

Fasted rats of either sex and of any strain should be infused s.c. for 24–48 h either with carbachol (0.5 μg kg^{-1} min^{-1}) and histamine (0.05 mg kg^{-1}min^{-1}) or carbachol and pentagastrin (2 μg kg^{-1}min^{-1}). In the guinea pig, histamine (90 μg kg^{-1}) is injected s.c. eight times at 30 min intervals.

The ulcers usually develop within 48 h and seem to originate from the superficial mucosa and to penetrate gradually through all of the duodenal layers[85–87]. They range from shallow erosions or ulcers (with ruptured muscularis mucosae) to perforation.

Because of the multiplicity of duodenal ulcers, ulcer count and diameter measurements should be standard procedures. The severity (depth) of ulcer may be evaluated semiquantitatively with a scale of 0–3, where 0 = normal mucosa, 1 = erosion, 2 = deep ulcer involving the muscularis propria (serosa is not ruptured but shows localized discoloration), and 3 = perforated ulcer (into free peritoneal cavity) or penetrating ulcer (into liver or pancreas). The intensity of the ulcer process and the degree of inflammation and healing should be evaluated by light microscopy.

Pathogenesis and pharmacology

The very few pathogenetic studies which have been performed with secretagogue models are essentially restricted to describing the natural history of this experimental duodenal ulcer[85,87]. It is assumed that the predominant pathogenetic factor here is enhanced gastric acid secretion.

These animal models are more important for screening drugs with antisecretory action. Duodenal ulcers induced by secretagogues can be prevented by antisecretory agents and antacids. However, drugs which promote ulcer healing have not been tested in this ulcer model. The widespread use of this model is probably precluded by the cumbersome techniques used in rats (e.g. s.c. infusion for 24–48 h).

Cysteamine and its derivatives

Cysteamine-induced duodenal ulcers are probably the most widely used animal models of acute and chronic duodenal ulcer. In addition to the simplicity of induction, the duodenal ulcer produced by cysteamine in rats is very similar to that seen in man, using functional and morphologic criteria[14.88].

The discovery of the cysteamine-induced duodenal ulcer was actually preceded by the observation that multiple injections of propionitrile (CH$_3$-CH$_2$-CN) induce solitary or double (often perforating) duodenal ulcers in 2–3 d in the rat (Figure. 4.5)[89]. Cysteamine (HS-CH$_2$-CH$_2$-NH$_2$), in a single dose, was subsequently found to produce perforating duodenal ulcers in rats within 24–48 h[90]. The ensuing structure-activity studies revealed several potent alkyl and aryl duodenal ulcerogens among which only cysteamine and n-butyronitrile are close in potency to cysteamine[91–94].

Induction of ulcers
For the cysteamine model, young adult rats of either sex and of any strain may be used. Our experience shows that female Sprague Dawley rats (170–200 g) are especially suitable. Cysteamine induces duodenal ulcers also in mice, cats and dogs, although not as rapidly as in rats[94–96]. It should be stressed that animals should not be fasted because food restriction increases toxicity, and, as a stressor, may cause gastric erosions and ulcer in addition to duodenal ulceration. Dose-response and comparative studies also revealed that the dose of cysteamine should be adjusted to local conditions (e.g. sex and strain, quality of food, tap water). Table 4.4 shows guidelines from our laboratory practice.

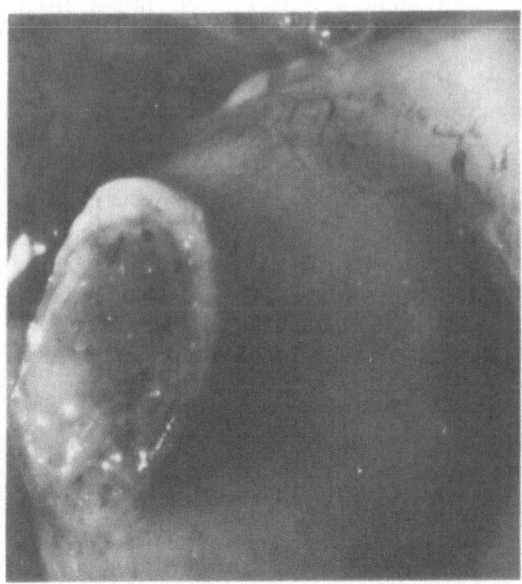

Figure 4.5 Propionitrile-induced perforated ulcer on the anterior wall of rat duodenum. The location (e.g. 3–5 mm from the pylorus), gross and microscopic appearance of this ulcer is indistinguishable from that induced by cysteamine. (Reprinted with permission from Szabo, S., and Selye, H. (1972). *Arch. Pathol.*, **93**, 390–391)

Table 4.4 Recommended models of duodenal ulcer

Type of disease	Duodenal ulcerogen Compound	Species	Dose
'Non-specific' duodenal ulcer	Cysteamine–HCl	Rat, mouse	$280-300$ mg kg^{-1} p.o. $\times 3$ (e.g. 9 am, 12 noon, 3 pm) *or* 400 mg kg^{-1} p.o. $\times 2$ *or* 700 mg kg^{-1} p.o. $\times 1$ *or* 400 mg kg^{-1} s.c. $\times 1$
Zollinger–Ellison and hypersecretory syndromes	Carbachol + histamine	Rat	0.5 μg kg^{-1} s.c. for $24-48$ h 0.05 mg kg^{-1} min^{-1} s.c. for $24-48$ h
	Carbachol + pentagastrin	Rat	0.5 μg kg^{-1} min^{-1} s.c. for $24-48$ h 2μg kg^{-1} min^{-1} s.c. for $24-48$ h
	Histamine	Guinea pig	90 μg kg^{-1} s.c. $\times 8$, 30 min apart

Cysteamine–HCl is prepared in distilled water as a 10% solution (100 mg ml^{-1}); $280-300$ mg kg^{-1} should be administered i.g. by rubber catheter (Rusch No. 8) three times at $3-4$ h intervals, or 400 mg kg^{-1} i.g. twice. The result is 100% incidence of severe duodenal ulcers in rats killed 48 h later, and the mortality is 20–30%[88]. This model is especially suitable to test antiulcer agents which can be administered 30 min before each dose of cysteamine. For pathogenetic studies where timing from the initial lesion is important, a single dose of 700 mg kg^{-1} i.g. or 400 mg kg^{-1} s.c. of cysteamine–HCl is optimal.

To obtain models of chronic duodenal ulcers, using cysteamine, two options are available. With one procedure, after receiving 280 mg kg^{-1} of cysteamine–HCl i.g. $\times 3$ on day one, rats are placed on 0.01% or 0.05% cysteamine–HCl in drinking water from the second day[88]. This low concentration of cysteamine is sufficient to maintain gastric hyperacidity and active duodenal ulcers which had been evaluated up to 60 days[88]. A similar method can be used with the *n*-butyronitrile-induced duodenal ulcer[93]. This method induces heterogeneous ulcers (e.g. scale 1–3), which heal at various rates[88,97]. The second procedure involves the elimination of rats with 0 or 1 grade duodenal lesions. Animals are laparotomized 48 hours after receiving cysteamine, (as described above) and only rats with severe (grade 2 or 3) duodenal ulcers are kept for further studies[97]. This method thus provides rather uniform duodenal ulcers which can be studied for weeks to months, and are especially suitable for testing antiulcer drugs which may accelerate ulcer healing.

Evaluation of ulcers
The ulcers develop mostly on the antimesenteric or anterior wall of the duodenum, 3–5 mm from the pylorus. They frequently perforate or penetrate into the liver or pancreas. These ulcers are sharply demarcated craters with a necrotic centre, acute and chronic inflammation, granulation tissue and re-epithelization on the edge of the crater.

Since the ulcer is usually most severe on the anterior wall of the duodenum, quantitative evaluation of lesions in this area is sufficient. Measurement of the largest diameter of the ulcer can be used to calculate the ulcer area, while the scale 0–3 (see above under 'Secretagogues') provides a semiquantitative evaluation of ulcer severity or intensity. Light microscopy is usually only confirmatory for the acute ulcers (up to 48 h), while the histological evaluation of chronic ulcers is essential to assess the healing process[88,97]

Pathogenesis
The mechanism of duodenal ulceration induced by cysteamine and its derivatives has been extensively investigated and its review is beyond the purpose of this chapter. Recent reviews[14,39,94] will be supplemented only by a brief description of new results (Figure 4.6). Most importantly, it should be stressed that the pathogenesis of this experimental duodenal ulcer (presumably like that in man) is a complex multifactorial (pluricausal) process which involves the interaction of several organs[14,15,94]. The initial neuroendocrine changes in the brain are apparently followed by similar alterations in the stomach and duodenum (Figure 4.6) and probably in the adrenals and pancreas. Subsequently, delayed gastric emptying, elevated serum gastrin and increased gastric acid secretion can be detected. The duodenum may also be affected by direct cytotoxicity of cysteamine[98] and increased vascular permeability[99]. Duodenal hypermotility interferes with the delivery of pancreatic bicarbonate from distal to proximal duodenum and creates an unusually high degree of hyperacidity[100–103]. The decreased bicarbonate secretion[104] and release of PAS-positive material from Brunner's glands[105] may be either a primary effect of cysteamine or a secondary response to duodenal dysmotility. The decreased availability of bicarbonate then aggravates the action of acid in the congested duodenal bulb and contributes to the necrosis of absorptive epithelial cells in the duodenum[106–108].

The cysteamine-induced duodenal ulcer is frequently accompanied by adrenocortical necrosis[14]. Clinically, one of the early endocrine complications of duodenal ulcer is adrenal lesions[14,109]. These observations suggest interactive factors in the aetiology of duodenal ulcer and of adrenal damage. Cysteamine induces both duodenal and adrenal damage, therefore providing a good model for studying the pathogenesis of human disease with similar organ malfunctions.

Other pathogenetic factors are also shared between cysteamine-induced duodenal ulcers and human duodenal disease. Cysteamine acutely increases serum gastrin levels in rats, and peptone or food administration further

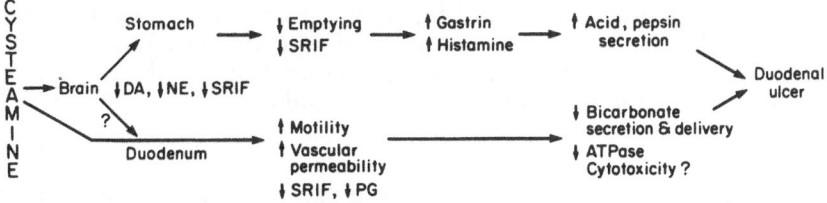

Figure 4.6 Pathogenesis of cysteamine induced duodenal ulcer

enhances this[110]. In duodenal ulcer patients, food-stimulated gastrin release is markedly higher than that of normal volunteers[111]. Furthermore, plasma secretin, a physiological inhibitor of gastric acid secretion, is decreased in rats after cysteamine administration[112]. Failure to release secretin as a consequence of duodenal acidification has been implicated as a factor in the pathogenesis of duodenal ulcer disease[113].

Although cysteamine and propionitrile produce an indistinguishable duodenal ulcer in rats, propionitrile is virtually ineffective in elevating serum gastrin levels and does not deplete tissue immune reactive somatostatin (an inhibitor of gastric acid secretion)[114]. These two animal models might thus represent two different pathogenetic pathways, even though the duodenal ulcers are the same both morphologically and in location. The cysteamine and propionitrile duodenal ulcer models support the clinical impression concerning the heterogeneity of chronic duodenal ulcers.

Pharmacology
Cysteamine- and propionitrile-induced duodenal ulcers are prevented by antacids and antisecretory agents acting at any of the three types of receptor on the parietal cells[14,94]. Although the chemical duodenal ulcerogens decrease PG production[11], cytoprotective doses of PG are not sufficient to reduce the cysteamine-induced duodenal ulcer[115], but PG in antisecretory doses are potent antiulcerogens in these models[116,117]. The cysteamine-induced duodenal ulcer is potentiated by indomethacin but decreased by hypertonic NaCl, probably because of an increase in PGE content[16]. This study indicates that the ulcerogenic effect of cysteamine may be due in part to inhibition of protective PG. The trophic properties of PGE_2 on gastrointestinal epithelium and the antitrophic effect of the PG-synthetase inhibitor, indomethacin, support this suggestion. Similar phenomena have also been demonstrated in duodenal ulcer patients in which the synthesis of PG in mucosa is diminished or lacking[13].

The models of acute and chronic duodenal ulcer produced by cysteamine and its derivatives may continue to serve as tools to investigate both the natural history of duodenal ulceration and the activity of new antiulcer drugs.

Mepirizole and MPTP

Mepirizole and MPTP (1-methyl-4-phenyl-1,2,3,6-tetrahydropyridine) are recently discovered duodenal ulcerogens[118,119]. It is of special pathogenetic interest that both of these compounds induce duodenal ulceration accompanied by decreased gastric acid output. Thus, both substances represent new models of duodenal ulcer disease where, instead of an excess of aggressive factors, perhaps a deficiency of protective mechanisms (e.g. bicarbonate, motility) might be a crucial factor in the pathogenesis of duodenal ulcer disease[36,118,119].

Induction and evaluation of ulcers
Mepirizole is a basic anti-inflammatory drug. There are species and strain differences in mepirizole-induced duodenal and gastric lesions[120]. Mepirizole

dose-dependently induces duodenal ulcers and superficial antral erosions in rats, duodenal lesions in rabbits and gastric superficial erosions in guinea pigs[118,120]. There is little or no damage to duodenum and stomach in mice and dogs[120]. Mepirizole, within three days, induces duodenal ulcers which gradually diminish in size and depth by the 15th day. Complete healing in rats occurs in 60 days.

The dopaminergic neurotoxin, MPTP, causes Parkinson's disease in humans and experimental animals. The toxin and its derivative and metabolite, reduced MPTP and MPP^+, are also ulcerogens in rats and mice[119,121]. MPTP is an analogue derived from the synthetic analgesic, alphaprodine, and, when given in multiple daily doses either i.g. or s.c., induces in a dose-dependent manner solitary or double (kissing) duodenal ulcers in rats. The most convenient model seems to be to prepare a $20\,mg\,ml^{-1}$ solution of the water-soluble MPTP–HCl and inject $20\,mg\,kg^{-1}$ (calcuated as free base) s.c. 3 times daily for four days and to kill the rats on the fifth day. This procedure results in 100% incidence of duodenal ulcers, some gastric erosions and some mortality.

Evaluation of ulcers should be similar to that described for cysteamine (see above).

Pathogenesis and pharmacology
The mechanisms of duodenal ulceration with these two new models have not been extensively investigated. Mepirizole decreases gastric acid output in most species and inhibits PG synthesis; yet the depressed PG level is not sufficient to cause duodenal ulcers[122]. Secretagogue inhibitors and antacids accelerate the healing of mepirizole-induced ulcers; however, oral 16,16-dm PGE_2 delays healing[118,120]. MPTP also decreases gastric secretion of acid and pepsin, as well as pancreatic bicarbonate, trypsin and amylase. The cerebral concentration of the dopamine metabolite, DOPAC, is also diminished and dopamine agonists and monoamine oxidase inhibitors prevent the duodenal ulcers[119,121]. This ulcer model represents a typical example of impaired defence in the duodenal bulb, which may be centrally mediated.

Other models

Acetic acid produces lesions in the duodenal wall after local injection or topical application[123] on the serosa of the duodenum. The initial damage is in the muscle and serosa which show severe congestion and haemorrhage. Eventually, a clearly defined, deep, round or oval ulcer develops and it usually penetrates into the adjacent organs (mainly liver). The topical application of acetic acid requires laparotomy, and its pathogenesis is unusual (see gastric ulcer models) but the ulcers are reproducible in size and depth. This method may be used to study the pathophysiology and pharmacology of healing of duodenal ulceration.

The unsaturated derivative of propionitrile, acrylonitrile, is a weak duodenal ulcerogen[124] despite its inhibition of PG synthesis[11]. Severe solitary or double duodenal ulcers develop if rats are pretreated with microsomal enzyme inducers, such as phenobarbital, before the administration of acrylonitrile[124].

This model may thus be useful in investigating the generation of ulcerogenic metabolites in the liver, stomach or duodenum.

If the inhibition of PG synthesis is followed by enhanced gastric acid output, duodenal ulcers will develop[125]. This new animal model is especially relevant to eicosanoids since PG are thought to be one of the modulators of bicarbonate and mucus secretion[125]. Suppression of defensive factors leads to duodenal ulceration only if accompanied by an enhanced load of acid into the proximal duodenum. The new animal models of duodenal ulcer disease thus provide new tools with which to study both the pathogenesis and new pharmacology of ulcer disease.

SUMMARY

This chapter reviews the animal models of acute gastric mucosal injury, as well as acute and chronic ulcers in the stomach and duodenum. Emphasis is placed on easily reproducible models in small rodents (e.g. rat, mouse, hamster) and their suitability for studying the pathogenetic mechanisms of ulceration and for testing new antiulcer drugs with either antisecretory or cytoprotective properties. Acute gastric mucosal injury is easily induced by i.g. administration of concentrated solutions of ethanol, HCl or NaOH in fasted rodents. The presence of endogenous gastric acid is not a prerequisite for the development of these acute haemorrhagic erosions which can be prevented by cytoprotective agents of the prostanoid or non-PG type. Multiple acute gastric ulcers are usually induced by aspirin, indomethacin or stress (e.g. restraint + cold) in the fasted rat while solitary. Often, perforating antral ulcers are induced by indomethacin in the normally fed hamster. Chronic gastric ulcer is produced by daily s.c. injection of indomethacin in the fed hamster, or local application of acetic acid in other animals. Duodenal ulcer models were rare until recently, but now models of non-specific duodenal ulcer with variable gastric secretion, hypersecretion (e.g. induced by secretagogues) or hyposecretory states (e.g. mepirizole, MPTP) are available. The most widely used model of non-specific acute and chronic duodenal ulcer is the cysteamine method in non-fasted rats. Virtually all the models of duodenal ulceration may be used to study both the pathogenesis and the pharmacology of ulcer disease. Some of the duodenal ulcerogens (e.g. acrylonitrile, cysteamine, mepirizole) decrease endogenous PG levels, providing especially valuable tools for investigating the role of eicosanoids in acute and chronic ulcer disease.

REFERENCES

1. Robert, A. (1987). Gastric antisecretory, antiulcer and cytoprotective properties of prostaglandins. In Szabo, S. and Mózsik, Gy. (eds.) *New Pharmacology of Ulcer Disease*, pp. 322–328. (New York: Elsevier)
2. Brooks, F.P. (1985). The pathophysiology of peptic ulcer disease. *Dig. Dis. Sci.*, **30**, 15S–19S
3. Szabo, A., Pihan, G. and Dupuy, D. (1987). The biochemical pharmacology of sulfhydryl

compounds in gastric mucosal injury and protection. In Szabo, S. and Mózsik, Gy. (eds.) *New Pharmacology of Ulcer Disease*, pp. 424–434. (New York: Elsevier)

4. Domschke, S. and Domschke, W. (1984). Gastroduodenal damage due to drugs, alcohol and smoking. *Clin. Gastroenterol.*, **13**, 405–436

5. Lam S.K. (1986). Review article. Prostaglandins for duodenal ulcer and gastric ulcer. *J. Gastroenterol. Hepatol.*, **1**, 471–481

6. Danon, A. and Ascouline, G. (1979). Antiulcer activity of hypertonic solutions in the rat: possible role of prostaglandins. *Eur. J. Pharmacol.*, **58**, 425–431

7. Peskar, B.M., Lange, K., Hoppe, U. and Peskar, B.A. (1986). Ethanol stimulates formation of leukotriene C_4 in rat gastric mucosa. *Prostaglandins*, **31**, 283–293

8. Boughton-Smith, N.K. and Whittle, B.J.R. (1987) Prostaglandin inhibition of ethanol-induced release of gastric mucosal leukotrienes. *Gastroenterology*, **92**, 1325

9. Rogers, C., Pihan, G., Raza, A. and Szabo, S. (1987). Possible participation of leukotrienes (LT) in the pathogenesis of gastric mucosal lesions and vascular injury induced by ethanol, HCl, NaOH, or aspirin (ASA) in the rat. Effect of eicosapentaenoic acid (EPA) or a lipoxygenase inhibitor L-651,392. *Gastroenterology*, **92**, 1808

10. Pihan, G., Rogers, C. and Szabo, S. (1988) Vascular injury in acute gastric mucosal damage: The mediatory role of leukotrienes. *Dig. Dis. Sci.* (In press)

11. Michel, F., Mercklein, L., Crastes, D.P.A., Dore, J.C., Gilbert, J. and Miguel, J.F. (1984). The effect of various acrylonitriles and related compounds on prostaglandin biosynthesis. *Prostaglandins*, **27**, 69–83

12. Assouline, G. and Danon, A. (1978). Gastric prostaglandins: antiulcer activity of hypertonic solutions. *Isr. J. Med. Sci.*, **14**, 493

13. Ahlquist, D.A., Dozois, R.R., Zinsmeister, A.N. and Malagelada, J.R. (1983). Duodenal prostaglandin synthesis and acid load in health and in duodenal ulcer disease. *Gastroenterology*, **85**, 522–528

14. Szabo, S. (1984). Biology of disease. Pathogenesis of duodenal ulcer disease. *Lab. Invest.*, **51**, 121–147

15. Szabo, S. and Mózsik, Gy. (1987). Foreward. In Szabo, S. and Mózsik Gy. (eds.) Ulcer Disease: Complex Pathology–Multifactorial Pharmacology. pp. 15–19. (New York: Elsevier)

16. Szabo, S. and Bynum, T.H. (1988) Alternatives to the acid-oriented approach to ulcer disease: does "cytoprotection" exist in man? *Scand. J. Gastroenterol.* (In press)

17. Lacy, E.R. and Ito, S. (1982) Microscopic analysis of ethanol damage to rat gastric mucosa after treatment with a prostaglandin. *Gastroenterology*, **82**, 619–625

18. Wallace, J.J., Morris, G.P., Krause, E.J. and Greaves, S.E. (1986). Reduction by cytoprotective agents of ethanol-induced damage to the rat gastric mucosa: a correlated morphological and physiological study. *Can. J. Physiol. Pharmacol.*, **60**, 1686–1699

19. Tarnawski, A., Hollander, D., Stachura, J., Krause, W.J. and Gergely, H. (1985). Prostaglandin protection of the gastric mucosa against alcohol injury – a dynamic time-related process. Role of the mucosal proliferative zone. *Gastroenterology*, **88**, 334–352

20. Bose, R. and Szabo, S. (1985). New macroscopic histochemical method to quantitate gastric mucosal injury in the rat. *Gastroenterology*, **88**, 1332

21. Szabo, S., Trier, J.S., Brown, A., Schnoor, J., Homan, H.D. and Bradford, J.C. (1985). A quantitative method for assessing the extent of experimental gastric erosions and ulcer. *J. Pharmacol. Meth.* **13**, 59–66

22. Cohen, M.M. (1975). Prostaglandins prevents gastric mucosal barrier damage. *Gastroenterology*, **68**, 876

23. Robert, A., Nezamis, J.E., Lancaster, C. and Hanchar, A.J. (1979). Cytoprotection by prostaglandins in rats: prevention of gastric necrosis produced by alcohol, HCl, NaOH, hypertonic NaCl and thermal injury. *Gastroenterology*, **77**, 433–443

24. Szabo, A., Trier, J.S., Brown, A. and Schnoor, J. (1985). Early vascular injury and increased vascular permeability in gastric mucosal injury caused by ethanol in the rat. *Gastroenterology*, **88**, 228–236

25. Wong, S.H., CHO, C.H. and Ogle, C.W. (1986). Protection by zinc sulphate against ethanol-induced ulceration and preservation of the gastric mucosal barrier. *Pharmacology*, **33**, 94–102

26. Lacy, E. and Ito, S. (1983). Rapid epithelial restitution of the rat gastric mucosa after ethanol injury. *Lab. Invest.*, **51**, 573–583

27. Lichtenberger, L.M., Graziani, L.A., Dial, E.J., Butler, B.D. and Hills, B.A. (1983). Role of surface active phospholipids in gastric cytoprotection. *Science*, **219**, 1327–1329

28. Whittle, B.J.R. and Steel, G. (1985). Evaluation of rat gastric mucosa by a prostaglandin analogue using cellular enzyme marker and histological techniques. *Gastroenterology*, **88**, 315–327

29. Guslandi, M. (1987). Effects of ethanol on the gastric mucosa. *Dig. Dis.*, **5**, 21–32

30. Szabo, S., Trier, J.S., Brown, A. and LaRocque, M. (1985). Prostaglandin- and sulfhydryl-sensitive vascular injury in the pathogenesis of acute gastric mucosal lesions. *Lab. Invest.*, **52**, 66A

31. Pihan, G., Majzoubi, D., Haudenschild, C., Trier, J.S. and Szabo, S. (1986). Early microcirculatory stasis in acute gastric mucosal injury in the rat and prevention by 16,16-dimethyl prostaglandin E_2 or sodium thiosulfate. *Gastroenterology*, **91**, 1415–1426

32. Leung, F.W., Robert, A. and Guth, P.H. (1985). Gastric mucosal blood flow in rats after administration of 16,16-dimethyl prostaglandin E_2 at a cytoprotective dose. *Gastroenterology*, **88**, 1948–1953

33. Guth, P.H., Poulsen, G. and Nagata, H. (1984). Histologic and microcirculatory changes in alcohol-induced gastric lesions in the rat: effect of prostaglandin cytoprotection. *Gastroenterology*, **87**, 1083–1090

34. Szabo, S. (1984). Role of sulfhydryls and early vascular lesions in gastric mucosal injury. *Acta Physiol. Hung.*, **64**, 203–214

35. Szabo, S., Pihan, G. and Trier, J.S. (1986). Alterations in blood vessels during gastric injury and protection. *Scand. J. Gastroenterol.*, **21** Suppl. 125, 92–96

36. Szabo, S. (1987). Mechanisms of mucosal injury in the stomach and duodenum: Time-sequence analysis of morphologic, functional, biochemical and histochemical studies. *Scand. J. Gastroenterol.*, **22**, Suppl. 127, 21–28

37. Miller, T.A. (1983). Protective effects of prostaglandins against gastric mucosal damage: current knowledge and proposed mechanisms. *Am J. Physiol.*, **245**, G601

38. Flemström, G. and Garner, A. (1982). Gastroduodenal HCO_3 transport: characteristics and proposed role in acidity regulation and mucosal protection. *Am. J. Physiol.*, **242**, G183–G193

39. Holt, K.M. and Hollander, D. (1986). Acute gastric mucosal injury: pathogenesis and therapy. *Annu. Rev. Med.*, **37**, 107–124

40. Roth, S.H. (ed.). (1985). *Rheumatic Therapeutics*. (New York: McGraw Hill)

41. Whittle, B.J.R. (1977). Mechanisms underlying gastric mucosal damage by indomethacin and bile salts and the actions of prostaglandins. *Br. J. Pharmacol.*, **60**, 455–460

42. Guth, P.H., Aures, S. and Poulsen, G. (1979). Topical aspirin plus HCl gastric lesions in the rat. Cytoprotective effect of prostaglandin, cimetidine and probanthine. *Gastroenterology*, **77**, 88–93

43. Selye, H. (1969). Prevention of indomethacin-induced intestinal ulcers by spironolactone and norbolethome. *Can. J. Physiol. Pharmacol.*, **47**, 981–983

44. Del Soldato, P. (1984). Nonsteroidal antiinflammatory drugs and their actions in the intestine: pharmacological, emotional, dietary, and microbial factors. In Rainsford K.D. and Velo, GP (eds.) *Advances in Inflammation Research*, Vol. 6, 89–101. (New York: Raven Press)

45. Hingeson, D.J. and Ito, S. (1971). Effects of aspirin and related compounds on the fine structure of mouse gastric mucosa. *Gastroenterology*, **61**, 156–177

46. Ligumsky, M., Golanska, E.M., Hansen, D.G. and Kauffman, G.L. Jr. (1983). Aspirin can inhibit gastric mucosal cyclo-oxygenase without causing lesions in rat. *Gastroenterology*, **84**, 756–761

47. Garay, G.L., Carter, H. and Annesley, P. (1985). The incidence and severity of experimentally induced gastroduodenal mucosal lesions by NSAIs or by analgesic compounds do not correlate with the degree of inhibition of prostaglandin (PG) biosynthesis in the monkey. *Dig. Dis, Sci.*, **30**, 376

48. Guth, P.H. and Poulsen, G. (1979). Effect of parenteral aspirin on the gastric mucosal barrier in the rat. *Digestion*, **19**, 93–98

49. Rowe, P.H., Starlinger, M.J., Kasdon, E., Hollands, M.J. and Silen, W. (1987). Parenteral aspirin and sodium salicylate are equally injurious to the rat gastric mucosa. *Gastroenterology*, **93**, 863–871

50. Bugat, R., Thompson, M.R., Aures, D. and Grossman, M.I. (1976). Gastric mucosal

lesions produced by intravenous infusion of aspirin in cats. *Gastroenterology*, **71**, 754–759

51. Hansen, D.G., Aures, D. and Grossman, M.I. (1978). Histamine augments gastric ulceration produced by intravenous aspirin in cats. *Gastroenterology*, **74**, 540–543

52. Pfeiffer, C.J. and Lewandewski, L.G. (1971). Comparison of gastric toxicity of acetylsalicylic acid with route of administration in the rat. *Arch. Int. Pharmacodyn. Ther.*, **190**, 5–13.

53. Kauffman, G.L. and Grossman, M.I. (1978). Prostaglandins and cimetidine inhibit the formation of ulcers produced by parenteral salicylates. *Gastroenterology*, **75**, 1099–1102

54. Selye, H. (1976). *Stress in Health and Disease*. (Boston: Butterworth)

55. Selye, H. (1936). A syndrome produced by diverse nocuous agents. *Nature (London)*, **138**, 32

56. Robert, A. and Szabo, S. (1983). Stress ulcers. In Selye H. (ed.) *Selye's Guide to Stress Research*, pp. 22–46. (New York: Van Nostrand Reinhold Company, Inc.)

57. Senay, E.C. and Levine, R.J. (1967). Synergism between cold and restraint for rapid productions of stress ulcers in rats. *Proc. Soc. Exp. Biol.*, **124**, 1221–1223

58. Kagi, K., Kasuya, Y. and Watanabe, K. (1964). Studies on the drugs for peptic ulcer, a reliable method for producing stress ulcer in rats. *Chem. Pharm. Bull.*, **12**, 465–472

59. Brodie, D.A. and Hanson, H.M. (1960). A study of the factors involved in the production of gastric ulcers by the restraint technique. *Gastroenterology*, **38**, 353–360

60. Skillman, J.J. and Silen, W. (1976). Stress ulceration in the acutely ill. *Annu. Rev. Med.*, **27**, 9–22

61. Garrick, T., Kolve, E., Kauffman, G.L. Jr. (1986). Prostaglandin requirements are greater for protection in cold-restraint-induced than alcohol-induced gastric mucosal injury. *Dig. Dis. Sci.*, **31**, 401–405

62. Hoult, J.R.S. and Moore, P.K. (1980). Effects of sulphasalazine and its metabolites in prostaglandin synthesis, inactivation and actions on smooth muscle. *Br. J. Pharmacol.*, **68**, 719–730

63. Ogle, C.N. and Cho, C.H. (1985). Effects of sulphasalazine in stress ulceration and mast cell degranulation in rat stomachs. *Eur. J. Pharmacol.*, **112**, 285–286

64. Ogle, C.W., Cho, C.H. and Dai, S. (1985). Sulphasalazine and experimental stress ulcers. *Agents Actions*, **17**, 153–157

65. Eagleton, G.B. and Watt, J. (1971). The selective production of gastric and duodenal ulceration using histamine. In Pfeiffer C.J. (ed.) *Peptic Ulcer*, pp. 34–44. (Philadelphia: Lippincott)

66. Cho, C.H., Ogle, C.W. and Dai, S. (1976). Acute gastric ulcer formation in response to electrical vagal stimulation in rats. *Eur. J. Pharmacol.*, **35**, 215–219

67. Kurotsu, T., Takeda, M. and Ban, T. (1951). Studies on the gastrointestinal motility and hemorrhage induced by the hypothalamic stimulation of rabbits. *Med. J. Osaka Univ.*, **2**, 443–449

68. Feldman, S., Behar, A.J. and Birnbaum, D. (1961). Gastric lesions following hypothalamic stimulation. *Arch. Neurol.*, **4**, 308–317

69. Takagi, K., Okabe, S. and Saziki, R. (1970). A new method for the production of chronic gastric ulcer in rats and the effect of several drugs on its healing. *Jpn. J. Pharmacol.*, **19**, 418–426

70. Okabe, S., Roth, J.L. and Pfeiffer, C.J. (1971). Differential healing periods of the acetic acid ulcer model in rats and cats. *Experientia*, **27**, 146–148

71. Okabe, S. and Pfeiffer, C.J. (1971). The acetic acid model. A procedure for chronic duodenal or gastric ulcer. In Pfeiffer C.J. (ed.) *Peptic Ulcer*, pp. 13–20. (Philadelphia: Lippincott)

72. Satoh, H., Inada, I., Hirata, T. and Maki, Y. (1981). Indomethacin produces gastric antral ulcers in the refed rat. *Gastroenterology*, **81**, 719–725

73. Szabo, S., Selye, H. and Mécs, I. (1971). Katatoxikus steroidok hatása az indomethacin és digitoxin mérgezésre hörcsögökben. *Kísérletes Orvostudomány*, **23**, 316–320

74. Kolbasa, K.P., Lancaster, C., Olafsson, A.S. and Robert, A. (1986). Indomethacin-induced gastric antral ulcers in hamsters. *Gastroenterology*, **90**, 1498

75. Satoh, H. and Guth, P.H. (1981). Gastric antral ulcers produced by indomethacin in the rat III. Role of acid and prostaglandins. *Gastroenterology*, **80**, 1272

76. Satoh, H., Guth, P.H. and Grossman, M.I. (1982). Role of food in gastrointestinal ulceration produced by indomethacin in the rat. *Gastroenterology*, **83**, 210–215

77. Wong, J. and Loewenthal, J. (1976). Chronic gastric ulcer in the rat produced by wounding at the fundo-antral junction. *Gastroenterology*, **71**, 416–420

78. Korynot, S.C,. Fam, F.S. and Kahn, D.S. (1971). Experience with production of experimental gastric ulcers by local thermal injury. In Pfeiffer, C.J. (ed.) *Peptic Ulcer*, pp. 138–142. (Philadelphia: Lippincott)

79. Ezer, E. (1988). A novel method for producing standard subacute gastric ulcer in rats and for the quantitative evaluation of the healing process. Effect of several drugs on healing. *J. Pharmacol. Meth.* (In press)

80. Kurata, J.H., Elashoff, J.D., Haile, B.M. and Honda, G.D. (1983). A reappraisal of time trends in ulcer disease: factors related to changes in ulcer hospitalization and mortality rates. *Am. J. Public Health*, **73**, 1066–1072

81. Berg, B.N., Zucker, T.F. and Zucker, L.M. (1949). Duodenal ulcers produced on a diet deficient in pantothenic acid. *Proc. Soc. Exp. Biol.*, **7**, 374–376

82. Zucker, T.F. (1958). Pantothenic acid deficiency and its effect on the integrity and functions of the intestines. *Am. J. Clin. Nutr.*, **6**, 65–74

83. Seronde, J.J. (1963). The pathogenesis of duodenal ulcer disease in the pantothenate-deficient rat. *Yale J. Biol. Med.*, **36**, 141–156

84. Thornton, G.H.M., Bean, W.B. and Hodges, R.E. (1955). The effect of pantothenic acid deficiency on gastric secretion and motility. *J. Clin. Invest.*, **34**, 1085–1091

85. Robert, A., Stout, T.J. and Dale, J.E. (1970). Production by secretatogues of duodenal ulcers in the rat. *Gastroenterology*, **59**, 95–102

86. Cho, C.H. and Pfeiffer, C.J. (1981). Gastrointestinal ulceration in the guinea pig in response to dimaprit, histamine, and H_1-and H_2-blocking agents. *Dig. Dis. Sci.*, **26**, 306–311

87. Joffe, S.H., Roberts, N.B., Taylor, W.H. and Baron, J.H. (1980). Exogenous and endogenous acid and pepsins in the pathogenesis of duodenal ulcers in the rat. *Dig. Dis. Sci.*, **25**, 837–841

88. Szabo, S. (1978). Animal model of human disease. Duodenal ulcer disease. Animal model: Cysteamine-induced acute and chronic duodenal ulcer in the rat. *Am. J. Pathol.*, **93**, 273–276

89. Szabo S. and Selye, H. (1972). Duodenal ulcers produced by propionitrile in rats. *Arch. Pathol.*, **93**, 390–391

90. Selye, H. and Szabo, S. (1973). Experimental model for production of perforating duodenal ulcers by cysteamine in the rat. *Nature (London)*, **244**, 458–459

91. Szabo, S., Reynolds, E.S. and Unger, S.H. (1982). Structure-activity relations between alkyl nucleophilic chemicals causing duodenal ulcer and adrenocortical necrosis. *J. Pharmacol. Exp. Ther.*, **223**, 68–76

92. Szabo, S., Horner, H.C. and Gallagher, G.T. (1982). Drug-induced duodenal ulcer: Structure-activity correlations and pathogenesis. In Pfeiffer, C.J. (ed.) *Drugs and Peptic Ulcer*, pp. 55–74. Vol. II, (Florida: CRC Press)

93. Szabo, S. and Gallagher, G.T. (1980). Acute and chronic duodenal ulcers produced by cysteamine or *n*-butyronitrile in the rat. In Umehara, S. and Ito, H (eds.) *Advances in Experimental Ulcer*, pp. 116–128. (Tokyo: 4th Int. Cong. Exp. Ulcer)

94. Szabo, S. and Pihan, G. (1987). Development and significance of cysteamine and propionitrile models of duodenal ulcer. *Chronobiol. Int.*, **6**, 31–42

95. Cahill, M.C., Gallagher, G.T. and Szabo, S. (1986). Cysteamine induces duodenal ulcer in the mouse. *Digestion*, **34**, 1–8

96. Malbert, C.H. and Ruckebusch, Y. (1987). Early myoelectrical activity changes during gastric or duodenal ulceration in dogs. *Dig. Dis. Sci.*, **32**, 737–742

97. Poulsen, S.S., Olsen, P.S and Kirkegaard, P. (1985). Healing of cysteamine-induced duodenal ulcers in the rat. *Dig. Dis. Sci.*, **30**, 161–167

98. Japundžić, I. and Levi, E. (1987). Mechanism of action of cysteamine on duodenal alkaline phosphatase. *Biochem. Pharmacol.*, **36**, 2489–2495

99. Yabana, T., Kondo, Y., Fujii, K., Yachi, A. and Szabo, S. (1985). Role of increased mucosal and vascular injury in pathogenesis of peptic ulcer. In Kasuya, Y., Tsuchiya, M., Nagao, F. and Matsuo, Y. (eds.) *Excerpta Medica Int. Congress Series, 704*, pp. 113–126. (Amsterdam: Excerpta Medica)

100. Pihan, G., Kline, T.J., Hollenberg, N.K. and Szabo, S. (1985). Duodenal ulcerogens cysteamine and propionitrile induce gastroduodenal motility alterations in the rat. *Gastroenterology*, **88**, 989–997
101. Pihan, G., Gallagher, G.T. and Szabo, S. (1985). Biliary and pancreatic influence experimental duodenal ulcer without affecting gastric secretion in the rat. *Dig. Dis. Sci.*, **30**, 240–246
102. Szabo, S., Pihan, G., Gallagher, G.T. and Brown, A. (1984). Role of local secretory and motility changes in the pathogenesis of experimental duodenal ulcer. *Scand. J. Gastroenterol.*, **19** Suppl. 92, 106–111
103. Gallagher, G.T. and Szabo, S. (1984). Direct measurement of duodenal acid–pepsin exposure at the site of ulceration in rats. *Am. J. Physiol.*, **246**, G660–G665
104. Bridén, S., Flemström, G. and Kivilaakso, E. (1985). Cysteamine and propionitrile inhibit the rise of duodenal mucosal alkaline secretion in response to luminal acid in rats. *Gastroenterology*, **88**, 295–302
105. Poulsen, S.S., Kirkegaard, P., Olsen, S. and Christiansen, J. (1981). Brunner's glands of the rat during cysteamine ulceration. *Scand. J. Gastroenterol.*, **16**, 459–464
106. Pfeiffer, D.C., Pfeiffer, C.J. and Szabo, S. (1987). Development of cysteamine-induced ultrastructural surface changes on duodenal mucosa. *Lab. Invest.*, (In press)
107. Pfeiffer, C.J., Pfeiffer, D.C. and Szabo, S. (1987). Early ultrastructural changes in rat duodenal mucosa associated with cysteamine-induced ulcer. *Exp. Mol. Pathol.*, **46**, 102–113
108. Poulsen, S.S. and Szabo, S. (1977). Mucosal surface morphology and histological changes in the duodenum of the rat following the administration of cysteamine. *Br. J. Exp. Pathol.*, **58**, 1–8
109. Ramos, A.R., Kirsner, J.B. and Plamer, I.V.L. (1960). Peptic ulcer in children. *Am. J. Dis. Child.*, **99**, 135–148
110 Lichtenberger, L.M., Szabo, S. and Trier, J.S. (1977). Duodenal ulcerogens, cysteamine and propionitrile stimulate serum gastrin levels in the rat. *Gastroenterology*, **73**, 1305–1308.
111. McGuigan, J.E. and Trudeau, W.L. (1973). Differences in rates of gastrin release in normal persons and patients with duodenal ulcer disease. *N. Engl. J. Med.*, **288**, 64–66
112. Narasaki, Y. and Yabana, T. (1979). Experimental studies on peptic ulcer: on the mechanism of duodenal ulcer formation after administration of cysteamine in rat. *Sapporo Med. J.*, **48**, 415–428
113. Fiddian-Green, R.G. (1977). Is peptic ulceration a hormonal disease? *Lancet*, **1**, 74–76
114. Szabo, S. and Reichlin, S. (1981). Somatostatin in rat tissues is depleted by cysteamine administration. *Endocrinology*, **109**, 2255–2257
115. Szabo, S. and Trier, J.S. (1984). Pathogenesis of acute gastric mucosal injury: sulfhydryls as a protector, adrenal cortex as a modulator, and vascular endothelium as a target. In Allen, A. et al. (eds.) *Mechanisms of Mucosal Protection in the Upper Gastrointestinal Tract.* pp. 287–293. (New York; Raven Press)
116. Robert, A., Nezamis, J.E., Lancaster, C. and Badalamenti, J.N. (1974). Cysteamine-induced duodenal ulcers: a new model to test antiulcer agents. *Digestion*, **11**, 199–214
117. Robert, A., Nezamis, J.E. and Lancaster, C. (1975). Duodenal ulcers produced in rats by propionitrile: factors inhibiting and aggravating such ulcers. *Toxicol. Appl. Pharmacol.*, **31**, 201–207
118. Okabe, S., Ishihara, Y., Inoo, H. and Matanaka, H. (1982). Mepirizole-induced duodenal ulcers in rats and their pathogenesis. *Dig. Dis. Sci.*, **27**, 242–249
119. Szabo, S., Brown, A., Pihan, G., Dali, H. and Neumeyer, J.L. (1985). Duodenal ulcer induced by MPTP (1-methyl-4-phenyl-1,2,3,6-tetrahydropyridine). *Proc. Soc. Exp. Biol. Med.*, **180**, 567–571
120. Ishihara, Y., Yamada, Y., Hata, Y. and Okabe, S. (1983). Species and strain differences in mepirizole-induced duodenal and gastric lesions. *Dig. Dis. Sci.*, **28**, 552–558
121. Marshall, F. and Szabo, S. (1987). Correlation between ulcerogenic and neurotoxic effects of 1-methyl-4-phenyl-1,2,3,6-tetrahydropyridine (MPTP) and its reduced derivative in rats. *Gastroenterology*, **92**, 2062
122. Robert, A., Tabata, K., Joffe, S.N., Jacobson, E.D. (1987). Prostaglandin deficiency by itself is not the cause of mepirizole-induced duodenal ulcers in rats. *Dig. Dis. Sci.*, **32**, 997–1003

123. Adler, R.S., Nafradi, J. and Szabo, S. (1985). Cysteamine-induced duodenal ulcer is not site-specific: Effect of local modulating factors. *J. Exp. Pathol.*, **2**, 111–122

124. Szabo, S., Silver, E.H., Gallagher, G.T. and Maull, E.A. (1983) Potentiation of duodenal ulcerogenic action of acrylonitrile by PCB or phenobarbital in the rat. *Toxicol. Appl. Pharmacol.*, **71**, 451–454

125. Takeuchi, K., Furukawa, O., Tanaka, H. and Okabe, S. (1986). A new model of duodenal ulcers induced in rats by indomethacin plus histamine. *Gastroenterology* **90**, 636–645

5
Protection against mucosal damage: mechanism of action of eicosanoids

A. Robert

In addition to inhibiting gastric acid secretion, several prostaglandins exert a protective effect on the gastrointestinal mucosa. This is a property by which prostaglandins, given at non-antisecretory doses, prevent gastric and intestinal mucosal necrosis produced by a variety of noxious agents. This property was first demonstrated in experimental animals and has been reproduced in humans. Gastric cytoprotection can be divided into three types: direct, adaptive and functional. We shall review the experimental evidence for each type of cytoprotection, present data on duodenal cytoprotection, and discuss hypotheses to explain the phenomenon.

GASTRIC CYTOPROTECTION

Direct cytoprotection

This type of cytoprotection is observed after exogenous administration of prostaglandins. A large number of prostaglandins, given orally or parenterally to experimental animals, prevented the formation of gastric mucosal necrosis produced by a variety of agents such as absolute ethanol, $0.6 \, mol \, L^{-1}$ HCl, $0.2 \, mol \, L^{-1}$ NaOH, $80 \, mmol \, L^{-1}$ acidified taurocholate and a hypertonic solution (25% sodium chloride)[1-3]. In each case, the protective effect was dose dependent. Histological examination revealed that the protection was not total. The surface epithelium, composed of a monocellular layer covering the mucosa, showed signs of damage after oral administration of absolute ethanol, with or without pretreatment with a prostaglandin[4]. However, the deeper layers, constituting more than 90% of the thickness of the gastric mucosa, were protected[4]. In control animals these layers were the site of massive necrosis, hyperaemia, oedema and haemorrhage; none of these pathological changes occurred in prostaglandin-pretreated animals. These studies were confirmed[5,6]. In addition, 16,16-dimethyl PGE_2 given orally at $20 \, \mu g \, kg^{-1}$, a non-anti-secretory dose, was reported to markedly reduce the damage produced to the surface epithelium by 98% ethanol[7]. Doses of 2.5 to 20 μg kg^{-1} strongly inhibited the release of cytoplasmic enzymes (lactic dehydrogenase) and lysosomal enzymes (acid phosphatase, β-glucuronidase) from the stomach after exposure to 98% ethanol[7].

What was unique in these various studies was that prostaglandins protected the stomach against injury without affecting gastric acid secretion. Moreover, pretreatment with antisecretory drugs, such as cimetidine, methscopolamine bromide (an anticholinergic), or omeprazole, at doses that totally inhibited acid secretion, did not protect the stomach against necrosis[1]. It was clear, therefore, that cytoprotection by prostaglandins was separate and independent from the antisecretory effect of such substances.

These same prostaglandins also protected the stomach against damage produced by a variety of non-steroidal anti-inflammatory compounds (aspirin, indomethacin)[8,9]. Again, the doses were non-antisecretory. Acute stress ulcers were also prevented by non-antisecretory doses of prostaglandins, as was shown for ulcers produced in dogs by a combination of sepsis and intraperitoneal administration of bile[10].

Adaptive cytoprotection

Since the gastric mucosa synthesizes relatively large amounts of prostaglandins, it was postulated that these endogenous prostaglandins may play a role in the natural defence of the stomach against damaging agents normally present in the lumen (e.g. acid–pepsin complex, foods at various pH and temperatures and spices, as well as other substances such as alcohol and irritating drugs). In favour of this hypothesis was the observation that inhibitors of prostaglandin synthesis, such as aspirin and indomethacin, are ulcerogenic[8,9,11,12], and that replacement therapy with exogenous prostaglandins prevents such ulcers[8,9]. To test this hypothesis, attempts were made to stimulate the formation of prostaglandins by the stomach over and above the normal production. It was surmised that the synthetic capacity of the mucosa for prostaglandins might be related to the concentration of luminal irritants. A series of irritants were given orally to rats, at various concentrations, prior to the oral administration of agents known to be necrotizing. The following results were obtained.

(1) Mild irritants such as 20% ethanol, 0.3 mol L^{-1} HCl, 0.075 mol L^{-1} NaOH, 3% NaCl and 5 mmol L^{-1} taurocholate, given orally, prevented gastric mucosal necrosis otherwise produced by very strong irritants such as absolute ethanol, 0.6 mol L^{-1} HCl, 0.2 mol L^{-1} NaOH, 25% NaCl and 80 mmol L^{-1} taurocholate[3,13]. Not only was a particular mild irritant protective against a higher concentration of the same substance (20% ethanol protecting against absolute ethanol, 0.3 mol L^{-1} HCl protecting against 0.6 mol L^{-1} HCl, a phenomenon called 'homocytoprotection'), but similar protection was demonstrated when the two agents were dissimilar (20% ethanol protecting against 0.6 mol L^{-1} HCl, 5 mmol L^{-1} taurocholate protecting against absolute ethanol, a phenomenon called 'cross-cyto-protection').

(2) Prior treatment with indomethacin, which blocks the formation of prostaglandins in the gastric mucosa by inhibiting the activity of the prostaglandin cyclo-oxygenase, prevented the protection afforded by mild irritants[3,13]. This suggested that the mechanism by which such protection occurred involved stimulation of prostaglandins by the gastric mucosa.

(3) Oral administration of mild irritants increased the actual synthesis of prostaglandins by the gastric mucosa, measured either in the mucosa itself or in gastric juice[13–15].

The phenomenon by which mild irritants protect against strong irritants was named 'adaptive cytoprotection', because it represents a response of the stomach to potential injury through the elaboration of protective substances[13]. Adaptive cytoprotection has also been demonstrated in humans[16].

Functional cytoprotection

Since the gastric mucosa is protected morphologically against the effect of necrotizing agents by either exogenous administration (direct cytoprotection) or endogenous formation of prostaglandins by mild irritants (adaptive cytoprotection), it was hypothesized that the gastric glands might also retain their capacity to secrete acid. To test this hypothesis, animals were given absolute ethanol, a necrotizing agent, and gastric secretion was measured at various time intervals thereafter, from 1 to 72 hours, using the pylorus ligation technique. In these animals, acid secretion stopped immediately after administration of ethanol, and near total anacidity persisted for eight hours, presumably because of destruction of or damage to most of the parietal cell mass. Thereafter, acid secretion gradually reappeared and reached normal values after 48 hours, presumably because of restoration of parietal cells. By contrast, in animals that had been pretreated, with either a prostaglandin (16,16-dimethyl PGE_2 given at non-antisecretory doses, $5\,\mu g\,kg^{-1}$ orally or subcutaneously) or a mild irritant (20% ethanol, $0.3\,mol\,L^{-1}$ HCl or $0.075\,mol\,L^{-1}$ NaOH), acid secretion was depressed immediately after ethanol, but quickly returned towards the normal baseline after six to eight hours. This indicated that certain prostaglandins, either given exogenously or formed endogenously, not only maintain the morphological integrity of the gastric mucosa, but also maintain its ability to secrete acid. This effect was called 'functional cytoprotection'[17].

DUODENAL CYTOPROTECTION

Duodenal ulcers, either in humans or produced experimentally in animals, are largely acid dependent. This statement is based on the facts that acid hypersecretion or acid perfused through the duodenum can lead to formation of duodenal ulcers, and that administration of antisecretory drugs prevents formation of experimentally-induced duodenal ulcers and recurrences of peptic ulcer in humans and accelerates ulcer healing. Recently, a new model of duodenal ulcer was developed in rats. Such ulcers are produced by ligating the bile duct and giving indomethacin as a single administration. Within two to three days, duodenal ulcers develop in nearly all animals, and in most cases these ulcers perforate[18]. Although the pathogenesis of this type of ulcer is not well understood, it is not associated with acid hypersecretion. Certain prostaglandins at non-antisecretory doses (e.g. 16,16-dimethyl PGE_2) and other prostaglandins that are not antisecretory at any dose (e.g. $PGF_{2\beta}$) prevent their formation. Since this antiulcer effect was observed without a reduction of gastric acid secretion, it was concluded that the prostaglandins can exert a cytoprotective effect on the duodenum.

Mechanism of cytoprotection

Several hypotheses have been suggested to explain the phenomenon of gastroduodenal cytoprotection. It is likely that there is no single explanation for the phenomenon. We will examine some of the most plausible hypotheses that have been proposed.

1. Mucus-bicarbonate secretion

Prostaglandins as well as mild irritants are potent stimulants of gastric and bicarbonate secretion by the stomach and the duodenum[19-21]. Although the amount of bicarbonate secreted by the stomach is relatively low compared with the amount of acid, much of the bicarbonate is trapped in the unstirred layer adherent to the surface epithelium[22]. This layer is thick and viscous because of the presence of mucus secreted by the surface epithelium and the mucus neck cells. It appears to serve as a physical barrier to some of the luminal contents, especially acid. It was determined that a gradient exists between the luminal pH of gastric juice and the pH recorded on the mucosal surface immediately under the unstirred layer. As long as the pH of the gastric lumen was 1.2 or above, the pH next to the mucosa was maintained at around 7. When, however, the pH fell below 1.2, the gradient was dissipated; acid could then come in contact with the mucosal cells and easily break the mucosal barrier[23]. By stimulating mucus and bicarbonate secretion, prostaglandins could help maintain an intact gradient.

Such a mechanism may play an important role in the protection against damaging agents that require acid in order to cause injury, as is the case for aspirin and bile salts. On the other hand, damage caused by strong irritants such as absolute ethanol is not acid dependent; it is unlikely that the mucus-bicarbonate layer exerts much of a barrier against such agents.

2. Increase in gastric mucosal blood flow

Several prostaglandins (PGE_1, PGE_2, 16,16-dimethyl PGE_2, PGI_2) increase gastric mucosal blood flow[24-29]. However, at cytoprotective doses, 16,16-dimethyl PGE_2 failed to increase gastric mucosal blood flow[30]. In fact, in anaesthetized rats, that particular prostaglandin caused a 15% decrease in gastric mucosal blood flow at a dose that prevented almost completely the formation of ethanol-induced mucosal lesions. Moreover, certain prostaglandins that constrict gastric mucosal blood flow, such as $PGF_{2\alpha}$, are also cytoprotective[8]. It is unlikely, therefore, that a change in gastric mucosal blood flow plays a role in the mechanism of cytoprotection by prostaglandins.

However, studies by Guth and co-workers showed that cytoprotective prostaglandins, although not actually increasing blood flow, maintain the flow of blood in the microcirculation despite the presence of a necrotizing agent such as absolute ethanol[31]. When the necrotizing agent is given alone, mucosal blood flow stops completely; the maintenance of flow in animals treated with a prostaglandin may explain the cytoprotective effect of these agents.

3. Lack of penetration of the damaging agent into the gastric mucosa
It was proposed that prostaglandins might prevent the entry of a damaging agent into the gastric mucosa. If this were the case, cells situated deep in the mucosa would be protected simply because they would never be in contact with the injurious agent. Such is not the case, however. Salicylates were measured in the gastric mucosa after oral administration of aspirin at doses producing deep erosions. The concentration of salicylates was the same in control animals, with ulcers, as in animals that had been protected by prior treatment with a prostaglandin[32]. Similar results were obtained with the necrotizing agent absolute ethanol which, unlike aspirin, does not require luminal acid to cause injury. [14C]ethanol was measured at various depths of the gastric mucosa. The amounts of ethanol present in the upper third as well as in the lower two-thirds of the mucosa were the same in control animals, in which necrosis was produced, as in animals that had been protected with a prostaglandin[33]. These results indicate that, in animals pretreated with a cytoprotective prostaglandin, cells located deep in the mucosa were protected in spite of the presence of either salicylate or ethanol. They suggest that the phenomenon of gastric cytoprotection is not related to a barrier between the damaging agent and the gastric mucosa, such as the unstirred layer of mucus-bicarbonate, since the damaging agent does penetrate freely. It appears that the cells themselves develop an increased resistance to noxious substances, by an unknown mechanism, if the animal has been treated with a prostaglandin.

4. Protection of the cells themselves
Studies performed with either isolated cells, isolated gastric glands or isolated gastric mucosa showed that damage produced *in vitro* by exposure to either aspirin, indomethacin, taurocholate or ethanol was reduced when a prostaglandin was added to the medium. The damage was assessed either by: (a) cell viability using dye exclusion, (b) the release of enzymes (LDH, glucuronidase, phosphatase, cathepsin), or (c) the release of ^{51}Cr from prelabelled cells. Although the protection was not as total as in *in vivo* experiments, the effect was clearly present regardless of the index of damage used[34-37].

5. Role of gastric phospholipids
The gastric mucosa, like the mucosa of the respiratory tract[38], contains phospholipids that render this mucosa hydrophobic[39]. As a consequence, a drop of water applied to the mucosal surface tends to bead up instead of spreading. Lichtenberger formulated the hypothesis that this hydrophobicity

may play a role in protecting the gastric mucosa against damaging agents. Instead of penetrating the mucosa, such agents might be repelled. In a series of publications, Lichtenberger et al. showed that:

(a) Oral administration of certain phospholipids prevents gastric mucosal necrosis produced by $0.6 \, mol \, L^{-1} \, HCl$[40,41];
(b) 16,16-dimethyl PGE_2, at a non-antisecretory but cytoprotective dose, increased the amount of these phospholipids in the gastric mucosa[40];
(c) Aspirin exerted the opposite effect[42];
(d) The surface hydrophobicity of the gastric mucosa was reduced by intraluminal administration of absolute ethanol, and this decrease was counteracted by 16,16-dimethyl PGE_2[43].

They concluded that the increase of phospholipids on the surface of the gastric mucosa may mediate the cytoprotective effect of prostaglandins.

CONCLUSIONS

Prostaglandins have been associated with the phenomenon of gastric and intestinal cytoprotection. The mechanisms appear to be multiple, and may involve the following effects of prostaglandins: stimulation of mucus and bicarbonate secretion, maintenance of blood flow of the microcirculation, stimulation of secretion of hydrophobic phospholipids, and increased resistance of the cell membrane to damage. Cytoprotection was demonstrated after exogenous administration (direct cytoprotection) as well as endogenous formation (adaptive cytoprotection) of prostaglandins. Morphological integrity of the mucosa as well as gastric secretion (functional cytoprotection) are maintained. Clinical implications of cytoprotection may include adjunct treatment of peptic ulcer, and gastritis caused by various agents, including non-steroidal anti-inflammatory drugs.

REFERENCES

1. Robert, A., Nezamis, J.E., Lancaster, C. and Hanchar, A.J. (1979). Cytoprotection by prostaglandins in rats: Prevention of gastric necrosis produced by alcohol, HCl, NaOH, hypertonic NaCl, and thermal injury. Gastroenterology, 88, 433–443
2. Robert, A. (1979). Cytoprotection by prostaglandins. Gastroenterology, 77, 761–767
3. Chaudhury, T.K. and Robert, A. (1980). Prevention by mild irritants of gastric necrosis produced in rats by sodium taurocholate. Dig. Dis. Sci., 25, 830–836
4. Lacy, E.R. and Ito, S. (1982). Microscopic analysis of ethanol damage to rat gastric mucosa after treatment with a prostaglandin. Gastroenterology, 83, 619–625
5. Guth, P.H., Paulsen, G. and Nagata, H. (1984). Histologic and microcirculatory changes in alcohol-induced gastric lesions in the rat: Effect of prostaglandin cytoprotection. Gastroenterology, 87, 1083–1090
6. Schmidt, K.L., Henagan, J.M., Smith, G.S., Hilburn, P.J. and Miller, T.A. (1985). Prostaglandin cytoprotection against ethanol-induced gastric injury in the rat. A histologic and cytologic study. Gastroenterology, 88, 649–659
7. Whittle, B.J.R. and Steel, G. (1985). Evaluation of the protection of rat gastric mucosa by a prostaglandin analogue using cellular enzyme marker and histologic techniques. Gastroenterology, 88, 315–317

8. Robert, A. (1976). Antisecretory, antiulcer, cytoprotective and diarrheogenic properties of prostaglandins. *Adv. Prostgl. Thromboxane Res.*, **2**, 507–520
9. Whittle, B.J.R. (1977). Mechanisms underlying gastric mucosal damage induced by indomethacin and bile-salts, and the actions of prostaglandins. *Br. J. Pharmacol.*, **60**, 455–460
10. Odonkor, P., Mowat, C. and Himal, H.S. (1981). Prevention of sepsis-induced gastric lesions in dogs by cimetidine via inhibition of gastric secretion and by prostaglandin via cytoprotection. *Gastroenterology*, **80**, 375–379
11. Djahanguiri, B. (1969). The production of acute gastric ulceration by indomethacin in the rat. *Scand. J. Gastroenterol.*, **4**, 265–267
12. Lee, Y.H., Cheng, W.D., Bianchi, R.C., Mollison, K. and Hansen, J. (1973). Effects of oral administration of PGE$_2$ on gastric secretion and experimental peptic ulcerations. *Prostaglandins*, **3**, 29–45
13. Robert, A., Nezamis, J.E., Lancaster, C., Davis, J.P., Field, S.O. and Hanchar, A.J. (1983). Mild irritants prevent gastric necrosis through 'adaptive cytoprotection' mediated by prostaglandins. *Am. J. Physiol.*, **245**, G113–G121
14. Konturek, S.J., Brzozowski, T., Piastucki, I., Radecki, T., Dembinski, A. and Dembinska-Kiec, A (1982). Role of locally generated prostaglandins in adaptive gastric cytoprotection. *Dig. Dis. Sci.*, **27**, 967–971
15. Assouline, G., Leibson, V. and Danon, A. (1977). Stimulation of prostaglandin output from rat stomach by hypertonic solutions. *Eur. J. Pharmacol.*, **44**, 271–273
16. Foschi, D., del Soldato, P., Ferrante, F., Toti, G.L. and Rovati, V. (1986). Adaptive cytoprotection: An endoscopical study in man. Presented at the *6th International Conference on Prostaglandins and Related Compounds*, June 3–6, Florence, Italy
17. Robert, A., Lancaster, C., Nezamis, J.E. and Hanchar, A.J. 1978). Cytoprotective prostaglandins, exogenous or endogenous, can maintain gastric secretory function. *Gastroenterology*, **74**, 1086
18. Robert, A., Nezamis, J.E. and Lancaster, C. (1975). Duodenal ulcers produced by nonsteroidal anti-inflammatory compounds plus bile duct ligation. *Fed. Proc.*, **34**, 442
19. Bolton, J.P. and Cohen, M.M. (1978). Stimulation of non-parietal cell secretion in canine Heidenhain pouches by 16,16-dimethyl prostaglandin E$_2$. *Digestion*, **17**, 291–299
20. Flemström, G. (1981). Gastric secretion of bicarbonate. In Johnson, L.R. (ed.) *Physiology of the Gastrointestinal Tract*, pp. 603–616. (New York: Raven Press)
21. Garner, A. and Heylings, J.R. (1979). Stimulation of alkaline secretion in amphibian isolated gastric mucosa by 16,16-dimethyl PGE$_2$ and PGF$_{2\alpha}$: A proposed explanation for some of the cytoprotective actions of prostaglandins. *Gastroenterology*, **76**, 497–503
22. Allen, A. and Garner, A. (1980). Gastric mucus and bicarbonate secretion and their possible role in mucosal protection. *Gut*, **21**, 249–262
23. Turnberg, L.A., Ross, I.N. and Bahari, H.M.M. (1984). pH Gradient across gastric mucus. In Allen, A. *et al.* (eds.) *Mechanisms of Mucosal Protection in the Upper Gastrointestinal Tract*, pp. 223–226. (New York: Raven Press)
24. Gerkens, J.F., Gerber, J.G., Shand, D.G. and Branch, R.A. (1978). Effect of PGI$_2$, PGE$_2$ and 6-keto-PGF$_{1\alpha}$ on canine gastric blood flow and acid secretion. *Prostaglandins*, **16**, 815–823
25. Konturek, S.J., Robert, A., Hanchar, A.J. and Nezamis, J.E. (1980). Comparison of prostacyclin and prostaglandin E$_2$ on gastric secretion, gastrin release, and mucosal blood flow in dogs. *Dig. Dis. Sci.*, **25**, 673–679
26. Cheung, L.Y. (1980). Topical effects of 16,16-dimethyl prostaglandin E$_2$ on gastric blood flow in dogs. *Am. J. Physiol.*, **238**, G514–G519
27. Gerber, J.G. and Nies, A.A. (1982). Canine gastric mucosal vasodilation with prostaglandins and histamine analogs. *Dig. Dis. Sci.*, **27**, 870–874
28. Konturek, S.J. and Robert, A. (1982). Cytoprotection of canine gastric mucosa by prostacyclin: Possible mediation by increased mucosal blood flow. *Digestion*, **25**, 155–163
29. Inatomi, N. and Maki, Y. (1983). Effect of prostaglandins on mucosal blood flow and aspirin-induced damage in the canine stomach. *Jpn. J. Pharmacol.*, **33**, 1263–1270
30. Leung, F.W., Robert, A. and Guth, P.H. (1985). Gastric mucosal blood flow in rats after administration of 16,16-dimethyl prostaglandin E$_2$ at a cytoprotective dose. *Gastroenterology*, **88**, 1948–1953
31. Guth, P.H., Paulsen, G. and Nagata, H. (1984). Histologic and microcirculatory changes in alcohol-induced gastric lesions in the rat: Effect of prostaglandin cytoprotection. *Gastroenterology*, **87**, 1083–1090

32. Guth, P.H. and Paulsen, G. (1979). Prostaglandin cytoprotection does not involve interference with aspirin absorption. *Proc. Soc. Exp. Biol. Med.*, **162**, 128–130
33. Robert, A., Lancaster, C., Davis, J.P., Field, S.O., Wickrema Sinha, A.J. and Thornburgh, B.A. (1985). Cytoprotection by prostaglandin occurs in spite of penetration of absolute ethanol into the gastric mucosa. *Gastroenterology*, **88**, 328–333
34. Terano, A., Mach, T., Stachura, J., Tarnawski, A. and Ivey, K.J. (1984). Effect of 16,16-dimethyl prostaglandin E_2 on aspirin-induced damage to rat gastric epithelial cells in tissue culture. *Gut*, **25**, 19–25
35. Terano, A., Mach, T., Stachura, J., Tarnawski, A. and Ivey, K.J. (1982). Prevention by prostaglandin of taurocholic acid-induced damage to rat gastric mucosal epithelial cells in tissue culture. *Clin. Res.*, **30**, 39A
36. Tarnawski, A., Brzozowski, T., Hollander, D., Krause, W.J. and Gergely, H. (1986). Prostaglandin protection of isolated gastric glands against ethanol-induced injury. Evidence for cytoprotection *in vitro*. *Gastroenterology*, **90**, 1658
37. Brzozowski, T., Tarnawski, A., Hollander, D., Sekhon, S., Krause, W.J. and Gergely, H. (1986). Comparison of prostaglandin and cimetidine in protection of isolated gastric glands against indomethacin injury. Histologic ultrastructural and functional assessment. *Gastroenterology*, **90**, 1360
38. Hills, B.A. (1982). Water repellency induced by pulmonary surfactants. *J. Physiol. (London)*, **325**, 175–186
39. Hills, B.A., Butler, B.D. and Lichtenberger, L.M. (1983). Gastric mucosal barrier: hydrophobic lining to the lumen of the stomach. *Am. J. Physiol.*, **7**, G561–G568
40. Lichtenberger, L.M., Graziani, L.A., Dial, E.J., Butler, B.D. and Hills, B.A. (1983). Role of surface-active phospholipids in gastric cytoprotection. *Science*, **219**, 1327–1329
41. Lichtenberger, L.M., Richards, J.E. and Hills, B.A. (1985). Effect of 16,16-dimethyl prostaglandin E_2 on the surface hydrophobicity of aspirin-treated canine gastric mucosa. *Gastroenterology*, **88**, 308–314
42. Goodard, P.J., Hills, B.A. and Lichtenberger, L.M. (1985). Does aspirin (ASA) damage the stomach by decreasing gastric mucosal surface hydrophobicity? *Gastroenterology*, **88**, 1714
43. Sierra, E.M. and Lichtenberger, L.M. (1986). Effect of ethanol (EtOH) and cytoprotective agents on the surface hydrophobicity (S-H) of rat gastric mucosa (GM) *in vivo*. *Gastroenterology*, **90**, 1633

6
Interplay between anti-inflammatory drugs and eicosanoids in gastro-intestinal damage

K. D. Rainsford

INTRODUCTION

Inhibition of the synthesis and production of prostaglandins (chiefly E_2 and I_2) has been considered a major factor in the development of gastrointestinal damage for some years now. Based on the original suggestion by Vane[1] in 1971 that 'aspirin-like' drugs exert their effects by inhibiting the biosynthesis of prostaglandins (PGs), it was proposed by Main and Whittle[2] and others that this property might underly the gastric mucosal damage caused by non-steroidal anti-inflammatory drugs (NSAIDs). Just before these suggestions were propounded, several workers became interested in the effects on acid-secretion[3], anti-ulcer[3] and smooth muscle contractile[4,5] actions of exogenous prostaglandins on the gastrointestinal (GI) tract and later on the involvement of PGs in the production of diarrhoea by cholera toxin[6]. Since these and other earlier studies, there has been an enormous upsurge in interest in the fundamental actions of PGs and other eicosanoids on the GI tract and the actions of NSAIDs and steroids on their generation and actions. It is the purpose of this review to focus on (a) the actions of anti-inflammatory drugs on eicosanoid metabolism, and (b) the possible relationship of these effects to the pathogenesis of mucosal damage in different regions of the GI tract. The pharmacological and physiological actions of the various eicosanoids, and their production in the GI tract, are discussed elsewhere in this book and in recent reviews[7-14]. Here, these aspects will only be considered as they relate to understanding the fundamental role of perturbing eicosanoid metabolism in the development of GI mucosal damage.

METHODOLOGY

Critical to understanding how anti-inflammatory agents affect eicosanoid metabolism *in vivo* and *in vitro* and the relationship of these effects to the development of GI damage, is the appreciation of what is being measured, and the relevance of these measurements in relation to the drug effects.

In vitro methods*

Several methods have been devised including:

(1) Measurement of the concentration of eicosanoids, (prostaglandins and leukotrienes) can be achieved by radioimmunoassay (RIA)[14,19], gas chromatography–mass spectrometry (GC–MS)[22,21], gas chromatography[22], or bioassay[23,24] following incubation of chopped slices, homogenates or microsomal (or other subcellular) components in the presence or absence of drug(s). Incubation times vary in different authors methods but usually they range from 30–60 min for homogenates or slices to 5–15 min for subcellular fractions. It is apparent that the optimal times for incubation and conditions thereof (including pH, type of buffer, presence of cofactors, O_2 etc.) have not been fully explored. The method of handling the tissue and preparation of homogenates can have marked effects on the results obtained. Thus, results can only be viewed as an act of faith in the author having satisfied himself that the optimal conditions have been fulfilled in his methods.

(2) Radiometric assay of the isolated products of the conversion of added ^{14}C-labelled arachidonic acid with thin layer chromatography following incubation as in (1) above. Separation of the PG products followed by scintillation counting of zones corresponding to PG standards[13,25]. Significant problems here derive from:

(a) The added labelled arachidonate being effectively diluted in tissue homogenates by unknown concentrations of the endogenous substrates (i.e. as derived from phospholipase activity stimulated by homogenizing the tissue),

(b) The incorporation of the labelled substrate into phospholipids which occurs to an appreciable extent ($\sim$ 80%) in homogenates and chopped tissue preparations, and

(c) The marked differences that are evident in pH optima required for synthesis of PGE_2 and 6-keto $PGF_{1\alpha}$ in homogenates and probably other systems.

(d) The low rate of conversion of labelled arachidonate to PGs etc. is a well known problem relating from the above mentioned factors[13].

It is clear from the above discussion that some doubts exist about data in the literature on *in vitro* effects of NSAIDs on production of oxygenated

---

*References cited are only intended to be a general guide to the main techniques and not an extensive coverage of all methods that have been published.

products of arachidonate metabolism in these systems. The most satisfactory way to examine the published data is to treat it in relative terms (i.e. drug effects relative to one another) and not in absolute terms.

Given these limitations, the data in Table 6.1 shows a comparison of the effects of a range of anti-inflammatory drugs in different *in vitro* systems. It will be seen that marked variations exist in the drug effects between preparations and from studies performed by different authors. This variation makes it difficult to compare drug rankings of the order of PG synthesis inhibitory potency (as IC_{50} or similar values) with their gastro-ulcerogenic effects. None-the-less some representative data are shown in Figure 6.1 for interest. This data is further discussed on pp. 7–14.

An important point to note in relation to drug effects in those *in vitro* systems where appreciable endogenous arachidonate is generated, is that those drugs which are reversible inhibitors of the cyclo-oxygenase (e.g. piroxicam), or indeed lipoxygenase, enzyme systems will show larger IC_{50} values reflecting the reversibility of drug-induced inhibitory effects. Irreversible or pseudoirreversible inhibitors (e.g. indomethacin) are not likely to show these effects. The whole question about the relative potencies of the NSAIDs as inhibitors of gastric mucosal cyclo-oxygenase *in vitro* may be limited by the concentration of arachidonate present in the incubation medium or tissue system (in the case of chopped preparations), for, not only will the potencies of reversible or irreversible inhibitors be so determined, but also the basic kinetics of the enzyme system.

In vivo and *ex vivo* systems

A variety of systems have been developed for the assay of the GI mucosal content or production of PGs and other eicosanoids. As with the *in vitro* methodologies, each has its limitations, though some are certainly somewhat more reliable and accurate than others.

Prepared mucosal extracts[18–23], aliquots of fluid from perfusion of organs[24], or collected luminal aspirates[26,27] are the usual sources for subsequent assays. Limitations on the accuracy of the methods depend on

(a) The ways in which these samples are prepared,
(b) Controls which are performed, including methods for correcting for recovery of PGs, and
(c) The methods employed in the subsequent PG assays.

For preparation of mucosal extracts, much will depend on the extent of metabolism of arachidonate and also that of the PGs during the homogenizing and extraction procedures. Many authors initially prepare mucosal homogenates in Tris or other buffers at about pH 7.0–8.4[28], and make no attempt to control the extensive conversion or metabolism of arachidonate, nor provide any estimates of recoveries from, for example, radiolabelled 'spiking' of samples[18,21]. Some do add aspirin or indomethacin to control the conversion of arachidonate which is at least a significant improvement. However, the efficiency of subsequent extractions with organic solvents (e.g. chloroform,

Table 6.1 Effects of NSAIDs on the production of PGE or PGI$_2$ in GI mucosae compared with other standard cell/microsomal systems *in vitro*

Drug/System	Guinea[62] pig 'gut' (†microsomes) IC$_{50}$	Rat[63] gastric mucosal PGI$_2$ IC$_{50}$	Rat[63] ileal homogenate PGI$_2$ IC$_{50}$	Rat[5] stomach 'resting tone' IC$_{50}$	Human[64] microsomes PGE % inhibition 10 μg/ml	Sheep seminal[43,65] vesicle microsomes IC$_{50}$	Chopped[42] guinea pig lung IC$_{50}$	Bovine[5,62] seminal vesicles PGE$_2$ IC$_{50}$	Mouse[65] macrophage PGE$_2$ IC$_{50}$
Piroxicam	0.3				39				0.10
Diclofenac		5.5	7.3			0.3[65]		1.6	0.0096
Ketoprofen						0.12			0.022
Indomethacin	8.4	3.9	5.8	0.6	88.3	0.4	0.9	1.0[5], 5.6	0.0017
Flurbiprofen		0.5	10.4	0.85		10.71[65]			0.0033
Meclofenamic acid		11.3			1.7	2.2		0.1[5]	0.0058
Sulindac–Sulphide						IA			3.7
–Sulphide (Prodrug)						IA			IA
Naproxen	6.5	3.9	6.3	10	63	6.17[65]		0.4[5], 5.7	0.28
Flufenamic acid	29					2.5[65]		11	0.016
Ibuprofen	32				54.7	1.5[65]		39	0.55
Phenylbutazone						12.9[65]		490	5.5
Fenbufen							IA		
–biphenylacetic acid							3.2		
Diflunisal	380				20.1	1.4[65]			1.4
BW 755C	3300		265						0.3
Aspirin			50				37.7	60[65], 330	6.6
Salicylate				1300		8.3[65]		8000[5]	
Paracetamol		1325	1000	2500	3.1				79.4

The data are arranged in approximate order of potency as inhibitors of PG cyclo-oxygenase. Data for paracetamol are included for comparison because it is an analgesic not regarded as an acute ulcerogenic agent.

It should be noted that differences exist between microsomal and whole cell or tissue (and even *in vivo*) systems with some drugs because they have specific metabolic patterns. For example, flurbiprofen, ketoprofen and ibuprofen are racemates and the $R(-)$ isomers are inactive as PG synthesis inhibitors. Thus *in vitro*, only the $S(+)$ form will be active. However, they will undergo some, albeit undetermined, conversion of $R(-)$ to $S(+)$ forms *in vivo* so that their potency may be expected to be increased substantially. Naproxen exists by comparison as 100% of the active $S(+)$ isomer. Likewise, the prodrugs, fenbufen and sulindac, will show low potency as PG synthesis inhibitors *in vitro* compared with their active metabolites (as shown in the data above) but their effects *in vivo* will depend on the extent of metabolic conversion[42,43]. Over 90% sulindac is converted to the sulphide form in the gastric mucosa of pigs when given orally and concomitantly reduces the levels of immunoreactive PGE_2 therein and produces microscopic signs of fundic injury[31]. Other such aspects are discussed in the text. The marked difference in relative potency of NSAIDs in the mouse macrophage system[65] probably reflects the fact that these cells were stimulated with the phorbol ester, 12-O-tetradecanoyl-phorbol, 13-acetate, so increasing the intracellular availability of the substrate arachidonic acid.

The main prostanoids formed by the GI mucosal cells and microsomes are: PGE_2, 6-keto, $PGF_{1\alpha}$ (the hydration product of PGI_2), $PGF_{2\alpha}$, TxA_2, with lesser quantities of PGD_2 and hydroxyacids[13,68,69]. The proportions vary somewhat according to species, location in GI tract and cell preparation[13,68,69]

IC_{50} = inhibitory concentration for 50% reduction in PG production/synthesis

BW755c = 3-amino-1(*m*-(trifluoro-methyl)-phenyl)-2-pyrazolone

References denoted by superscript numbers

All data are μ mol L^{-1} except where stated

IA = inactive at concentrations equal to or greater than 1 m mol L^{-1}

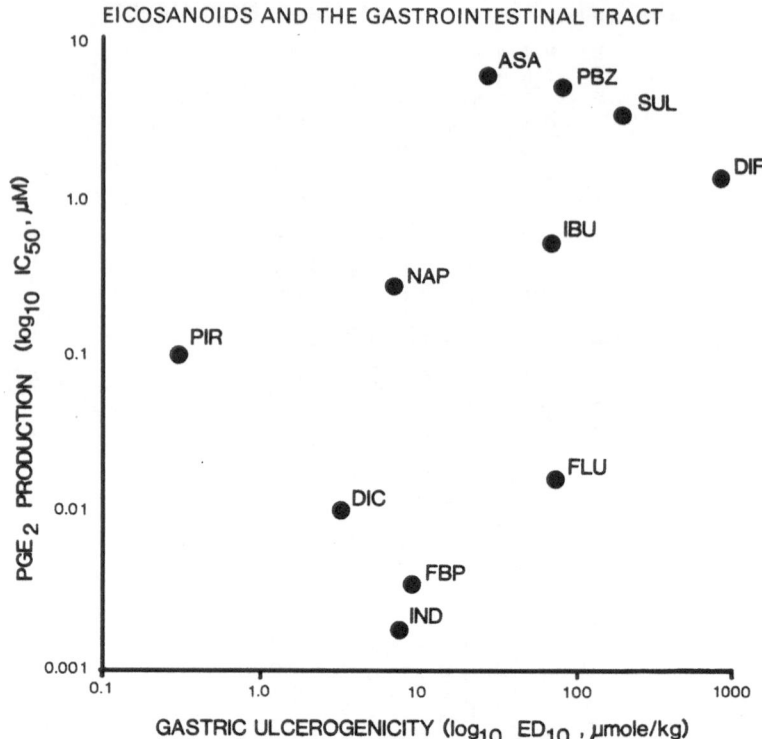

Figure 6.1 Relationship between gastric ulcerogenicity of non-steroidal anti-inflammatory drugs (NSAIDs) to their inhibitory effects on the synthesis of prostaglandin E$_2$ *in vitro*.

There does not appear to be a correlation between the two parameters. It should be noted that sulindac is a prodrug and accordingly the value for PGE$_2$ production is that of the parent sulphoxide compound and not the active sulphide metabolite. Also, ibuprofen, like most propionic acids (with the exception of naproxen) is a mixture of active PG synthesis inhibitory and non-inhibitory diastereoisomers. Thus these two drugs would be expected to deviate from any correlation which is attempted.

Abbreviations for drugs: ASA = aspirin (acetylsalicylic acid), DIC = diclofenac, DIF = diflunisal, FLU = flufenamic acid, FBP = flurbiprofen, IBU = ibuprofen, IND = indomethacin, NAP = naproxen, PBZ = phenylbutazone, PIR = piroxicam, and SUL = sulindac.

Data on gastric ulcerogenicity from ref. 44, these studies being performed in fasted and cold-stressed rats. Data on the inhibition of PGE$_2$ synthesis from studies in phorbol ester stimulated mouse peritoneal macrophages as cited in ref. 65

ethyl acetate or ether) from homogenates at pH 7.8–8.4 will be severely limited because the PGs and other eicosanoids are all organic acids, and, thus, will be charged under the pH conditions employed during the extraction; a situation which will inevitably lead to poor recoveries. A simple solution to both the problem of uncontrolled conversion of arachidonate and obtaining homogenates at the required pH for most efficient extraction into organic acids, is use of 0.2 mol L^{-1} citrate, pH 3.0, or an acid of similar pKa, for the preparation of the homogenates[13]. If the extracts are prepared ice cold (*ca* 4°C) and the subsequent organic extractions performed rapidly, there is relatively little metabolism which occurs, or PGE$_2$ chemically converted to PGA$_2$, such as occurs under strongly acidic conditions[26]. 'Spiking' samples with radiolabelled eicosanoids ensures reliable estimates of recovery[18].

The only condition under which acidic extracts cannot be prepared is for the assay of (PGI_2) prostacyclin. Here Tris or similar buffers at pH 8.4 or thereabouts must be employed for preparation of extracts, as PGI_2 is converted to its hydration metabolite, 6-oxo-$PGF_{1\alpha}$ (6-keto-$PGF_{1\alpha}$) under acidic conditions[29]. Also, PGI_2 can only be determined by bioassay using the inhibition of platelet aggregation method. It is difficult to work out recoveries where such methods are used to prepare mucosal extracts for the assay of PGI_2, though, as Whittle and Boughton-Smith have pointed out, the bioassay does give comparable *relative* values quite consistently[13].

Another misplaced belief (e.g. see ref 14) is the reporting of tissue 'content' of PGs, which is not really 'content' at all but that which is formed during the homogenizing process. While no doubt the results reported by many authors do in fact reflect the contribution due to homogenizing, workers have attempted to minimise this; rapid extraction from tissues collected following freeze-clamping of the mucosa[21,30] represents an attempt to (a) minimize post-sampling conversion of arachidonate to PGs, and (b) reduce inherant variability in the content of PGs and other eicosanoids; measured amounts may then approach basal levels of the products of arachidonate metabolism, although these may not be stored as such in mucosal or other tissues.

The belief that, as PGs are extracellular products they can be determined by measurements of their content in gastric juice, has to be treated with much caution. Aside from the need to perform careful controls in obtaining luminal samples and subsequent assays, it is possible that products of arachidonate metabolism find their way to the GI circulation so that the 'unidirectional' measurement of PG content in the gastric juice is only one of the compartments into which these products can be released.

Table 6.2 shows a compilation of published data on the effects, *in vivo* or *ex vivo*, of NSAIDs on the content of PGs in the gastric mucosal tissue of some laboratory species and man. Some considerable variability is noted in the relative effects which can be ascribed to both technique and the source of tissue.

Most data reported has been on the effect of drugs on PG synthesis; however, attempts to measure products of the 5-lipoxygenase pathway have shown that 5-HETE can be assayed in reasonable quantity[22,31]. However, the leukotrienes (LTs) cannot be detected in normal gastric mucosal tissues which are obtained freeze-clamped from rats[22], although it appears that they can be detected following oral administration of ethanol[10]. Possibly, the actions of irritants, such as ethanol, are sufficient to cause endogenous stimulation of LTs through an overall enhanced production of all arachidonate metabolites.

CORRELATIONS OF GI MUCOSAL INJURY WITH INHIBITION OF PGs

The *in vitro* and *ex vivo* potency of the inhibitory effects of NSAIDs on PG production or mucosal content show some rough correspondence with their

Table 6.2 Comparison of *in vivo* and *ex vivo* effects of NSAIDs on prostaglandin production or levels in GI mucosa

Drug	PGI$_2$ ex vivo[63] rat stomach		PGE ex vivo *in rat stomach*[66]		PGE *in vivo rat*[67] stomach
	Dose (mg/kg)	Effect % Inhibition	Dose (mg/kg)	Effect % Inhibition	Dose (mg/kg) for inhibition at 3 h
Indomethacin	5	90	20	63	28.8
Flurbiprofen	0.5	83			19.6
Naproxen	5	87			
Flufenamic acid			100	Ca.70	
Ibuprofen					16.4
BW 755c	100	5			
Aspirin	50	73	10	78	
Paracetamol			800	180*	12.0

* % stimulation

Values shown in the left and middle columns are the dose of drug and inhibition of PGI$_2$ (prostacyclin) or PGE production, achieved. The data in the right-hand column shows the dose at which significant inhibition of PGE production was achieved. The latter data do not indicate the extent of inhibition. Also, it should be noted that, in this study[67], the tissues were allowed to 'incubate' by standing at room temperature for 60 min, during which time the extent of arachidonic acid released and subsequently metabolized is virtually uncontrolled. Thus, this is strictly an *ex vivo* system, though it is described in the paper by the authors as an *in vivo* system.

It should be appreciated that the published reports on the effects of NSAIDs on PG production *in vivo* often fail to consider the dose-response characteristics (but see references 30 and 63). In some cases, the product ascribed to a particular prostaglandin has not been adequately characterized nor quantitative recoveries stated gastric mucosal irritancy or ulcerogenicity in laboratory animals and man (Tables 6.1 and 6.2, Figures 6.1 and 6.2). There are some notable exceptions, and discussion of the importance of these will be taken up in detail later. For the moment, the so-called 'reasonable correlation' between this biochemical change and the development of gastric injury has been a powerful impetus in generating the widespread belief that an induced deficiency in the gastric content of so-called 'cytoprotective' PGs by NSAIDs will *per se* lead to gastric mucosal injury. Such a view has been strongly criticized[11,21,23].

There are several intrinsic flaws in this thesis, namely:

(1) That prostaglandins are indeed 'cytoprotective'[34]. This aspect has, of itself, been subject to much scrutiny and skepticism[11,35,36]. The overall consensus is that, while PGs may exhibit some protective effects against mucosal injury caused by NSAIDs and other noxious agents, they may not exhibit true protection of all cells in the gastric mucosa. Indeed, some of the effects of PGs in mediating mucosal protection may be due to actions on blood flow and mucus production or secretion, which could be considered special pharmacological effects of these agents and not necessarily physiological as such.

(2) A deficiency in prostaglandins created by NSAID administration necessarily means that this drug action is related to its influence upon intrinsic functions. Needleman[37] has been especially critical of this aspect, and has, in fact, devised a set of criteria which should be satisfied in order for a prostaglandin-related effect to be considered as an intrinsic factor in any physiopathological process. It is true to say that, although considerable evidence exists for the role of prostaglandins in regulating certain gastric functions, such as the secretion of acid[34–36,38], bicarbonate[35,39] and mucus[35], as well as influences on blood flow[35], the exact role of endogenous PGs on these functions has not been proven.

(3) The inhibition of PG production by NSAIDs is the sole biochemical action of these drugs of importance in the development of mucosal injury by these drugs. As shown in Table 6.3, a whole range of effects has been implicated in the pathogenesis of NSAID-induced gastric mucosal injury. Furthermore, in relation to ulcer development and haemorrhage associated with NSAID ingestion in man, there are a large number of environmental factors which contribute to the ulcerogenic actions of NSAIDs. (See refs 32 and 33 for extensive review.) Thus, the development of peptic ulcer in man may have a variety of causative factors, not just the inhibition of PG production.

Studies with stereoisomers and prodrugs

Evidence that inhibition of PG production is a major factor in the pathogenesis of NSAID-induced gastric lesions will be considered.

Aside from the broad correlations noted in Tables 6.1 and 6.2 and Figures 6.1 and 6.2, probably the most compelling data in favour of this concept

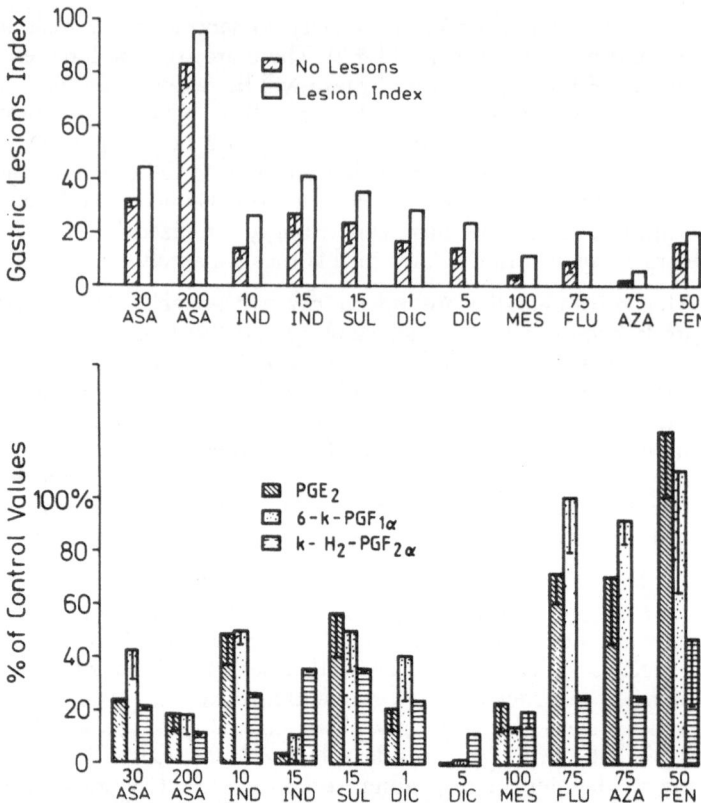

Figure 6.2 Relationship between content of prostaglandins in the fundus of pigs (upper graph) and gastric lesion development (lower graph) following repeated oral administration of NSAIDs for 10 days. From reference 30 (reproduced with permission). PGE$_2$ and 6-keto-PGF$_{1\alpha}$ refer to the gastric (fundic) mucosal content (expressed as a percentage of control values of prostaglandins E$_2$ and 6-keto-F$_{1\alpha}$ respectively). k-H$_2$-PGF$_{2\alpha}$ denotes the plasma content (as % control) of 15-keto-13, 14-dihydroprostaglandin F$_{2\alpha}$ (the stable metabolite of PGF$_{2\alpha}$) which was assayed as a guide to *in vivo* effects of the NSAIDs. The pigs were dosed with the following drugs: 30 mg kg^{-1} day^{-1} and 200 mg kg^{-1} day^{-1} aspirin (= 30 ASA, 200 ASA); 10 mg kg^{-1} day^{-1} and 15 mg kg^{-1} day^{-1} indomethacin (= 10 IND, 15 IND); 15 mg kg^{-1} day^{-1} sulindac (= 15 SUL); 5 mg kg^{-1} day^{-1} and 1 mg kg^{-1} day^{-1} diclofenac (= 1 DIC); and 100 mg kg^{-1} day^{-1} meseclazone (= 100 MES). A good correlation was apparent between mucosal damage and reduction in mucosal prostaglandin content of pigs dosed with all the above drugs except meseclazone. No statistically significant changes were observed in the mucosal prostaglandin content of animals dosed with 75 mg kg^{-1} day^{-1} flufenamic acid (= 75 FLU), 75 mg kg^{-1} day^{-1} azapropazone (= 75 AZA), and 50 mg kg^{-1} day^{-1} fenclofenac (= FEN), but the plasma k-H$_2$-PGF$_{2\alpha}$ content was significantly reduced in pigs dosed with flufenamic acid and azapropazone

$$\text{Lesion Index} = \sum \text{No. of lesions} + \text{Severity} + \frac{\text{Percent animals with lesions}}{10}$$

(Method of Robert et al., reference 3)

Table 6.3 Summary of physiopathological and biochemical implications in the pathogenesis of GI mucosal injury by NSAIDs

Factor	Principal consequences
Acidity of drug (organic acid)	Loss of membrane integrity

Inhibition of PGI$_2$ and PGE$_2$ synthesis	Altered blood flow → anoxia
	Platelet-vessel adhesion promoted
	Microvascular injury
	Reduced 'cyto'-protection by:
	    decreased mucus production
	    decreased HCO$_3^-$ secretion

Release of lysosomal hydrolases	Local cellular autolysis
Cholinergic activation	Acid/pepsin secretion enhanced in stomach
Histamine release from mast cells	Promotes acid secretion, vasodilatation (stomach)
Enhanced oxyradical production*	Localized tissue destruction
Reduced sulphydryls	Possible loss of reductive protection by mucosal biomolecules against oxyradical damage and perturbed eicosanoid metabolism*
Enhanced motility (amplitude)	Altered GI transit ? relation to prostaglandin control of smooth muscle functions*
Inhibition of ATP production	Reduced capacity to resist cell injury from mucus and other synthetic reactions*
Altered cAMP levels (? from phosphodiesterase inhibition)	Altered cell metabolism, including effects on acid and mucus secretion (stomach)
Sloughing of surface mucus layer and inhibition of mucus biosynthesis (at enzyme level)	Impaired surface mucus protection

It should be emphasized that some of these drug actions* are rather speculative at the present state of knowledge

From reference 33

have been from studies with stereoisomers of NSAIDs. These show varying activity as inhibitors of PG production, and, with prodrugs, the comparison of an inactive PG synthesis prodrug compared with its 'active' metabolite can be made.

Gaut and co-workers[40] showed that the $l(-)$ isomer of the NSAID, d,l-6-chloro-α-methyl carbazole-2-acetic acid, was both inactive as an inhibitor or prostaglandin production *in vitro* and produced negligible gastric irritancy in the rat, whereas the $d(+)$ isomer of this drug was both a potent PG synthesis inhibitor and a powerful gastric ulcerogen. Incidently, these correlations could also be extended to inhibitory effects on platelet aggregation. This aspect has particular revelance in view of correlations observed with other NSAIDs between their propensity to induce gastric mucosal microvascular injury and their effects on platelet aggregation[31]. Such correlations may have a basis in that impairment of platelet aggregation may enhance blood loss from damaged mucosal capillaries (Table 6.3).

Similar suggestions have been made with some phenylpropionic acids which, except for naproxen, have been marketed as an equal mixture of inactive (i.e. with respect to PG synthesis inhibition) $R(-)$ and active $S(+)$ isomers. Conversion of R to S isomers occurs *in vivo*, so, in this respect, these drugs can be considered to be 50% prodrugs. The exact relationship between the effects of these propionic acid isomers and their gastro-irritancy remains, however, to be fully determined.

Sulindac and fenbufen are both prodrugs which are inactive as PG synthesis inhibitors but which undergo *in vivo* metabolism to form sulindac sulphide[41] and biphenyl acetic acid[42], respectively. Both prodrugs produce much less gastric mucosal injury, in various experimental animal models and in man, than their active PG synthesis inhibitory metabolites[41-44].

Furthermore, some esters of aspirin and related NSAIDs, alkyl (e.g. aspirin methyl ester) and cyclic aryl derivative (e.g. meseclazone), are themselves inactive as PG synthesis inhibitors and cause negligible gastric irritancy in rats. These drugs are metabolized *in vivo* to their acidic forms and so can be considered prodrugs, as with sulindac and fenbufen[45-49].

Time-course studies

Another approach has been to look at the time-sequence of gastric mucosal injury from NSAIDs in relation to their effects in causing changes in the mucosal content of prostaglandins. This approach attempts to discriminate whether the inhibition of PG production precedes, accompanies or follows the appearance of mucosal lesions.

In one such study, Whittle[50] purported to show that there was a so-called 'temporal' relationship between the inhibition of prostacyclin (PGI_2) production and the appearance of mucosal lesions in the gastric mucosal and jejuno-ileum of rats following subcutaneous administration of indomethacin. The time scale of the experiment, which covered times of 3, 24 and 48 h, really precluded precise relationships between these two measurements, especially that concerning the appearance of mucosal injury. The latter point is particularly important since this author, like many, only determined mucosal injury by the visual assessment of mucosal lesions or ulcers. It is, however, well known that microscopic injury to surface mucosal and other cells of the GI mucosa, appear long before the visual appearance of lesions and ulcers[21,30,31,51]. Thus, to describe such a 'temporal' relationship based on visual assessment of gross lesions is inadequate.

In other studies in pigs[30] and rats[22,31,32], fine structural changes in the gastric mucosa were determined and related to changes in mucosal content of PGE_2 and 6-keto-$PGF_{1\alpha}$, determined by GC–MS[22] or radioimmunoassay[30,31,32] in freeze-clamped mucosa at time intervals ranging up to 1 h following oral administration of several NSAIDs. These measurements were related to the rate of uptake of radioactively labelled drugs into the gastric mucosa. The

122

overall conclusions were that there was a good correlation between all three parameters with the known ulcerogenic drugs, such as aspirin and indomethacin. However, the lesser ulcerogenic NSAIDs showed quite variable effects on PG production even though it appeared that they were well absorbed. Some showed reduction in PG content without detectable, or at least with minimal, mucosal injury, while others failed to depress PG content with little or no effects on PGs.

In another study by Ligumsky and co-workers[52], the mucosal PG content was shown to be reduced following a single low dose of aspirin given orally or parenterally to rats without visible gastric lesions being produced. While the procedures used to determine gastric injury were somewhat crude, these results are interesting in that they show that, in gross pathological terms, the inhibition of PG production may be quite independent of mucosal damage.

Diversion of arachidonic acid

It is theoretically possible that the inhibition of PG cyclo-oxygenase (CO) by NSAIDs might cause diversion of arachidonic acid (AA) through the 5- or other lipoxygenases (LO) pathway, so leading to a relative excess of LO products, e.g. leukotrienes (LTs), and an oxygen radical (Ox·) as a product of peroxidative cleavage of hydroperoxyeicosatetraenoic acids (HPETEs). Such a possibility has been demonstrated in other tissues, e.g. lungs, and their importance is seen in relationship to asthma[54].

This hypothetical situation has begun to be investigated recently[55]. Some initial results have shown that inhibitors of 5-LO activity, as well as some LT antagonists, reduce the number and severity of gastric lesions induced by both oral or parenteral indomethacin in mice[55]. While more work is required to extend these initial findings, they provide an interesting lead towards understanding the consequence of inhibiting PG cyclo-oxygenase by NSAIDs.

The Ox· produced from the peroxidative cleavage of HPETEs when forming their corresponding hydroxy acids (HETEs) has been suggested to cause tissue injury[55,56] Antioxidants (e.g. buylated hydroxytoluene), which might be expected to scavenge such oxygen radicals (as well as superoxide) when given orally, ameliorate the gastric injury caused by NSAIDs in rats[56,57]. While this indicates that the Ox· species might have some role in NSAID-induced gastric injury, it is known that many of these antioxidants have, in addition, effects on the 5-LO pathway. Thus, the amelioration of NSAID-induced gastric injury might result from inhibition of the excess production of 5-LO products.

Long-term effects of perturbing PG synthesis

One of the many puzzling features about the (inter)actions of NSAIDs in the gastric mucosa centres around the question of the long-term consequences of inhibiting PG production. For instance, does the repeated administration of PG synthesis inhibitors simply lead to a situation where all the endogenous

PGs have been depleted to such low levels that the mucosa is incapable of retaining any 'protective' capacity?

The puzzling feature about this aspect is that it is possible to identify mucosal adaptive processes in both man and laboratory species following repeated oral ingestion of aspirin and other NSAIDs[30,59,60]. With aspirin (an irreversible cyclo-oxygenase inhibitor), it seems that repeated inhibition of PG production can proceed without the appearance of mucosal damage; this is in contrast to that seen soon after single doses of aspirin and other NSAIDs.

An understanding of the causes of this adaptive effect may be obtained from the data of Halter and co-workers[61]. They found that the mitotic index of the gastric mucosa of rats given repeated doses of indomethacin was markedly increased. It is hard to explain the mechanism underlying this observation. It is unlikely to be prostaglandin related since oral administration of E type PGs has, paradoxically, also been shown to enhance mucosal cell proliferation.

CONCLUSIONS

It is clear from the critical evaluation of the published work that there is overall a crude correlation between inhibitory effects of NSAIDs on PG production and their gastric irritancy or ulcerogenic potency. However, examination of this relationship in greater detail indicates that there are considerable gaps in our knowledge about:

(1) The relationship between inhibition of PG production and the development of mucosal injury, and

(2) The consequence of PG inhibition on different functions in various cells of the gastric mucosa.

The latter aspect has not been considered in appreciable detail since no measuring techniques have been derived to examine the changes in PG content in individual cell types in the gastric mucosa.

Most of the emphasis in this review has been on studies in the gastric mucosa. Relatively little is known about NSAID-induced changes in the intestinal tract and the relationship of this to the pathogenesis of mucosal injury in this region by indomethacin and fenamates which are known to cause small intestinal injury.

Based on a variety of published work, it is possible to speculate on the consequences of inhibition of PG production for gastric mucosal protective mechanisms. In the case of drugs which inhibit PG production without producing mucosal damage in the short term, it is possible that environmental influences (e.g. stress, disease state, ingestion of alcohol or cigarettes) may then exacerbate conditions in this PG 'deficient' state. Thus, generally, the consequences of NSAIDs might be to prime the mucosa leading to a range of biochemical and cellular consequences which could be described as part of the PG-deficient state. Additional exposure to untoward environmental influences might then enhance ulcerogenic responses, e.g. acid and pepsin secretion, impairment of blood flow etc.

REFERENCES

1. Vane J.R. (1971). Inhibition of prostaglandin biosynthesis as a mechanism of action of aspirin-like drugs. *Nature (London) New Biol.*, **231**, 232–235
2. Main, I.H.M. and Whittle, B.J.R. (1974). Prostaglandins and prostaglandin synthetase inhibitors in gastrointestinal function and disease. In Robinson, H.J. and Vane, J.R. (eds.) *Prostaglandin Synthetase Inhibitors*, pp. 363–372. (New York: Raven Press)
3. Robert, A., Nezamins, J.E. and Phillips, J.P. (1968). Effects of prostaglandin E₁ on gastric secretion and ulcer formation in the rat. *Gastroenterology*, **55**, 481–487
4. Bennett, A., Eley, K.G. and Scholes, G.B. (1968). Effects of prostaglandins E₁ and E₂ on human, guinea pig and rat isolated small intestine. *Br. J. Pharmacol.*, **34**, 630–638
5. Collier, H.O.J. (1974). Prostaglandin synthetase inhibitors and the gut. In Robinson, H.J. and Vane, J.R. (eds.) *Prostaglandin Synthetase Inhibitors*, pp. 121–133. (New York: Raven Press)
6. Bennett, A. (1971). Cholera and prostaglandins. *Nature (London)*, **232**, 536
7. Bennett, A. (1976). Prostaglandins and the alimentary tract. In Karim, S.M.M. (ed.). *Prostaglandins: Physiological Pharmacological and Pathological Aspects*, pp. 247–276. (Baltimore: University Park)
8. Whittle, B.J.R. (1976). Gastric antisecretory and antiulcer activity of prostaglandin E₂ methyl analogs. In Samuelsson, B. and Paoletti, R (eds.). *Advances in Prostaglandin and Thromboxane Research*. Vol. II, p. 948. (New York: Raven Press)
9. Robert A. (1977). Prostaglandins and the digestive system. In Ramwell, P.W. (ed.). *The Prostaglandins*, pp. 225–266. (New York: Plenum)
10. Dreyling, K.W., Hoppe, U., Kleine, A., Kozuschek, W. and Peskar, B.M. (1987) Leukotriene formation in the gastrointestinal tract and effects of anti-inflammatory drugs. In Rainsford, K.D and Velo, G.P. (eds.). *Side Effects of Anti-inflammatory Drugs*, pp. 101–112. (Lancaster, MTP Press)
11. Rainsford, K.D. (1979). Prostaglandins and the development of gastric mucosal damage by anti-inflammatory drugs. In Rainsford, K.D. and Ford-Hutchinson, A.W. (eds.). *Prostaglandins and Inflammation, Agents Actions*, Suppl. 6, pp. 193–210. (Basel: Birkaeuser)
12. Miller, T.A. (1983). Protective effects of prostaglandins against gastric mucosal damage: current knowledge and proposed mechanisms. *Am. J. Physiol.*, **245**, G601–G623
13. Whittle, B.J.R. and Boughton-Smith, N.K. (1984). Biosynthesis of exogenous arachidonate products involved in gastric damage and protection. In Paton, W., Mitchell, J. and Turner, P. (eds.) *Proceedings of the 9th International Pharmacology Congress, IUPHAR*, London, Vol. 3, pp. 345–354. (London: Macmillan)
14. Hawkey, C.J. and Rampton, D.S. (1985). Prostaglandins and the gastro-intestinal mucosa: are they important in its function, disease or treatment? *Gastroenterology*, **89**, 1162–1168
15. Jobke, A., Peskar, B.A. and Peskar, B.M. (1973). On the specificity of prostaglandins A₂ and E₂. *FEBS Lett.*, **37**, 192–196
16. Peskar, B. M. (1978). Radioimmunoassay fur prostaglandine. *Z. Gastroenterologie*, **16**, 1–8
17. Peskar, B.M. Seybert, H.W. and Peskar, B.A. (1980). Synthesis and metabolism of endogenous prostaglandins by human gastric mucosa. In Samuelsson, B., Ramwell, P.W. and Paoletti, R. *Advances in Prostaglandin and Thromboxane Research*, Vol. 8, pp. 1511–1551. (New York: Raven Press)
18. Lee, D.K.H., Cohen, R., Gilliar, J., Muller, B. and Smith, T. (1986). A subchronic study of the effect of etodolac on the gastric mucosal prostaglandin levels in the rat. *Agents Actions*, **19**, 228–232
19. Hoppe, U., Hoppe, E.M., Peskar, B.M. and Peskar, B.A. (1986). Radioimmunoassay for leukotriene E₄. Use of determination of total sulfidopeptide–leukotriene release from rat gastric mucosa. *FEBS Lett.*, **208**, 26–30
20. Pace-Asciak, C.R. and Rangaraj, G. (1977). Distribution of prostaglandin biosynthetic pathways in several rat tissues. Formation of 6-ketoprostaglandin F₁ₐ. *Biochim. Biophys. Acta*, **486**, 579–582
21. Rainsford, K.D., Fox, S.A. and Osborne, D.J. (1984). Comparative effects of some non-steroidal anti-inflammatory drugs on the ultrastructural integrity and prostaglandin levels in the rat gastric mucosa: Relationship to drug uptake. *Scand. J. Gastroenterol.*, **19** (Suppl. 101), 35–68

22. Goswanni, S., Mai, J., Bruckner, G. and Kinsella, J. E. (1981). Extraction and purification of prostaglandins and thromboxane from biological samples for gas-chromatographic analysis. *Prostaglandins*, **22**, 693–702
23. Moncada, S., Salmon, J.A., Vane, J.R. and Whittle, B.J.R. (1977). Formation of prostacyclin and its product 6-oxo-PGF$_{1\alpha}$ by the gastric mucosa of several species. *J. Physiol.*, **275**, 4P–5P
24. Konturek, S.J., Piastucki, I., Brozozowski, T., Radecki, T., Dembinska-Kiec, A., Zmuda, A. and Gryglewski, R. (1981). Role of prostaglandins in the formation of aspirin-induced gastric ulcers. *Gastroenterology*, **80**, 4–9
25. Green, K., Aly, A. and Johansson, C. (1981). Measurements of prostaglandin biosynthesis in the gastrointestinal tract: biochemical and technical problems. *Prostaglandins*, **21**, (Suppl. I), 1–7
26. Peskar, B.M., Holland, A. and Peskar, B.A. (1974). Quantitative determination of prostaglandins in human gastric juice by radioimmunoassay. *Clin. Chim. Acta*, **55**, 21–27
27. Minuz, P., Cavallin, G., Brocco, G., Degan, M., Jeunet, F., Kunorits, G., Riela, A. and Velo, G.P. (1986). Effect of carprofen and indomethacin on gastric function and the content of prostaglandins E$_2$ and F$_{2\alpha}$ in the human gastric juice. *Hepato-gastroenterology*, **33**, 20–22
28. Whittle, B.J.R. (1983). The potentiation of taurocholate-induced rat gastric erosions following parenteral administration of cyclo-oxygenase inhibitors. *Br. J. Pharmacol.*, **80**, 545–551
29. Pace-Asciak, C.R. and Carrara, M.C. (1978). Stability of authentic PGI$_2$ during routine extraction. Clarification of the nature and sequences of products formed by the rat stomach including the origin of ozonolysis products reported in 1971. *Prostaglandins*, **16**, 397–410
30. Rainsford, K.D. and Willis, C. (1982). Relationship of gastric mucosal damage induced in pigs by anti-inflammatory drugs to their effects on prostaglandin production. *Dig. Dis. Sci.*, **27**, 624–635
31. Rainsford, K.D., Fox, S.A. and Osborne, D.J. (1985). Relationship between any absorption, inhibition of cyclooxygenase and lipoxygenase pathways and the development of gastric mucosal damage by non-steroidal anti-inflammatory drugs in rats and pigs. In Bailey, M. J. (ed.) *Advances in Prostaglandins, Leukotrienes and Lipoxins*, pp. 639–653. (New York: Plenum Press)
32. Rainsford, K.D. (1987). Mechanisms of gastric contrasted with intestinal damage by non-steroidal anti-inflammatory drugs. In Rainsford, K.D. and Velo, G.P. (eds.) *Side Effects of Anti-inflammatory Drugs*, pp. 3–26. (Lancaster: MTP Press)
33. Rainsford, K.D. (1987). Mechanisms of gastrointestinal damage by non-steroidal anti-inflammatory drugs. In Szabo, S. and Pfeiffer, C.J. (eds.) *Experimental Gastric Ulcer*. (Boca Raton: CRC Press) (In press)
34. Robert, A. (1984). Mechanisms of cytoprotection. In Paton, W., Mitchell, J. and Turner, P. (eds.) *Proceedings of the 9th International Congress of Pharmacology, IUPHAR*, Vol. 3 pp. 355–359. (London: Macmillan)
35. Miller, T.A. (1983). Protective effects of prostaglandins against gastric mucosal damage: current knowledge and proposed mechanisms. *Am. J. Physiol.*, **245**, G601–G623
36. Jacobson, E.D. (1986). Direct and adaptive cytoprotection. *Dig. Dis. Sci.*, **31** (Suppl.), 28S–31S
37. Needleman, P. (1978). Experimental criteria for evaluating prostaglandin biosynthesis and intrinsic function. *Biochem. Pharmacol.*, **27**, 1515–1518
38. Baker, R., Jaffe, B.M., Read, J.D., Shaw, B. and Venables, C.W. (1978). Endogenous prostaglandins and gastric secretion in the cat. *J. Physiol.*, **278**, 451–460
39. Flemstrom, G., Briden, S. and Kivilaakso, E. (1984). Stimulation by BW 755 C and inhibition by cysteamine of duodenal epithelial alkaline secretion suggest a role of endogenous prostaglandin in mucosal protection. *Scand. J. Gastroenterol.*, **19** (Suppl. 92), 101–105
40. Gaut, Z.N., Baruth, H., Randall, L.O., Ashley, C. and Paulsrud, J.R. (1975). Steroisomeric relationships among anti-inflammatory activity, inhibition of platelet aggregation, and inhibition of prostaglandin synthetase. *Prostaglandins*, **10**, 1–8
41. Shen, T.Y. (1985). Indomethacin, sulindac and their analogs. In Rainsford, K.D. (ed.) *Anti-inflammatory and Anti-rheumatic Drugs*, Vol. 1, pp. 149–159. (Boca Raton, CRC Press)
42. Greenberg, B.P. and Bernstein, J. (1985). Fenbufen. In Rainsford, K.D. (ed.) *Anti-inflammatory and Anti-rheumatic Drugs*, Vol. II. pp. 87–103. (Boca Raton: CRC Press)

43. Shen, T.Y. and Winter, C.A. (1977). Chemical and biological studies on indomethacin, sulindac and their analogs. *Adv. Drug Res.*, **12**, 89–245
44. Rainsford, K.D. (1981). Comparison of the gastric ulcerogenic activity of new non-steroidal anti-inflammatory drugs in stressed rats. *Br. J. Pharmacol.*, **73**, 79c–80c
45. Rainsford, K.D. and Whitehouse, M. W. (1976). Gastric irritancy of aspirin and its congeners: Anti-inflammatory activity without this side effect. *J. Pharm. Pharmacol.*, **28**, 599–601
46. Whitehouse, M.W., Rainsford, K.D., Young, T.G. Ardlie, N.G. and Brune, K. (1977). Alternatives to aspirin derived from biological sources. *Agents Actions, Suppl. 1*, 43–47
47. Whitehouse, M.W. and Rainsford, K.D. (1980). Esterification of acidic anti-inflammatory drugs suppresses their gastrotoxicity without adversely affecting their anti-inflammatory activity in rats. *J. Pharm. Pharmacol.*, **32**, 795–796
48. Rainsford, K.D., Schweitzer, A., Green, P., Whitehouse, M.W. and Brune, K. (1980). Biodistribution in rats of some salicylates with low gastric ulcerogenicity. *Agents Actions*, **20**, 452–464
49. Rainsford, K.D., Schweitzer, A. and Brune, K. (1981). Autoradiographic and biochemical observations on the distribution of non-steroidal anti-inflammatory drugs. *Arch. Int. Pharmacodyn.*, **250**, 180–194
50. Whittle, B.J.R. (1981) Temporal relationship between cyclo-oxygenase inhibition, as measured by prostacyclin biosynthesis, and the gastrointestinal damage induced by indomethacin in the rat. *Gastroenterology*, **80**, 94–98
51. Rainsford, K.D. (1975). Electronmicroscopic observations on the effects of orally administered aspirin and aspirin–bicarbonate mixtures on the development of gastric mucosal damage in the rat. *Gut*, **16**, 514–527
52. Ligumsky, M., Golanska, E.M., Hansen, D.G. and Kauffman, G.L. (1985). Aspirin can inhibit mucosal cyclo-oxygenase without causing lesions in the rat. *Gastroenterology*, **84**, 756–61
53. Reinhardt, M.C. and deWeck, A.L. (1984). Immunological actions of aspirin in relation to hypersensitivity reactions. In Rainsford, K.D. and Velo, G.P. (eds.) *Side-effects of Anti-inflammatory/Analgesic Drugs*, pp. 209–217. (New York: Raven Press)
54. Rainsford, K.D. (1984). *Aspirin and the Salicylates*, pp. 238–239. (London: Butterworths)
55. Rainsford, K.D. (1987). Effects of modulation of the 5-lipoxygenase pathway on the development of gastric mucosal lesions induced by nonsteroidal anti-inflammatory drugs in cholinomimetic treated mice. *Agents Actions*, **21**, 316–319
56. Rainsford, K.D. (1984). The mechanisms of gastro-intestinal ulceration by non-steroidal anti-inflammatory drugs. In Rainsford, K.D. and Velo, G.P. (eds.) *Side Effects of Anti-inflammatory/Analgesic Drugs*, pp. 51–64. (New York: Raven Press)
57. Van Kolfschoten, A.A., Hagelin, F. and van Noordwijk, J. (1984). Butyl hydroxy toluene antagonizes the gastric toxicity but not the pharmacological activity of acetylsalicylic acid in rats. *Naunyn-Schmeidebergs Arch. Pharmacol.*, **325**, 283–285
58. Swingle, K.F., Bell, R.L. and Moore, G.G.I. (1985). Anti-inflammatory activity of antioxidants. In Rainsford, K.D. (ed.) *Anti-inflammatory and Anti-rheumatic Drugs*, Vol. 3, pp. 105–126. (Boca Raton, CRC Press)
59. Hurley, J.W. and Crandall, L.A. (1963). The effects of salicylates upon the dog's stomach: A gastroscopic photographic evaluation. In Dixon, A.St.J., Martin, B.K., Smith, M.J. H. and Wood, P.H.N. (eds.) *Salicylates, an International Symposium*. pp. 213–216. (London: Churchill)
60. Graham, D.Y., Lacey Smith, J. and Dobbs, S.M. (1983). Gastric adaptation occurs with aspirin administration in man. *Dig. Dis. Sci.*, **28**, 1–6
61. Halter, F., Baumgartner, A., Varga, L. and Koelz, H.R. (1987). Both E-prostaglandins and prolonged indomethacin treatment exert trophic effects on the gastric mucosa. In Rainsford, K.D. and Velo, G.P. (eds.) *Side Effects of Anti-inflammatory Drugs*. pp. 133–142. (Lancaster MTP Press)
62. Krupp, P., Menasse, R., Riesterer, L. and Ziel, R. (1976). The biological significance of inhibition of prostaglandin synthesis. In Lewis, G.P. (ed.) *The Role of Prostaglandins in Inflammation*, pp. 106–115. (Berne: Hans Huber)
63. Boughton-Smith, N.K. and Whittle, B.J.R. (1983). Stimulation and inhibition of prostacyclin formation in the gastric mucosa and ileum *in vitro* by anti-inflammatory agents. *Br. J. Pharmacol.*, **78**, 173–180

64. Collins, P.O., Tavares, I.A. and Bennett, A. (1987). Inhibition of prostanoid synthesis by anti-inflammatory drugs in human gastric mucosa. In Rainsford, K.D. and Velo, G.P. (eds.) *Side Effects of Anti-inflammatory Drugs*, Vol. II, pp. 97–100. (Lancaster, MTP Press)
65. Brune, K., Rainsford, K.D., Wagner, K. and Peskar, B.A. (1981). Inhibition by anti-inflammatory drugs of prostaglandin production in cultured macrophages. Factors influencing the apparent drug effects. *Naunyn-Schmeidebergs Arch. Pharmacol.*, **315**, 269–276
66. Danon, A., Leibsen, V. and Assouline, G. (1983). Effects of aspirin, indomethacin, flufenamic acid and paracetamol on prostaglandin output from rat stomach and renal papilla *in vitro* and *ex vivo. J. Pharm. Pharmacol.*, **35**, 576–579
67. Fitzpatrick, F.A. and Wynalda, M.A. (1976). *In vivo* suppression of prostaglandin biosynthesis by non-steroidal anti-inflammatory agents. *Prostaglandins*, **12**, 1037–1051
68. Le Duc, L.E. and Needleman, P. (1979). Regional localization of prostacyclin and thromboxane synthesis in dog stomach and intestinal tract. *J. Pharmacol. Exp. Ther.*, **211**, 181–188
69. Skoglund, M.L., Gerber, J.G., Murphy, R.C. and Nies, A.S. (1980). Prostaglandin production by intact isolated gastric parietal cells. *Eur. J. Pharmacol.*, **66**, 145–148

7
Alkaline secretion by the stomach and intestine: Effects of eicosanoids and anti-inflammatory drugs

A. Aly and G. Flemström

INTRODUCTION

Bicarbonate is secreted by the gastroduodenal mucosa into the unstirred layer of mucus that adheres to this epithelium. This mucus-bicarbonate surface layer is impermeable to pepsin and prevents or retards diffusion of luminal acid to the epithelial cells. The surface pH gradient is maintained at luminal acidities as high as pH 2 in the rat stomach[1] and duodenum[2], and a similar gradient has been demonstrated in the human stomach[3]. At higher luminal acidities the gradient is overwhelmed with consequent acidification of the surface. In humans, the luminal pH in the stomach is below 2 during some periods of the day but acidities below this pH seldom occur in the duodenum[4]. It therefore seems likely that the mucosal bicarbonate secretion constitutes, along with the mucus layer, a first line of defence against acid in the stomach, and it is probably a principal protective mechanism in the duodenum[5]. In addition, bicarbonate secretion by the duodenal mucosa is considerably greater (per unit surface area) than in the stomach[6,7].

The aim of this chapter is to describe recent studies on the physiological control of gastroduodenal mucosal alkaline secretion and protection and the effects of exogenous prostaglandins and anti-inflammatory drugs on this secretion. Some of the methods developed for these studies are also summarized.

METHODS OF STUDYING BICARBONATE SECRETION BY THE GASTRODUODENAL MUCOSA

Control of the preoperative handling and feeding of the animals and control of the experimental procedure are important in studies of gastric and duodenal mucosal bicarbonate secretion. Feeding as well as intraluminal acid increases alkaline secretion in both the stomach and duodenum[6-9]. Furthermore, sham-feeding has been demonstrated to increase gastric bicarbonate secretion in humans[10,11], and duodenal secretion in animals has been reported to be under α_2-adrenergic inhibition[12]. This makes it important to avoid any teasing with food or stress situations in experiments in humans and conscious animals. It must be stressed that in acute experiments with isolated preparations or in anaesthetized animals operative handling and stretching of the tissue may increase mucosal endogenous synthesis of prostaglandins or (in vivo) elicit local neural reflexes.

Measurement of gastric bicarbonate secretion

The use of isolated mucosa in vitro facilitates the determination of the nature of the ion transport processes. Antral and fundic mucosa from amphibia[5,13], rabbits[14], guinea-pigs[15,16] and dogs[17] have been mounted in in vitro chambers. Luminal alkalinization by antral mucosa can be titrated directly, and the antrum has been used in some studies as a model for gastric non-parietal ion transport. In most species the fundus secretes acid spontaneously. Neither histamine H_2-receptor antagonists[5] nor the H^+/K^+ ATPase inhibitor, ome-prazole[15,16], affect gastric alkaline secretion, and these and some other agents have been used to inhibit fundic acid secretion for studies on alkaline secretion. Basal rates of in vitro secretion disclosed by H^+ inhibition amount to 0.1 to 0.5 μEq cm^{-2} h^{-1} in amphibian preparations and 0.3 to 1.0 μEq cm^{-2} h^{-1} in mammalian ones.

Various methods, including the use of histamine H_2-receptor antagonists and omeprazole, have been used to inhibit fundic H^+ secretion in vivo for studies on alkaline secretion. Methods for simultaneous estimations of gastric acid and alkali secretion have also been developed. Studies have been performed in a variety of species[18,21], including man[22,23]. The occurrence of gastric alkaline secretion as well as stimulation and/or inhibition of this secretion has been demonstrated in all species tested.

In simultaneous determination of acid and alkaline secretions, the rates of secretion have been calculated either from intragastric pH and pCO_2, using the Henderson–Hasselbalch equation[21,22], or from measurements of intragastric osmolality[23]. The former technique is based on the assumption that the CO_2 appearing in the gastric lumen is formed during the reaction between secreted bicarbonate and acid, and the latter is based on the fact that this reaction reduces the osmolality of the gastric juice. A prerequisite for these methods is that the permeability of the gastric mucosa to CO_2 and water, respectively, is relatively low. The two methods provide very similar results qualitatively, but rates estimated from osmolality measurements are higher.

Measurement of duodenal mucosal alkaline secretion

In early studies Florey and co-workers measured the volume and alkalinity of the secretion from duodenal segments containing Brunner's glands and suggested that the secretion, including its content of bicarbonate, originated from these glands[24]. Later studies have demonstrated that duodenal mucosa from species devoid of these glands[25,26] and mucosal segments distal to the Brunner's glands area[7,9] secrete bicarbonate. The sensitivity to inhibitors and stimulants of this secretion by the mucosa alone appears to be indistinguishable from that of the area containing Brunner's glands. Secretion of some bicarbonate by Brunner's glands cannot be ruled out, but it seems likely that the origin of bicarbonate is mainly the duodenal mucosa itself.

The duodenal mucosal alkaline secretion has been measured by continuous titration of recirculating perfusate using pH-stat equipment[7,25] or by determining the bicarbonate content of the effluent of duodenal segments[27,28]. Studies have been performed in amphibian mucosae *in vitro* and in a variety of mammalian species, including man, *in vivo*. It should be noted that there is a gradient in the capacity to secrete alkali in that rates in proximal duodenum are higher than those in distal duodenum, which are higher than those in jejunum. This gradient has been demonstrated in amphibians[26], rats[27] and humans[29]. Studies in amphibians and in the rat suggest that it is an inherent property of the duodenal epithelium.

TRANSPORT PROCESSES FOR BICARBONATE

The secretion that creates a pH gradient across the surface (mucus) layer adherent to the gastric and duodenal surfaces is dependent on tissue metabolism and exhibits sensitivity to a variety of stimulants and inhibitors[2,3,30,31]. This secretion must be distinguished from the leakage (or ultrafiltration) of bicarbonate across previously damaged epithelium[5]. In all probability, the latter process is important in mucosal repair, however[32].

The process of metabolic-dependent bicarbonate secretion by the *gastric* mucosa has been studied in epithelium isolated from amphibia. The results suggest that both bicarbonate produced endogenously by cell metabolism and bicarbonate entering the cell via a Na^+-dependent transport mechanism at the nutrient membrane are secreted across the luminal membrane by electroneutral Cl^-/HCO_3^- exchange. Carbonic anhydrase activity, which has been demonstrated in the luminal membrane of the surface epithelial cell, is probably important in this process[5].

The secretion of bicarbonate by the *duodenal* mucosa is more complex in that both electroneutral Cl^-/HCO_3^- exchange and electrogenic transport have been demonstrated in isolated amphibian preparations[33]. The former process is inhibited by furosemide and stimulated by some gastrointestinal hormones. The latter transport process is the quantitatively superior one and is stimulated by prostaglandins and cyclic AMP. Evidence has been presented that these two processes for secretion of bicarbonate also operate in the mammalian duodenal mucosa[5].

BICARBONATE SECRETION AND EICOSANOIDS

Effect of exogenous eicosanoids

The effect of various naturally occurring eicosanoids or of synthetic prostanoid analogues on gastroduodenal mucosal bicarbonate secretion has been studied in different species, including humans. The results of these studies are summarized in Tables 7.1 (*in vivo* studies) and 7.2 (*in vitro* studies).

Bicarbonate responses in *in vivo* studies were considerably stronger following topical (luminal) application of the compounds than on intravenous administration[18,34]. Prostaglandin E_2 (PGE_2) was, on a molar basis, the most potent stimulant among the natural prostaglandins[34]. Increased bicarbonate

Table 7.1 *In vivo* studies on the effect of some exogenous eicosanoids on gastroduodenal bicarbonate secretion

	Substance					
					Synthetic analogues of	
Species	PGE_2	$PGF_{2\alpha}$	PGI_2	Arachidonic acid	PGE	PGI_2
Stomach						
Rat	+[74]				+[72]	+[40]
Cat	+[20,75]	+[75]			+[20,75]	
Dog	+[34]	0[34]	0[34]	+[37]	+[18,19,34]	+[34,40]
Humans	+[35]				+[22,35]	
	0[36]					
Duodenum						
Guinea-pig	0[7]*				0[7]	
Rabbit	0[7]*					
Rat	+[2,7,27,28]	+[2]			+[2]	
Cat	+[7,20]				+[20]	
Dog	+[7,34]	+[34]	0[34]	+[37]	+[34]	+[34]
Humans					+[29]	

The substances have in most studies been applied topically. + = stimulation, 0 = no effect. Numbers indicate references.
*A response to PGE_2 is observed after treatment with cyclo-oxygenase blocking drugs

Table 7.2 *In vitro* studies on the effect of some exogenous prostanoids on gastroduodenal bicarbonate secretion

		Substance			
Species	Organ	PGE_2	$PGF_{2\alpha}$	PGI_2	16,16-dimethyl-PGE_2
Rana temporaria	Corpus	0[42]	+[76]	0[42]	+[76]
	Antrum		+[76]		+[76]
Rana catesbeiana	Corpus				0[77]
	Antrum				0[77]
	Duodenum	+[25,78]	+[25,78]		+[25,78]
Rabbit	Corpus	0[14]	0[14]		+[14]
	Antrum	0[14]	0[14]		0[14]

+ = stimulation, 0 = no effect. Numbers indicate references

secretion was observed in denervated gastric corpus pouches in the dog with topically applied PGE_2 at a concentration of 2.8×10^{-6} mol L^{-1}. A still lower concentration $(2.8 \times 10^{-7}$ mol $L^{-1})$ was effective in duodenal pouches[34]. In segments of rat[27,28] and cat[20] duodenum, 10^{-5} mol L^{-1} PGE_2 stimulated bicarbonate secretion. The bicarbonate secretion increased dose-dependently (Figure 7.1), and the highest observed bicarbonate response in the rat duodenum was of the same magnitude as the response observed in this preparation after mucosal exposure to 150 mmol L^{-1} HCl^{28} (Figure 7.2). In humans, topical PGE_2 $(5.6 \times 10^{-3}$ mol $L^{-1})$ significantly increased gastric bicarbonate secretion[35], whereas lower doses were ineffective[36]. However, the reduction of basal bicarbonate following aspirin administration was partly reversed by as little as 5×10^{-7} mol L^{-1} PGE_2[36].

Topical $PGF_{2\alpha}$ was a weak stimulant of gastric[34] and duodenal[2,34] bicarbonate secretion, whereas PGI_2 had no effect[34]. Topical application of arachidonic acid increased gastric and duodenal bicarbonate output in the dog[37], and the increase of bicarbonate secretion was paralleled by increased luminal levels of PGE_2. Pretreatment of the animals with indomethacin prevented the rise of both bicarbonate output and luminal PGE_2, indicating that arachidonic acid itself does not stimulate bicarbonate secretion.

Synthetic analogues of PGE_2, which are more resistant to enzymatic degradation, are considerably more potent stimulants of gastroduodenal bicarbonate secretion than natural PGE_2. 16,16-dimethyl-PGE_2 has been

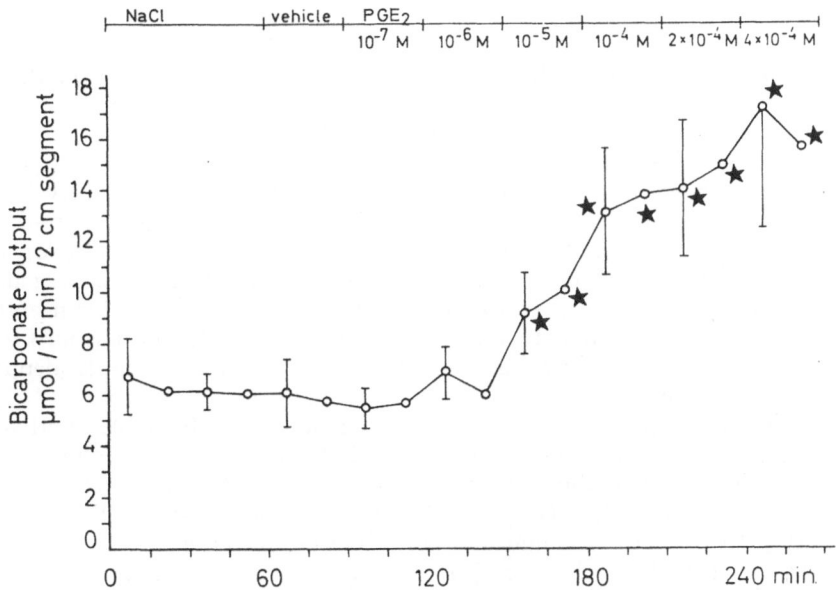

Figure 7.1 Bicarbonate secretion in the proximal duodenal loop of unanaesthetized rats increased dose-dependently in response to perfusion of the lumen with graded doses of prostaglandin E_2 (mean ± SEM, $^*p < 0.05$ vs. basal). Reproduced with the kind permission of the authors and *Gastroenterology*[28]

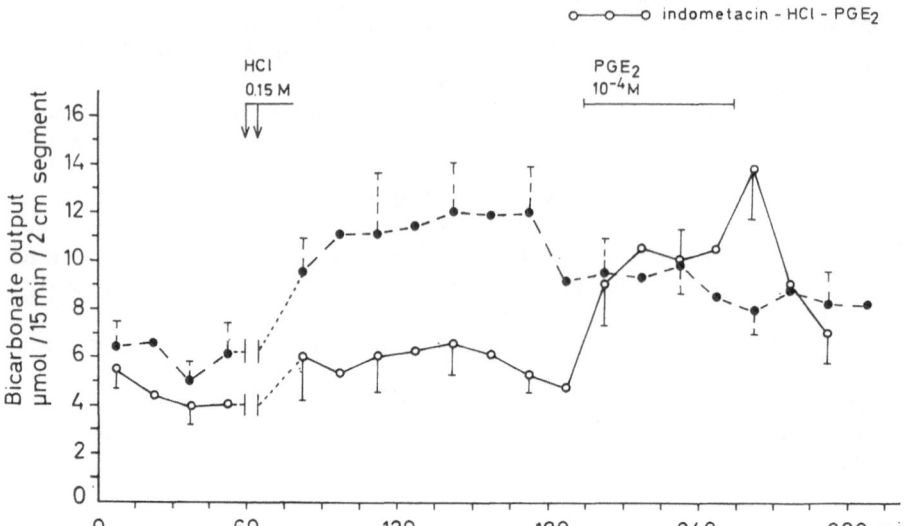

Figure 7.2 Bicarbonate output in the proximal duodenal loop of unanaesthetized rats increased significantly following 5 minutes' exposure of the mucosa to 150 mmol L^{-1} HCl (solid circles). Pretreatment with indomethacin inhibited the effect of HCl. However, perfusion of the lumen with prostaglandin E$_2$ caused a significant bicarbonate response (mean $\pm$ SEM, $p < 0.05$ vs. basal). Reproduced with the kind permission of the authors and *Gastroenterology*[28]

studied most intensely and has been shown to stimulate gastric and duodenal bicarbonate output in various experimental animals (Table 7.1). This analogue of PGE$_2$ has been reported to be up to 200 times more effective than the natural compound; it induces a bicarbonate response at lower doses as well as higher maximal rates of secretion[2,20,34]. It should be noted that very high doses of 16,16-dimethyl-PGE$_2$ ($> 3 \times 10^{-5}$ mol L^{-1}) have been reported to induce mucosa damage[34,38] and that under such conditions, ultrafiltration of tissue bicarbonate may contribute to the luminal alkalinization. In humans, 16,16-dimethyl-PGE$_2$ at a concentration of 1×10^{-6} mol L^{-1} significantly increased gastric bicarbonate output[22,35]. The PGE$_1$ analogue, misoprostol, dose-dependently increased mucosal bicarbonate secretion in the duodenum of rats[39] and humans[29].

While natural prostacyclin (PGI$_2$) exerted no effect, its stable synthetic analogues had been found to stimulate both gastric[34,40] and duodenal[34] bicarbonate output in the dog. In *in vivo* studies of guinea-pig and rabbit duodenum neither PGE$_2$ (1–10 $\times$ 10^{-6} mol L^{-1} nor 16,16-dimethyl-PGE$_2$ (2–10 $\times$ 10^{-6} mol L^{-1}) stimulated bicarbonate secretion[7]. It has been suggested that the lack of response may be due to high endogenous levels of prostaglandins. In fact, after probable reduction of endogenous prostaglandin formation by pretreatment of the animals with aspirin or indomethacin, topical PGE$_2$ dose-dependently increased the bicarbonate output. High endogenous levels of prostaglandins might also explain the failure of different prostaglandins to stimulate gastric bicarbonate secretion in some *in vitro* experiments (Table 7.2). The manipulation of the tissues in such experiments can be presumed to cause increased local prostaglandin formation. However, in duodenal mucosa isolated from amphibians, all tested prostaglandins were effective (Table 7.2)[25]. The effects of a large variety of other eicosanoids on bicarbonate secretion in this preparation have been reported recently[41]. PGE_2 was the most potent stimulant, but PGE_1, PGI_2, $PGF_{2\alpha}$, PGD_2, 6-keto-$PGF_{1\alpha}$ (the stable metabolite of PGI_2), leukotriene D_4, PGA_2, arachidonic acid and thromboxane B_2 (10^{-5} mol L^{-1}) also increased duodenal bicarbonate secretion. Linoleic acid and leukotriene B_4 were inactive.

The role of endogenous eicosanoids in gastroduodenal bicarbonate secretion

Effect of drugs influencing the metabolism of arachidonic acid
Non-steroidal anti-inflammatory drugs (NSAID) have been widely used in a variety of experiments to test the effect of cyclo-oxygenase blockade on gastroduodenal bicarbonate secretion. In judging such studies, one must remember that it has very rarely been determined whether, under the experimental conditions, the employed dose of NSAID causes a significant inhibition of cyclo-oxygenase activity in the organ under study. Furthermore, the observed effects, attributed to cyclo-oxygenase blockade, may be secondary to increased formation of lipoxygenase products or to other pharmacological effects of NSAID not related to arachidonic acid metabolism.

Effect of NSAID on gastric bicarbonate secretion
Acetylsalicylic acid (ASA) as well as indomethacin lowered basal bicarbonate secretion from isolated amphibian[42,43] and mammalian[14] gastric mucosa, and luminally applied ASA (10^{-2} mol L^{-1}) diminished the pH gradient across the layer of gastric mucus in the anaesthetized rat[1,44]. Basal bicarbonate output in amphibian gastric mucosa was also sensitive to fenclofenac[42]. The basal gastric bicarbonate secretion in unanaesthetized dogs[9] and cats[20] was not affected, however, by intravenous indomethacin (2.5–5 mg kg^{-1}), whereas the rise in bicarbonate secretion in response to luminal HCl was inhibited[9]. The reduction by indomethacin of acid-stimulated bicarbonate secretion in the dog was associated with a decreased output of PGE_2 (radioimmunoassay) into the lumen[9].

In humans, high concentrations of luminal ASA (2×10^{-2} mol L^{-1}) lowered the basal gastric bicarbonate output[36], while intravenous[11] or oral[45] indomethacin (50 mg) had no effect. The peak increase of bicarbonate secretion in response to sham-feeding was lower after indomethacin than in control experiments, but this difference did not attain statistical significance[11]. Thus, under conditions presumably involving increased formation of endogenous prostaglandins (such as *in vitro* experiments or following exposure of the mucosa to acid) both indomethacin and ASA decreased the bicarbonate output. Basal bicarbonate secretion *in vivo*, seems, however, to be less dependent on endogenous prostaglandin formation. The inhibitory effect of ASA (but not indomethacin) in this situation is probably due to other factors unrelated to cyclo-oxygenase blockade.

The effect of NSAID on duodenal bicarbonate secretion

Indomethacin decreased spontaneous bicarbonate secretion in isolated amphibian duodenum[25] as well as in proximal and distal duodenal segments from dogs[9] and humans[46]. Basal bicarbonate secretion in rat duodenum was not affected by indomethacin[47]. In the case of cat duodenum, indomethacin has been reported both to exert no effect[7] and to decrease[20] basal bicarbonate secretion. Bicarbonate secretion in the duodenum of the guinea-pig was sensitive to indomethacin[7]. The different effects of NSAID on basal bicarbonate output are probably due to species differences and to different experimental conditions.

Luminal acid is a potent and presumably physiological stimulant of duodenal mucosal bicarbonate secretion. Pretreatment with indomethacin reduced the post-acid bicarbonate response in all tested mammals[7,9,28], including humans[46]. This has been observed in both proximal and more distal duodenal segments[9,46]. In the duodenum of conscious rats, indomethacin completely abolished the bicarbonate response to $150 \, mmol \, L^{-1}$ of HCl^{28} (Figure 7.2). In anaesthetized rats and cats, pretreatment with indomethacin decreased the duration of the alkaline response to $10 \, mmol \, L^{-1} \, HCl$ but did not affect the peak bicarbonate output[7]. The possibility that the difference in acid load on the duodenum may be of particular importance is suggested by another study: intravenous ASA lowered the bicarbonate response in the duodenum of the rat when the luminal pH was decreased from 7.6 to 2.0 but had no effect on the response at pH 5.0^2. These studies suggest that basal and particularly acid-stimulated duodenal bicarbonate secretion is partly dependent on mucosal cyclo-oxygenase activity. The observation that low doses of exogenous PGE_2 ($5 \times 10^{-7} - 10^{-4} \, mol \, L^{-1}$) reversed the depressive effect of NSAID on both spontaneous[7,25] and acid-induced[7,28] bicarbonate secretion constitutes further support for this hypothesis.

The effect of other drugs influencing the metabolism of arachidonic acid

Low doses of the dual cyclo-oxygenase–lipoxygenase inhibitor BW755C have been reported to increase *in vitro* production of prostacyclin by gastrointestinal tissues[48]. On intravenous administration, this drug ($20 \, mg \, kg^{-1}$) caused an increase in mucosal bicarbonate secretion in rat duodenum[47,49]. This effect could be prevented by pretreatment of the animal with indomethacin, which indicates that the stimulating effect of BW755C might be secondary to increased endogenous prostaglandin formation (Figure 7.3). At higher doses of BW755C a decrease in duodenal bicarbonate secretion was observed[47], which might indicate inhibition of endogenous cyclo-oxygenase activity. Sucralfate[50] and antacids containing aluminium[51] increase gastroduodenal mucosal prostaglandin formation in the rat as indicated by radioimmunological measurements of PGE_2 in gastric luminal contents. Both sucralfate[52] and these antacids[53] have been shown to stimulate bicarbonate secretion from isolated amphibian gastroduodenal mucosa. It has also been reported that sucralfate increased gastric bicarbonate output in humans[54].

Measurement of endogenous prostaglandins in relation to gastroduodenal bicarbonate secretion

Prostaglandin contents of mucosal biopsies and the formation of prostaglandins in incubated specimens do not reflect mucosal prostaglandin synthesis *in vivo*

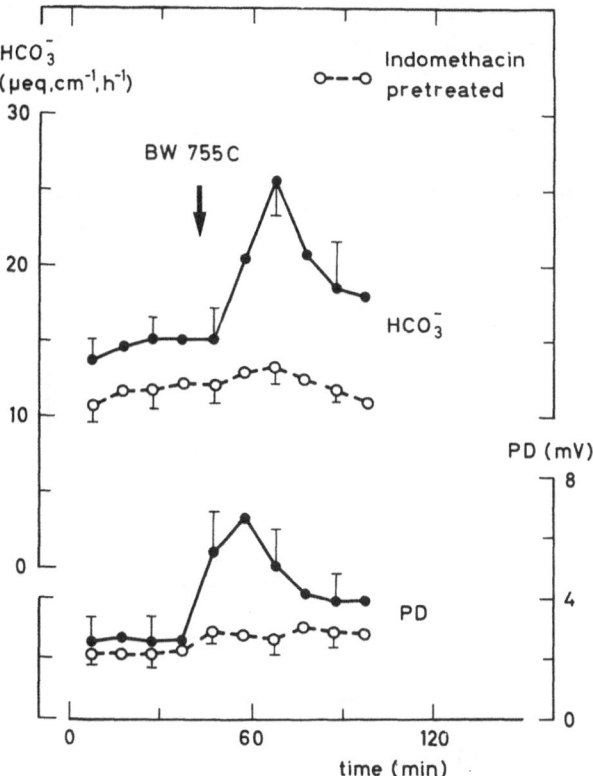

Figure 7.3 Bicarbonate secretion and the transmucosal electrical potential difference in duodenal segments from anaesthetized rats increased significantly following intravenous BW 755C (20 mg kg^{-1}). Indomethacin, given intravenously 40 min prior to BW 755C, prevented this effect ($n = 6$, mean $\pm$ SEM). Reproduced with the kind permission of the authors and *Scand. J. Gastroenterol.*[49]

because of the rapid activation of arachidonic acid metabolism by the sampling procedure. The measurement of eicosanoids in luminal secretions is one approach to following mucosal prostaglandin formation during an experiment. Samples can then be obtained atraumatically. Luminal levels of prostaglandins are assumed to reflect mucosal synthesis[55]. Radioimmunoassays (RIA) have been most widely used, but the risk of non-specific cross-reactivity has to be considered. Measurements with gas chromatography–mass spectrometry (GC–MS) combine high specificity with high sensitivity.

Instillation of acid (100 mol L^{-1}) in canine denervated fundic pouches increased outputs of bicarbonate and PGE$_2$ (determined by RIA)[9]. Pretreatment of the animals with indomethacin (2.5 mg kg^{-1}) decreased bicarbonate and PGE$_2$ concurrently. In humans, 5 minutes' exposure of the gastric mucosa to 150 mmol L^{-1} HCl increased luminal levels of PGE$_2$ (GC–MS)[56]. Cell shedding to the lumen was monitored by measurements of DNA in luminal contents, and no increase was observed following this acid exposure. The gastric secretion of bicarbonate was not measured in this study. Histamine-H$_2$-blockers were used in these studies to suppress gastric acid secretion.

Recent studies have provided clear evidence that spontaneous bicarbonate secretion by isolated amphibian duodenum is dependent on endogenous formation of type E prostaglandins[8]. PGE$_2$ accumulated in the serosal bathing fluid under basal conditions and replacement with a prostaglandin-free solution caused a significant decrease in bicarbonate secretion (Figure 7.4). When the original bathing fluid was re-applied, bicarbonate secretion returned to the

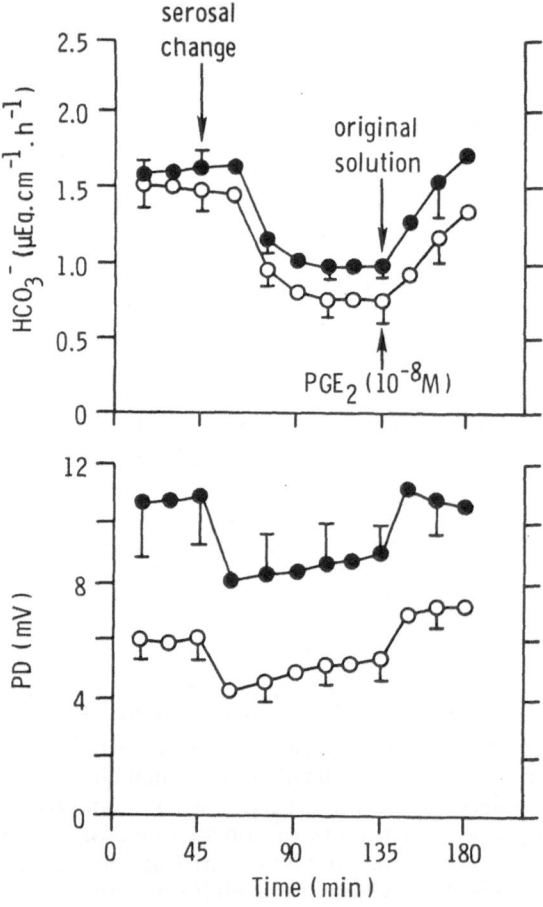

Figure 7.4 Spontaneous alkaline secretion by amphibian duodenum *in vitro* and the transmucosal potential difference decreased when the serosal bathing solution was replaced by fresh solution. The PGE concentration had increased to 8.5×10^{-9} mol L^{-1} immediately before replacement. Re-application of the original solution (solid circles) or addition of 10^{-8} mol L^{-1} PGE$_2$ to the serosal solution (open circles) restored the initial values for bicarbonate secretion and potential difference (mean ± SEM). Reproduced with the kind permission of the authors and *Gastroenterology*[8]

initial values.

Simultaneous measurement of mucosal outputs of bicarbonate and PGE_2 have been performed *in vivo* in the duodenum of dogs (RIA)[9] and humans (GC–MS)[57]. Basal secretion of bicarbonate, as well as outputs of PGE_2, decreased following treatment with indomethacin. Acid stimulation of duodenal bicarbonate secretion was paralleled by increases in levels of PGE_2 in the lumen of both dogs and humans. The rise in bicarbonate secretion as well as in luminal PGE_2 was partly prevented by indomethacin in both species. Topical acid also increased bicarbonate secretion and luminal PGE_2 levels in anaesthetized cats[7]. Measurements of mucosal PGE_2 formation *in vivo* thus provide direct evidence that basal duodenal bicarbonate secretion in mammals is at least partly regulated by local prostaglandin formation. Furthermore, both the gastric and duodenal bicarbonate responses to topical acid are highly dependent on mucosal prostaglandin generation.

NEURAL AND HUMORAL CONTROL OF GASTRODUODENAL BICARBONATE SECRETION

In addition to the local (tissue) control by endogenous prostaglandins, gastric and duodenal mucosal bicarbonate secretion is under neural and humoral influence. Sham-feeding stimulates gastric bicarbonate secretion in humans and antimuscarinic drugs inhibit this response[10,11]. This finding is in line with previous observations that carbachol increases alkaline secretion by gastric mucosa in experimental animals *in vitro*[13] and *in vivo*[21]. Furthermore, electrical stimulation of the vagal nerves in cats[58] and rats[59] increases not only gastric secretion of acid but also the secretion of bicarbonate by gastric and duodenal mucosa. The duodenal response is abolished by hexamethonium but is only partly inhibited by atropine, suggesting that transmission is, in part, non-cholinergic. The duodenal response suggests the occurrence of duodenal mucosal anticipatory protection against acid discharged from the stomach. It has been recently observed that intrahypothalamic injection of corticotropin releasing factor[60] or intravenous administration of pirenzepine[61] increases gastric and duodenal bicarbonate secretion respectively in the rat. These responses are abolished by vagotomy, thus providing evidence that the secretions are under central neural control.

Luminal acid stimulates bicarbonate secretion in both the stomach and the duodenum, and tissue prostaglandin synthesis is important in mediating this response[6,7,9,28,29,62]. However, strong evidence has been produced that humoral factors and neural mechanisms are also involved in the mediation (Figure 7.5). Exposure of the lumen of one isolated mucosa *in vitro* to acid thus stimulates the alkaline secretion by a second (non-acid-exposed) mucosa mounted in parallel[6]. Exposure of human mucosa to luminal acid increases the release of vasoactive intestinal peptide[63] and β-endorphin[64]. Both of these peptides stimulate duodenal mucosal alkaline secretion *in vivo*[65–67] and may have a role in humoral mediation of the alkaline response. Hexamethonium and atropine inhibit the rise in duodenal mucosal alkaline secretion in response to luminal acid, thus indicating the involvement of neural control in the mediation.

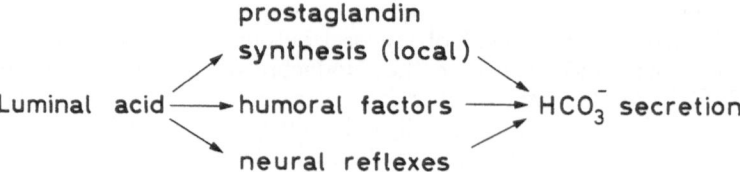

Figure 7.5 Summary of the factors mediating the increase in mucosal bicarbonate secretion in response to luminal acid

SUMMARY AND OUTLOOK

Amphibian and mammalian gastric and duodenal mucosa is capable of actively secreting bicarbonate into the lumen. The unstirred layer consisting of bicarbonate and mucus covers the gastroduodenal epithelial surface and is considered to be the first line of defence against agressive luminal factors like acid and pepsin. The increase of bicarbonate secretion following exposure of the mucosa to acid is dependent on the formation of prostaglandins by the mucosa, but neural and hormonal factors are also involved in this defensive mechanism. Further studies are needed to elucidate the interrelationship between these different regulatory factors.

There has been a recent report of decreased basal and acid-stimulated bicarbonate secretion in the duodenal bulb of duodenal ulcer patients without an active ulcer[68]. It remains to be established whether this is due to a decrease in the capacity of the bicarbonate transport systems (primary or secondary to recurrent ulcers) or to decreased activity of the above-mentioned mediators. Further research in this field, including *in vivo* measurements of prostaglandin formation will contribute to a better understanding of the pathogenesis of duodenal ulcers.

The protective effect of exogenous prostaglandins against experimental damage to the gastroduodenal mucosa may partly reflect stimulation of mucosal secretion of bicarbonate (and mucus)[69]. However, in several damage models in which prostaglandins were protective[70] and in particular when absolute ethanol is used as the damaging agent, other mechanisms must be involved[71,72]. In the treatment of peptic ulcers, the protective and bicarbonate-stimulating properties of prostaglandin E analogues seem less important. Thus, doses with a strong gastric acid inhibitor effect seem needed to achieve healing rates comparable to those obtained with histamine-H_2-blockers[73]. However, future studies may identify subgroups of peptic ulcer patients who may benefit more from drugs that stimulate endogenous defence mechanisms rather than inhibiting aggressive factors.

ACKNOWLEDGEMENTS

The authors thank Mrs Eva Hendig for excellent secretarial assistance.

This work was supported by the Nanna Swartz foundation, Uppsala, Sweden and the Swedish Medical Research Council (grant O4X-3515), Stockholm, Sweden.

REFERENCES

1. Ross, I.N., Bahari, H.M.M. and Turnberg, L.A. (1981). The pH gradient across mucus adherent to rat fundic mucosa *in vivo* and the effect of potential damaging agents. *Gastroenterology*, **81**, 713–718
2. Flemström, G. and Kivilaakso, E. (1983). Demonstration of a pH gradient at the luminal surface of rat duodenum *in vivo* and its dependence on mucosal alkaline secretion. *Gastroenterology*, **84**, 787–794
3. Quigley, E.M.M. and Turnberg, L.a. (1987). pH of the microclimate lining human gastric and duodenal mucosa in vivo. Studies in control subjects and in duodenal ulcer patients. *Gastroenterology*, **92**, 1876–1884
4. Archambault, A.P., Rovelstad, R.A. and Carlson, H.C. (1967). In situ pH of duodenal bulb contents in normals and duodenal ulcer subjects. *Gastroenterology*, **52**, 940–947
5. Flemström, G. and Turnberg, L.A. (1984). Gastroduodenal defence mechanisms. *Clin. Gastroenterol.*, **13**(2), 327–354
6. Heylings, J.R., Garner, A. and Flemström, G. (1984). Regulation of gastroduodenal HCO_3^- transport by luminal acid in the frog *in vitro*. *Am. J. Physiol.*, **246**, G235–242
7. Flemström, G., Garner, A., Nylander, O., Hurst, B.C. and Heylings, J.R. (1982). Surface epithelial HCO_3^- transport by mammalian duodenum *in vivo*. *Am. J. Physiol.*, **243**, G348–358
8. Heylings, J.R., Hampson, S.E. and Garner, A. (1985). Endogenous E-type prostaglandins in regulation of basal alkaline secretion by amphibian duodenum *in vitro*. *Gastroenterology*, **88**, 290–294
9. Konturek, S.J., Bilski, J., Tasler, J. and Laskiewics, J. (1984). Gastroduodenal alkaline response to acid and taurocholate in conscious dogs. *Am. J. Physiol.*, **247**, G149–154
10. Feldman, M. (1985). Gastric H^+ and HCO_3^- secretion in response to sham-feeding in humans. *Am. J. Physiol.*, **248**, G188–191
11. Forssell, H., Stenquist, B. and Olbe, L. (1985). Vagal stimulation of human gastric bicarbonate secretion. *Gastroenterology*, **89**, 581–586
12. Nylander, O. and Flemström, G. (1986). Effects of alpha-receptor agonists and antagonists on duodenal surface epithelial HCO_3^- secretion in the rat *in vivo*. *Acta Physiol. Scand.*, **125**, 433–442
13. Flemström, G. (1977). Active alkalinization by amphibian gastric fundic mucosa *in vitro*. *Am. J. Physiol.*, **233**, E1–12
14. Rees, W.D.W., Gibbons, L.C. and Turnberg, L.A. (1984). Alkali secretion by isolated rabbit gastric mucosa: effects of non-steroidal anti-inflammatory drugs and prostaglandins. *Scand. J. Gastroenterol.*, **19** (Suppl. 92), 63–68
15. Mattsson, H., Carlsson, K. and Carlsson, E. (1984). Omeprazole is devoid of effect on alkaline secretion in isolated guinea-pig antral mucosa. In Allen, A., Flemström, G., Garner, A., Silen, W. and Turnberg, L.A. (eds.) *Mechanisms of Mucosal Protection in the Upper Gastrointestinal Tract*, pp. 141–146. (New York: Raven Press)
16. Flemström, G. and Mattsson, H. (1986). Effects of omeprazole on gastric and duodenal bicarbonate secretion. *Scand. J. Gastroenterol.*, **21** (Suppl. 118), 65–67
17. Kuo, Y.J., Shanbour, L.L. and Miller, T.A. (1983). Effects of 16,16-dimethyl-prostaglandin E_2 on alkaline secretion in isolated canine gastric mucosa. *Dig. Dis. Sci.*, **12**, 1121–1126
18. Kauffman, G.L., Reeve, J.J. and Grossman, M.I. (1980). Gastric bicarbonate secretion: Effect of topical and intravenous 16,16-dimethyl-prostaglandin E_2. *Am. J. Physiol.*, **239**, G44–48
19. Miller, T.A., Kraemer, B.B., Henagan, J.M. and Foucar, C.E. (1983). Topical 16,16-dimethyl-prostaglandin E_2. Effects on gastric morphology, hydrogen ion loss and bicarbonate secretion. *Dig. Dis. Sci.*, **28**, 641–648
20. Smeaton, L.A., Hirst, B.H., Allen, A. and Garner, A. (1983). Gastric and duodenal HCO_3^- transport *in vivo*: influence of prostaglandins. *Am. J. Physiol.*, **245**, G751–759
21. Garner, A. and Flemström, G. (1978). Gastric HCO_3^- secretion in the guinea-pig. *Am. J. Physiol.*, **234**, E535–545
22. Forssell, H. and Olbe, L. (1985). Continuous computerized determination of gastric bicarbonate secretion in man. *Scand. J. Gastroenterol.*, **20**, 767–774
23. Feldman, M. (1983). Gastric bicarbonate secretion in humans. Effect of pentagastrin, bethanechol, and 11,16,16-trimethyl-prostaglandin E_2. *J. Clin. Invest.*, **72**, 295–303

24. Florey, H.W. and Harding, H.E. (1934). Further observations on the secretion of Brunner's glands. *J. Pathol. Bacteriol.*, **39**, 255–276
25. Flemström, G. (1980). Stimulation of HCO_3^- transport in isolated proximal bullfrog duodenum by prostaglandins. *Am. J. Physiol.*, **239**, G198–204
26. Simson, J.N.L., Merhav, A. and Silen, W. (1981). Alkaline secretion by amphibian duodenum. I. General characteristics. *Am. J. Physiol.*, **240**, G401–408
27. Isenberg, J.I., Flemström, G. and Johansson, C. (1984). Mucosal bicarbonate secretion is significantly greater in the proximal versus distal duodenum in the rat *in vivo*. In Allen, A., Flemström, G., Garner, A., Silen, W. and Turnberg, L.A. (eds.) *Mechanisms of Mucosal Protection in the Upper Gastrointestinal Tract*, pp. 175–180. (New York: Raven Press)
28. Isenberg, J.I., Smedfors, B. and Johansson, C. (1985). Effect of graded doses of intraluminal H^+, prostaglandin E_2, and inhibition of endogenous prostaglandin synthesis on proximal duodenal bicarbonate secretion in the unanaesthetized rat. *Gastroenterology*, **88**, 303–307
29. Isenberg, J.I., Hogan, D.L., Koss, M.A. and Selling, J.A. (1986). Human duodenal mucosal bicarbonate secretion: evidence for basal secretion and stimulation by hydrochloric acid and a synthetic prostaglandin E_1 analogue. *Gastroenterology*, **91**, 370–378 .
30. Kivilaakso, E. and Flemström, G. (1984). Surface pH gradient in gastroduodenal mucosa. *Scand. J. Gastroenterol.*, **19** (Suppl. 105), 50–52
31. Takeuchi, K., Magee, D., Critchlow, J., Matthew, J. and Silen, W. (1983). Studies of the pH gradient and thickness of frog gastric mucus gel. *Gastroenterology*, **84**, 331–40
32. Svanes, K., Ito, S., Takeuchi, K. and Silen, W. (1982). Restitution of the surface epithelium of the *in vitro* frog gastric mucosa after damage with hyperosmolar sodium chloride. Morphologic and physiologic characteristics. *Gastroenterology*, **82**, 1409–1426
33. Flemström, G., Heylings, J.R. and Garner, A. (1982). Gastric and duodenal HCO_3^- transport *in vitro*: Effects of hormones and local transmitters. *Am. J. Physiol.*, **242**, G100–110
34. Konturek, S.J., Tasler, J., Bilski, J. and Kania, J. (1983). Prostaglandins and alkaline secretion from oxyntic, antral, and duodenal mucosa of the dog. *Am. J. Physiol.*, **245**, G539–546
35. Johansson, C., Aly, A., Nilsson, E. and Flemström, G. (1983). Stimulation of gastric bicarbonate secretion by E_2 prostaglandins in man. *Adv. Prostagl. Thromboxane Leukotriene Res.*, **12**, 395–401
36. Rees, W.D.W., Gibbons, L.C., Warhurst, G. and Turnberg, L.A. (1984). Studies of bicarbonate secretion by the normal human stomach *in vivo*: Effect of aspirin, sodium taurocholate, and prostaglandin E_2. In Allen, A., Flemström, G., Garner, A., Silen, W. and Turnberg, L.A. (eds.) *Mechanisms of Mucosal Protection in the Upper Gastrointestinal Tract*, pp. 119–122. (New York: Raven Press)
37. Konturek, S.J., Tasler, J., Bilski, J., Kaminska, A. and Laskiewicz, J. (1984). Role of prostaglandins in alkaline secretion from the gastroduodenal mucosa exposed to acid and taurocholate. *Scand. J. Gastroenterol.*, **19** (Suppl. 92), 69–74
38. O'Brien, P.E. and Carter, D.C. (1975). Effect of gastric secretory inhibitors on the gastric mucosal barrier. *Gut*, **16**, 437–442
39. Smedfors, B. and Johansson, C. (1986). Stimulation of duodenal bicarbonate secretion by misoprostol. *Dig. Dis. Sci.*, **31** (Suppl.), 96S–100S
40. Whittle, B.J.R., Kauffman, G.L. Jr. and Boughton-Smith, N.K. (1984). Stimulation of gastric alkaline secretion by stable prostacyclin analogues in rat and dog. *Eur. J. Pharmacol.*, **100**, 277–283
41. Keogh, J.P., Stanier, A.M., Heylings, J.R., Allen, A. and Garner, A. (1985). Effects of eicosanoids on amphibian duodenal luminal alkaline secretion *in vitro*. *Gut*, **26**, A1110
42. Garner, A., Flemström, G. and Heylings, J.R. (1979). Effects of anti-inflammatory agents and prostaglandins on acid and bicarbonate secretions in the amphibian-isolated gastric mucosa. *Gastroenterology*, **77**, 451–457
43. Garner, A. (1977). Effects of acetylsalicylate on alkalinization, acid secretion and electrogenic properties in the isolated gastric mucosa. *Acta Physiol. Scand.*, **99**, 281–291
44. Ross, I.N. and Turnberg, L.A. (1983). Studies on the mucus-bicarbonate barrier on rat fundic mucosa: the effects of luminal pH and a stable prostaglandin analogue. *Gut*, **24**, 1030–1033
45. Feldman, M. and Colturi, T.J. (1984). Effect of indomethacin on gastric acid and bicarbonate secretion in humans. *Gastroenterology*, **87**, 1339–1343
46. Selling, J.A., Hogan, D.L., Koss, M.A. and Isenberg, J.I. (1985). Human proximal versus

distal duodenal bicarbonate secretion: effect of endogenous prostaglandin synthesis. *Gastroenterology*, **88**, 1580

47. Flemström, G., Bergman, A. and Bridén, S. (1984). Stimulation of mucosal bicarbonate secretion in rat duodenum *in vivo* by BW755C. *Acta Physiol. Scand.*, **121**, 39–43

48. Boughton-Smith, N. and Whittle, B.J.R. (1983). Stimulation and inhibition of prostacyclin formation in the gastric mucosa and ileum *in vitro* by anti-inflammatory agents. *Br. J. Pharmacol.*, **78**, 173–180

49. Flemström, G., Bridén, S. and Kivilaakso, E. (1984). Stimulation by BW755C and inhibition by cysteamine of duodenal epithelial alkaline secretion suggest a role of endogenous prostaglandin in mucosal protection. *Scand. J. Gastroenterol.*, **19** (Suppl. 92), 101–105

50. Hollander, D., Tarnawski, A., Gergely, H. and Zipser, R.D. (1984). Sucralfate protection of the gastric mucosa against ethanol-induced injury: a prostaglandin-mediated process? *Scand. J. Gastroenterol.* **19**, (Suppl. 101), 97–102

51. Szelenyi, I., Postius, S. and Engler, H. (1983). Evidence for a functional cytoprotective effect produced by antacids in the rat stomach. *Eur. J. Pharmacol.*, **88**, 403–406

52. Crampton, J.R., Gibbons, L.C. and Rees, W.D.W. (1985). Effect of sucralfate on isolated amphibian gastroduodenal bicarbonate secretion. *Gut*, **26**, A1119

53. Crampton, J.R., Gibbons, L.C. and Rees, W.D.W. (1985). Effect of aluminium on bicarbonate secretion by isolated amphibian gastroduodenal mucosa. *Gut*, **26**, A1150

54. Guslandi, M. (1985). Sucralfate and gastric bicarbonate. *Pharmacology*, **31**, 298–300

55. Aly, A. (1985). Studies on prostaglandin formation in gastroduodenal mucosa of man. *Thesis*. (Stockholm: Karolinska Institute)

56. Aly, A., Gréen, K. and Johansson, C. (1985). Acid instillation increases gastric luminal prostaglandin E_2 output in man. *Acta Med. Scand.*, **218**, 505–510

57. Selling, J.A., Hogan, D.L., Aly, A., Koss, M.A. and Isenberg, J.I. (1987). Indomethacin inhibits duodenal mucosal bicarbonate secretion and endogenous prostaglandin E_2 output in human subjects. *Ann. Intern. Med.*, **106**, 368–371

58. Nylander, O., Fändriks, L., Delbro, D. and Flemström, G. (1985). Effect of vagal nerve stimulation on gastroduodenal HCO_3^- secretion in the cat. *Acta Physiol. Scand.*, **123**, 30A

59. Jönsson, C., Nylander, O., Flemström, G. and Fändriks, L. (1986). Vagal stimulation of duodenal HCO_3^- secretion in the rat. *Acta Physiol. Scand.* (In press)

60. Gunion, M.W., Taché, Y. and Kauffman, G.L. (1985). Intrahypothalamic corticotropin-releasing factor (CRF) increases gastric bicarbonate content. *Gastroenterology*, **88**, 1407

61. Säfsten, B. and Flemström, G. (1986). Stimulatory effect of pirenzepine on mucosal bicarbonate secretion in rat duodenum *in vivo*. *Acta Physiol. Scand.* (In press)

62. Takeuchi, K., Furukawa, O., Tanaka, H. and Okabe, S. (1986). A new model of duodenal ulcers induced in rats by indomethacin plus histamine. *Gastroenterology*, **90**, 636–645

63. Bloom, S.R., Mitchell, S.J., Greenberg, G.R., Christofides, N., Domschke, W., Domschke, S., Mitznegg, P. and Demling, L. (1978). Release of VIP, secretin and motilin after duodenal acidification in man. *Acta Hepato-gastroenterol.*, **25**, 365–368

64. Matsumura, M., Wada, H. and Saito, S. (1983). Effect of solution of low pH on releases of β-endorphin-like immunoreactivity and ACTH-like immunoreactivity from human gastric antral mucosa *in vitro*. *Gastroenterol. Jpn.*, **18**, 210–215

65. Isenberg, J.I., Wallin, B., Johansson, C., Smedfors, B., Mutt, V., Takemoto, K. and Emås, S. (1984). Secretin, VIP, and PHI stimulate rat proximal surface epithelial bicarbonate secretion *in vivo*. *Regul. Pept.*, **8**, 315–320

66. Flemström, G., Kivilaakso, E., Bridén, S., Nylander, O. and Jedstedt, G. (1985). Gastroduodenal bicarbonate secretion in mucosal protection. Possible role of vasoactive intestinal peptide and opiates. *Dig. Dis. Sci.*, **30** (Suppl.), 63S–68S

67. Flemström, G., Hedstedt, G. and Nylander, O. (1986). β-endorphin and enkephalins stimulate duodenal mucosal alkaline secretion in the rat *in vivo*. *Gastroenterology*, **90**, 368–372

68. Isenberg, J.I., Selling, J.A., Hogan, D.L., and Koss, M.A. (1987). Impaired proximal duodenal mucosal bicarbonate secretion in patients with duodenal ulcer. *N. Engl. J. Med.*, **316**, 374–379

69. Kollberg, B., Aly, A. and Johansson, C. (1981). Protection of the rat gastric mucosa by prostaglandin E_2: Possible relation to stimulation of the alkaline secretion. *Acta Physiol. Scand.*, **113**, 189–192

70. Robert, A., Nezamis, J.E., Lancaster, C. and Hanchar, A.J. (1979). Cytoprotection by prosta-glandins in rats. *Gastroenterology*, **77**, 433–443
71. Johansson, C., Aly, A., Befrits, R., Smedfors, B. and Uribe, A. (1985). Protection of the gastroduodenal mucosa by prostaglandins. *Scand. J. Gastroenterol.*, **20** (Suppl. 110), 41–48
72. Reichstein, B.J. and Cohen, M.M. (1984). Effect of acetazolamide on rat gastric mucosal protection and stimulated bicarbonate secretion with 16,16-dimethyl PGE_2. *J. Lab. Clin. Med.*, **104**, 797–804
73. Aly, A. (1987). Prostaglandins in clinical treatment of gastroduodenal mucosal lesions: a review. *Scand. J. Gastroenterol.*, **22**, (Suppl. 137), 43–49
74. van Kolfschoten, A.A., Hagelen, F., Hillen, F.C., Jager, L.P., Zandberg, P. and van Noord-wijk, J. (1983). Protective effects of prostaglandins against ulcerogenic activity of indomethacin during different stages of erosion development in rat stomach. Role of acid and bicarbonate secretion. *Dig. Dis. Sci.*, **28**, 1127–1132
75. Gascoigne, A.D. and Hirst, B.H. (1981). Prostaglandins alter the relationship between gastric hydrogen ion concentration and flow: evidence for stimulation of non-parietal secretion in the cat. *J. Physiol.*, **316**, 427–438
76. Garner, A. and Heylings, J.R. (1979). Stimulation of alkaline secretion in amphibian-isolated gastric mucosa by 16,16-dimethyl PGE_2 and $PGF_{2\alpha}$. *Gastroenterology*, **76**, 497–503
77. Schiessel, R., Allison, J.G., Barzilai, A., Fluscher, L.A., Matthews, J.B., Merhav, A., Simson, J. and Silen, W. (1980). Failure of 16,16-dimethyl-prostaglandin E_2 to stimulate alkaline secretion in the isolated amphibian gastric mucosa. *Gastroenterology*, **78**, 1513–1517
78. Simson, J.N.L., Merhav, A. and Silen, W. (1981). Alkaline secretion by amphibian duodenum. III. Effects of DBcAMP, theophylline, and prostaglandins. *Am. J. Physiol.*, **241**, G528–536

8
Eicosanoids and gastrointestinal motility

P. K. Moore

INTRODUCTION

The effect on gastrointestinal motility of prostaglandins, thromboxanes and more recently the leukotriene family has been enthusiastically researched ever since Kurzrok and Lieb[1] first demonstrated the contractile effect of seminal 'prostaglandin' on the isolated rabbit gut preparation. In the space of the last fifty years the gastrointestinal tract has been shown to be an excellent source of the enzymes responsible for the synthesis and break-down of eicosanoids and this, coupled with their potent biological effects on gut motility and secretions, has prompted a search for their physiological role(s) in this part of the body.

This chapter summarizes current knowledge concerning the function of eicosanoids in the control of gut motility in health and disease. Several excellent reviews have already appeared on this subject[2-6].

METHODS FOR STUDYING THE EFFECT OF EICOSANOIDS ON MOTILITY

The effect of eicosanoids on gastrointestinal motility has been studied both in vitro using isolated segments of oesophagus, stomach, ileum, colon or rectum and in vivo following injection or infusion into conscious or anaesthetized animals including man.

Each of these procedures have their advantages and their disadvantages. For in vitro experiments, preparations are either suspended in physiological salt solution and mounted in a thermostatically-controlled organ bath or superfused with anticoagulated blood or oxygenated salt solution as part of a superfusion cascade experiment[7]. In either case, drug-induced contractions or relaxations of the preparation are monitored by means of force transducers connected to a pen recorder.

The major benefits of *in vitro* experiments are:

(1) That the longitudinal and circular muscle layers of the gut may be studied independently,

(2) Results obtained are not complicated by factors such as the release of other local hormones (or hormones) or changes in blood flow to the gut, and,

(3) Such preparations will respond to unstable eicosanoids (e.g. PGI_2 and TxA_2) which, because of their chemical evanescence, cannot be studied directly in intact animals.

Additionally, *in vitro* preparations, set up either in the organ bath or as part of a superfusion cascade arrangement, are normally sensitive to nanogram (and sometimes picogram) amounts of eicosanoids, and are inexpensive and simple to prepare and work with. Since gastrointestinal smooth muscle will respond to a variety of other local hormones and neurotransmitters, their selectivity towards prostanoids may be increased by including a mixture or 'cocktail' of antagonist drugs in the bathing solution. In this way it is frequently possible to detect nanogram quantities of eicosanoid in the presence of microgram quantities of substances like acetylcholine, 5-hydroxytryptamine or histamine.

In contrast, the major drawbacks of *in vitro* experiments are:

(1) Because there is no intact blood supply to gut smooth muscle *in vitro*, the central region of particularly thick tissues may well become hypoxic during the experiment thereby altering responsiveness to drugs.

(2) Drugs administered into an organ bath or over a cascade of tissues diffuse into the muscle in a physiologically abnormal manner, i.e. directly across the membrane of the cells and not via the bloodstream.

(3) Possibly because of the reasons outlined above, it is not unknown for drugs to affect gastrointestinal motility differently *in vivo* and *in vitro*.

The second procedure, estimation of the effect of drugs on gut motility *in vivo*, requires more complicated and time-consuming techniques but does provide an invaluable pointer to what happens in the intact animal. Numerous *in vivo* techniques are available. The very earliest attempts to study the effect of eicosanoids on gut motility *in vivo*, for example, were made by direct observation through an abdominal window in anaesthetized rabbits[8]. Subsequently, more accurate and quantifiable procedures have been developed. Intraluminal pressure in a particular part of the gastrointestinal tract of either anaesthetized animals or conscious humans may be measured by means of air-filled balloons connected to pressure transducers and inserted into the ileum, colon or rectum. In recent years, less invasive techniques such as radiotelemetry have been used. This procedure involves using a scintillation counter coupled to a ratemeter to monitor the position in the alimentary tract of a swallowed capsule containing a radioactive source. Similarly, capsules containing a radio-opaque source or radiotransmitter which may be easily detected on passage through the gut have become increasingly used in the last few years to determine the effect of drugs (including eicosanoids) on gastrointestinal propulsion in intact animals.

146

EFFECT OF EICOSANOIDS ON MOTILITY *IN VITRO*

Longitudinal muscle

As a general rule, prostanoids contract longitudinal smooth muscle of all parts of the gut *in vitro*. In the majority of species this effect is most obvious in the stomach[9–11], ileum[2,12–14] and colon[2,11,15] with only feeble or no observable contractions of the oesophagus or rectum even at high doses. The exception is the chick rectum which responds to as little as 1–5 ng of PGE_2 or $PGF_{2\alpha}$[16].

For obvious reasons, those preparations which have been routinely employed to bioassay prostaglandins in tissue extracts, perfusates etc. have been most used to study the structure–activity relationship of different eicosanoids. The rank order of contractile potency of '2' series prostanoids on 5 commonly used gut smooth muscle preparations is shown in Table 8.1. In each tissue the most potent prostanoid was PGE_2.

However, the biological activity of unstable eicosanoids like PGI_2 and TxA_2 may be underestimated using *in vitro* experiments of this type. Both PGI_2 and TxA_2 decompose spontaneously into products, 6-oxo-$PGF_{1\alpha}$ and TxB_2 respectively, which have little or no effect on gut contractility. In contrast, the chemical break-down products of PGG_2/PGH_2 are PGE_2, $PGF_{2\alpha}$ and PGD_2 which have potent spasmogenic activity on longitudinal muscle. Furthermore, the major prostanoid formed enzymatically from PGG_2 in the gut is likely to be PGI_2 which also contracts longitudinal muscle of the gastrointestinal tract[17]. For these reasons, the biological activity of prostaglandin endoperoxides on the gut relative to other eicosanoids may be overestimated.

The extreme chemical lability of TxA_2 ($t_{1/2} = 30$–35 s) provides further problems for the prostanoid researcher since reproducible dose-response curves for this prostanoid cannot be constructed in the normal way using tissues mounted in organ baths. The biological activity of TxA_2 may be measured using superfused preparations set up in cascade. For this purpose TxA_2 may be generated in situ, either from perfused guinea-pig lungs challenged with arachidonic acid or following incubation of arachidonic acid with a mixture of ram seminal vesicle and human platelet microsomes. Experiments of this sort have revealed that although TxA_2 potently contracts vascular tissue it has little action on commonly-used gut tissues such as the guinea-pig ileum or rat stomach strip[18].

An alternative approach to studying the pharmacology of TxA_2 has been

Table 8.1 Potency of some prostanoids and their chemical analogues on 5 commonly-used bioassay preparations

Rat stomach strip	PGE_2 > U46619 > U44049 > PGH_2 > $PGF_{2\alpha}$ > PGD_2 > PGI_2 > 6-oxo-$PGF_{1\alpha}$ > 6,15-dioxo-$PGF_{1\alpha}$ > TxB_2
Guinea-pig stomach	PGE_2 > PGI_2 > $PGF_{2\alpha}$ > PGD_2 = U46619
Guinea-pig ileum	PGE_2 > U46619 > $PGF_{2\alpha}$ > PGD_2 > PGI_2 > 6-oxo-$PGF_{1\alpha}$ > TxB_2
Dog stomach	PGE_2 > PGI_2 > PGD_2 > $PGF_{2\alpha}$ > U46619
Chick ileum	PGE_2 > PGI_2 > $PGF_{2\alpha}$ > PGD_2 = U46619

the use of U46619 and its isomer U44019. These stable epoxymethano derivatives of PGG_2 behave pharmacologically as TxA_2 agonists. On guinea-pig ileum preparation, U46619 produced contraction but was some three orders of magnitude less potent than PGE_2[19].

Prostanoids containing 1 or 3 double bonds have also been assessed for biological activity on longitudinal smooth muscle *in vitro*[11,20]. In general, prostanoids of the '1' and '3' series have relatively similar contractile potency to the '2' series metabolites of arachidonic acid shown in Table 8.1. The order of potency within each series varies as follows: $E_1 = E_2 > E_3$.

Prostanoid metabolites lacking the C15-hydroxyl moiety (e.g. 15-oxo-PGE_2, 13,14-dihydro-15-oxo-PGE_2) are several orders of magnitude less potent than the parent prostanoids[21]. In contrast, those metabolites which retain the C15-hydroxyl group such as 6-oxo-PGE_1, produced from PGI_2 by action of a selective prostaglandin 9-hydroxydehydrogenase enzyme and 13,14-dihydro prostaglandins of the E, F and I series exhibit considerable spasmogenic activity *in vitro*[22,23]. Of the other arachidonic acid metabolites which have been studied, prostaglandins of the A, B and C series and their 19-hydroxy derivatives have only weak spasmogenic activity on longitudinal (and circular) muscle. However, it is now widely accepted that these prostaglandins do not occur naturally in the body, rather they are formed by dehydration of PGEs following chemical extraction in an acid environment.

As in laboratory animals, longitudinal smooth muscle of the human gut is also contracted by the so-called 'classical' prostanoids, like PGE_2, $PGF_{2\alpha}$ and PGD_2, as well as stable epoxymethano PGG_2 derivatives[24–26]. In contrast, PGI_2 reportedly relaxes human stomach longitudinal muscle strips[25]. A similar atypical relaxation of gut longitudinal smooth muscle has been observed with PGE_1 on the human stomach[27], and rat and frog intestine mounted in organ baths[28,29].

Leukotrienes also contract longitudinal muscle of the gut[30,31]. Unlike prostanoids, the leukotrienes produce a characteristic slowly developing contraction. LTC_4, LTD_4 and LTE_4 are at least three orders of magnitude more potent than histamine on the isolated intact guinea-pig ileum and stripped guinea-pig ileum smooth muscle (GPISM) preparations. The rank order of potency on the guinea-pig ileum is $D_4 > C_4 > E_4$. However, LTC_4 is rapidly converted to LTD_4 by the enzyme γ-glutamyltranspeptidase present in the ileum and thus these 2 leukotrienes may appear to be equipotent on this tissue. The rat stomach strip is also contracted by leukotrienes but is considerably less responsive than the guinea-pig ileum.

Circular muscle

In vitro, the response of circular smooth muscle may be investigated using spirally cut strips of ileum, duodenum or colon[32]. The relaxant effects of eicosanoids may be assessed directly in preparations which exhibit spontaneous tone (e.g. guinea-pig colon) or indirectly by the ability to inhibit KCl-induced contractions in tissues without tone (e.g. guinea-pig ileum). Alternatively, stomach preparations cut transversely across the longitudinal layer to expose the circular muscle may be used[25].

The response of circular muscle to eicosanoids is more variable than that of the longitudinal layer. In general, prostanoids of the E series cause relaxation while PGFs contract circular muscle. However, the effect of other prostanoids depends upon the tissue being studied and the conditions of the experiment.

Rabbit and rat stomach circular muscle strips relax in the presence of PGE_2 and PGD_2 (1–10 ng) but are contracted by $PGF_{2\alpha}$ and PGI_2 (20–50 ng)[25]. In contrast, prostacyclin and its stable methyl ester analogue have been reported to inhibit the spontaneous contractility of the guinea-pig stomach[33]. Dose-response curves for several prostanoids on dog stomach antral circular muscle strips are shown in Figure 8.1. Prostaglandin endoperoxides and their stable chemical analogues have little or no effect on stomach circular smooth muscle.

Circular muscle from other parts of the gut have also been investigated. Guinea-pig colon preparations were contracted by PGD_2, $PGF_{2\alpha}$, PGI_2 and U46619, but relaxed by PGE_2, whereas each of these prostanoids antagonized KCl-induced contractions of the spirally cut ileum of the same species[34,35].

To date, the effects (if any) of leukotrienes on circular smooth muscle of the gut have not been reported.

Gastrointestinal sphincters

Considerably less attention has been paid to the action of eicosanoids on contractility of gut sphincters than has been devoted to their actions on longitudinal/circular muscle. Indeed, the majority of published research has concentrated upon a single example, the lower oesophageal sphincter.

Eiscoanoids have little or no effect on upper oesophageal sphincter pressure or upon oesophageal peristaltic movements. Administration of E-type prostanoids has repeatedly been found to relax the lower oesophageal sphincter, both in animals and in man, while prostanoids of the F series produce constriction[36,37]. Similarly, intravenous infusion of PGE_2 or oral administration of 16,16-dimethyl PGE_2 in human volunteers inhibited contractions of the lower oesophageal sphincter induced by pentagastrin[38].

In man, indomethacin treatment results in an increase in lower oesophageal sphincter pressure suggesting that endogenous prostanoids formed locally in this region of the oesophagus normally exhibit a tonic inhibitory effect[39].

Taken together, these results suggest that certain eicosanoids may play a physiological role in controlling the calibre of the lower oesophageal sphincter.

EFFECT OF EICOSANOIDS ON MOTILITY *IN VIVO*

An important effect of prostanoids on gastrointestinal motility *in vivo* was first suggested over 20 years ago when Bergstrom and his colleagues infused PGE_1 or PGE_2 intravenously into human volunteers, and observed, among other things, that several of the subjects experienced painful abdominal cramps[40]. This finding has subsequently been confirmed in other studies in man[41–43] and may be caused by an increase in intestinal motility. Furthermore, administration of a variety of eicosanoids and their chemical analogues to

149

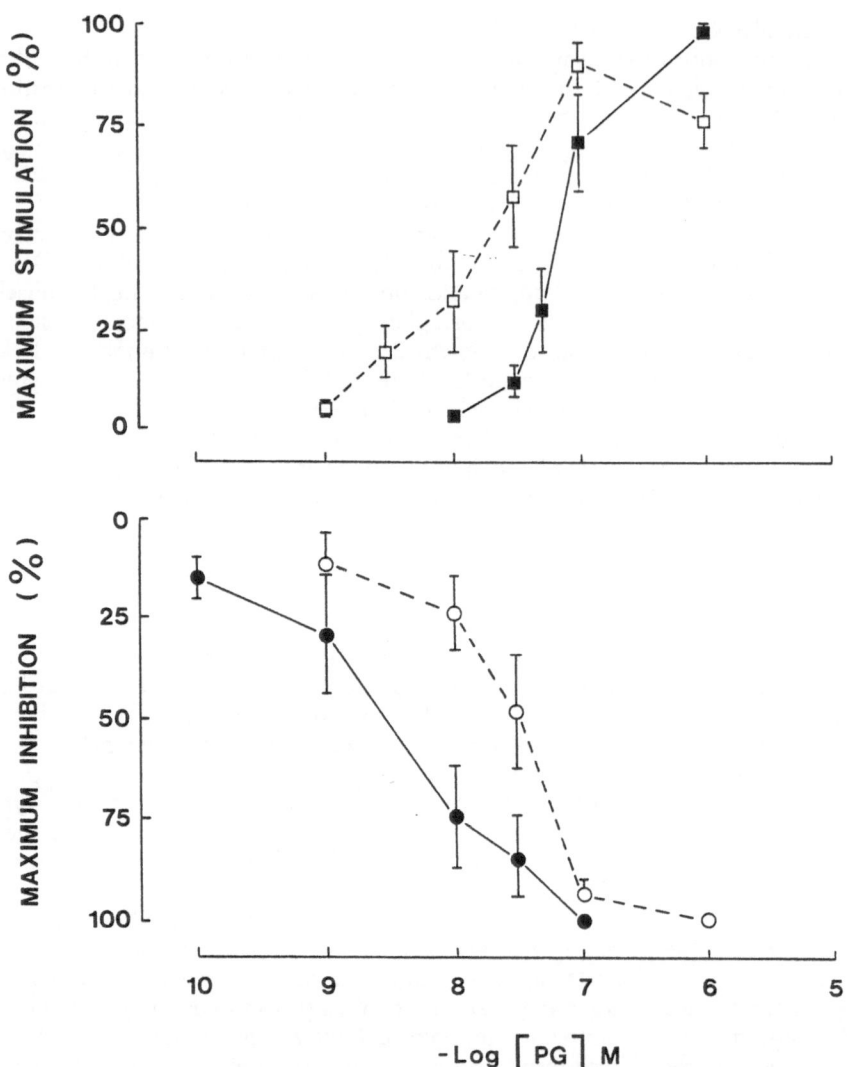

Figure 8.1 Response of dog ileum circular smooth muscle to prostaglandins. PGD_2 (open squares) and $PGF_{2\alpha}$ (closed squares) produced contraction of indomethacin (10^{-5} M) treated preparations (upper graph). PGE_2 (closed circles) and PGI_2 (open circles) caused relaxation (lower graph). Data are means $\pm$ SE, $n = 6$; taken from Sanders, K.M. (1984). *Am. J. Physiol.*, **246**, G361, with permission

pregnant women to induce labour/abortion is associated with a high incidence of vomiting[44–46] which again may reflect augmented gastric motility. Finally, eicosanoids administered orally, intravenously, intra-amniotically or into the vagina cause profuse, watery diarrhoea in humans and experimental animals. The mechanism of action of this diarrhoeagenic effect of eicosanoids is discussed in detail later in this chapter.

The subjective observations outlined above have been supported by carefully controlled scientific studies. Misiewicz et al.[47] measured intraluminal pressure in the small intestine, proximal colon and distal colon in human volunteers by a radiotelemetry technique. Approximately 2 h after oral administration of 2 mg PGE_2, all volunteers experienced gastrointestinal discomfort in the form of colic, desire to defaecate and the passage of loose, watery stools. Simultaneously, a marked increase in propulsive activity of both the small and the large intestine was observed compared with activity in the intestines of placebo-treated controls.

Similar experiments using other prostanoids and other species have produced variable results. Intravenous infusion of $PGF_{2\alpha}$ in man increased motility of the antral portion of the stomach, while similar administration of PGE_2 had the opposite effect[48]. Furthermore, intravenously injected PGE_2 inhibited propulsive activity in the human colon while $PGF_{2\alpha}$ was inactive[49]. Conflicting results have also been obtained using chemically and metabolically stable prostanoid analogues. 16,16-dimethyl PGE_2, for example, has been reported to accelerate[50] or reduce[51] gastric emptying in man, while, in conscious Rhesus monkeys, 15-methyl PGE_2 enhanced gastric[52] but inhibited duodenal[53] motility.

There have been few reports on the effect of chemically labile prostanoids on gut motility in vivo. Prostacyclin, adminstered intravenously or intra-arterially to monkeys or rats, reduced gastric emptying but had little effect on intestinal transit time[54]. This result is in agreement with clinical observations that PGI_2 does not produce the nausea, vomiting and diarrhoea in human volunteers which is such a common side effect of E and F series prostanoids.

Thus, although eicosanoids have potent and, for the most part, reproducible activity on gastrointestinal muscle in vitro, their effects on gut motility in the intact animal are much more variable. As a general rule, $PGF_{2\alpha}$, prostaglandin endoperoxides and PGE_2 analogues appear to stimulate motility of most parts of the gut in most species, whilst naturally occurring prostanoids of the E series and PGI_2 are inhibitory.

MECHANISM OF ACTION

Prostanoids interact directly with receptors on the membranes of gut smooth muscle cells. These receptors are not blocked by atropine, hexamethonium, mepyramine, methysergide, propranolol or phentolamine[55]. Thus, in most cases, the effect of prostanoids on gut motility are not mediated by the release of acetylcholine, histamine, 5-hydroxytryptamine or catecholamines. An exception to this general rule is the guinea-pig ileum preparation where prostanoid-induced contractions may be partially inhibited by atropine and tetrodotoxin, suggesting that a component of the effect is likely to be stimulation of postganglionic cholinergic nerves in the myenteric plexus[56,57]. In addition, the rat duodenum set up in an organ bath may, occasionally, respond to PGE_1 with a relaxation which is blocked by a combination of propranolol and phentolamine suggesting the intermediacy of catecholamines[29].

Gastrointestinal smooth muscle cells are equipped with receptors which respond to different groups of eicosanoids. The relative proportions and number of these receptors varies with the part of the gut under study, the species and the type of smooth muscle (i.e. longitudinal or circular). No single means of classifying prostanoid receptors has been universally accepted. However, according to the classification proposed by Kennedy and his colleagues[58], the predominant receptor on longitudinal muscle is of the EP type. Thus, prostanoids of the E series are the most potent agonists and the responses obtained are antagonized by SC19220[59] and AH6809[60] but unaffected by thromboxane A_2 receptor antagonists such as AH19283 and EPO-45. The pA_2 values for SC19220 and AH6809 on the guinea-pig ileum, using PGE_2 as agonist, are 5.4 and 6.8 respectively.

Presumably the circular muscle layer contains both EP receptors which mediate relaxation and FP receptors which, when occupied by prostanoids of the F series, produce contraction. The lack of effect of TxA_2, U46619 and PGD_2 on longitudinal and circular muscle both *in vitro* and *in vivo* would imply a scarcity of so-called TP and DP receptors in the gut.

Little is known of the events which take place within gut smooth muscle cells after combination of prostanoid with prostanoid receptor. However, it may be assumed that changes in resting membrane potential occur which ultimately lead to an increase or decrease in the amount of calcium available to the contractile proteins. Although the effect of selected prostanoids on electrical activity of circular and longitudinal muscle cells has been reported (and discussed below), it is important to point out that the ionic basis of these events and the way in which they change intracellular free calcium concentrations has not been satisfactorily explained.

The majority of electrophysiological studies have concentrated on the effect of prostanoids on circular muscle. For example, intracellular recording of electrical activity in dog ileum circular muscle cells reveals that the membrane rhythmically depolarizes and repolarizes. These so-called 'slow waves' have a frequency of approximately 10 Hz and an amplitude of about 17 mV. Similar slow waves occur in many other gut smooth muscle cells. In such cells, spontaneous action potentials do not normally arise, contraction of the muscle cell occurring after the depolarization phase of each slow wave. When dog ileal cells are exposed to PGE_2 or PGI_2, each of which is known to reduce contractility in this part of the gut, the amplitude and frequency of slow waves declines. Resting membrane potential also decreases[61].

Prostaglandins of the E series similarly decrease the amplitude and duration of slow waves in dog stomach antral circular smooth muscle[62] and produce hyperpolarization both in this preparation and in antral smooth muscle cells of the guinea-pig stomach[63]. It is likely that the hyperpolarization of circular muscle cells by E and I series prostanoids identified in these experiments follows an increase in membrane conductance to potassium ions.

The effect of prostanoids on electrical properties of longitudinal muscle membranes has also received some attention. PGE_2, $PGF_{2\alpha}$ and PGI_2, which contract the stomach of most species *in vitro* and *in vivo* (see before), produced a depolarization or increase in resting membrane potential in muscle cells of the dog stomach antrum[64-66].

Similarly, prostanoids like $PGF_{2\alpha}$, which contract circular muscle of the gut, produce membrane depolarization when applied to tissues such as the guinea-pig stomach antrum[63].

Thus, one may conclude from these studies that contraction, either of longitudinal or circular muscle of the gut, by prostanoids is associated with membrane depolarization and increased availability of free calcium ions, while relaxation follows membrane hyperpolarization and reduced availability of calcium to the contractile proteins. As previously stated, the ionic base of these effects is largely unknown.

PHYSIOLOGICAL ROLES OF EICOSANOIDS

Numerous chemicals influence gastrointestinal motility. These include substances released from autonomic nerves (i.e. acetylcholine, noradrenaline, purines, substance P and vasoactive intestinal polypeptide), histamine and 5-hydroxytryptamine from mast cells and enterochromaffin cells respectively and finally metabolites of arachidonic acid which are formed on demand by the smooth muscle cells.

Each of these substances no doubt plays a part in the physiological regulation of gut contractility and a derangement in the formation/activity of any of them may have clinical consequences in the form of diarrhoea, constipation and/or colic. The evidence that eicosanoids have a regulatory function in gastrointestinal motility comes from three main sources.

(1) The gastrointestinal tract is an excellent source of enzymes which synthesize and break down eicosanoids[24,25,67–69]. Microsomes prepared from longitudinal and circular muscle convert arachidonic acid to a range of different eicosanoids[70].

(2) As detailed previously, at concentrations which may well occur locally *in vivo*, exogenous eicosanoids (particularly PGI$_2$ and PGE$_2$) have profound effects on the contractility of both muscle layers of the gut.

(3) Inhibitors of eicosanoid biosynthesis alter gut smooth muscle electrical activity and motility which suggests that endogenous prostanoids may be influential.

Experiments using drugs which inhibit arachidonic acid metabolism have suggested that naturally occurring prostanoids have diametrically opposite functions in the two muscle layers of the gut.

Longitudinal muscle: effect of cyclo-oxygenase inhibitors

Non-steroid anti-inflammatory drugs, such as aspirin or indomethacin, have been shown to diminish or, in some preparations, produce complete cessation of the pendular motility of the rabbit small intestine[13]. This effect on contractility was correlated with a reduction in the spontaneous release of prostanoids from the tissue into the organ bath.

Similar results have also been obtained using isolated guinea-pig ileum in which indomethacin treatment reduced the contractile response to exogenous acetylcholine and to electrical (field) stimulation[71,72]. The effect of indomethacin, aspirin and 5,8,11,14-eicosatetraynoic acid (EYA) on the resting tension and spontaneous contractile activity of the isolated guinea-pig taenia coli has also been investigated[73]. In this study, mechanical activity was measured along with alterations in membrane potential determined by a sucrose gap procedure. After 15–20 min exposure to one of the above cyclo-oxygenase inhibitors, both the frequency and the amplitude of the slow-wave contractions were reduced by approximately 70% and in some preparations mechanical activity was abolished altogether. These effects were irreversible. Measurement of membrane potential in these tissues revealed that all three inhibitors produced a consistent and marked reduction in (1) spontaneous spike activity, (2) rhythmic slow changes in resting membrane potential, and (3) bursts of high-frequency spikes which, in this tissue, are associated with mechanical contraction. Thus, results obtained from electrophysiological studies are consistent with the reduction in contractility which follows inhibition of gut prostanoid biosynthesis.

Similar results have been obtained with human tissue. Indomethacin, for example, reduced the spontaneous activity of longitudinal muscle strips of human stomach[74], intestine[75] and colon[76].

Circular muscle: effect of cyclo-oxygenase inhibitors

Unlike the results with longitudinal muscle, exposure of gastrointestinal circular muscle preparations *in vitro* to cyclo-oxygenase-blocking concentrations of indomethacin increases (not decreases) the frequency and force of spontaneous contractions. Additionally, the contractile response to spasmogens such as acetylcholine is augmented. To date, such conclusions have been drawn from experiments using muscle strips prepared from dog and guinea-pig stomach antrum[63,77], dog ileum[62,78] and cat ileum[79]. In each case, the increased mechanical activity following inhibition of prostanoid biosynthesis took about 1 hour to develop fully. The effect of indomethacin on circular muscle has been examined electrophysiologically. The membrane potential of single antral muscle cells was measured with an implanted microelectrode. Continuous recording from these cells revealed three important consequences of indomethacin treatment:

(1) Depolarization of the membrane potential by 3 mV,
(2) Maximum depolarization achieved during normal rhythmic slow waves was increased by an average of 4 mV, and
(3) Duration of slow waves was increased by in excess of 1 s.

These changes are shown in Figure 8.2.

Thus, measurement of both electrophysiological and mechanical properties of stomach and ileal circular smooth muscle suggests an excitatory action of indomethacin on motility implying that the predominant arachidonic acid metabolite in these parts of the gut must normally act to reduce contractility in the circular muscle layer.

The identity of this endogenous prostanoid in circular muscle is not clear. However, the finding that PGE_2 (10^{-8} mol L^{-1}) and PGI_2 (10^{-6} mol L^{-1}) reversed the electrophysiological changes in indomethacin-treated dog antral

A B

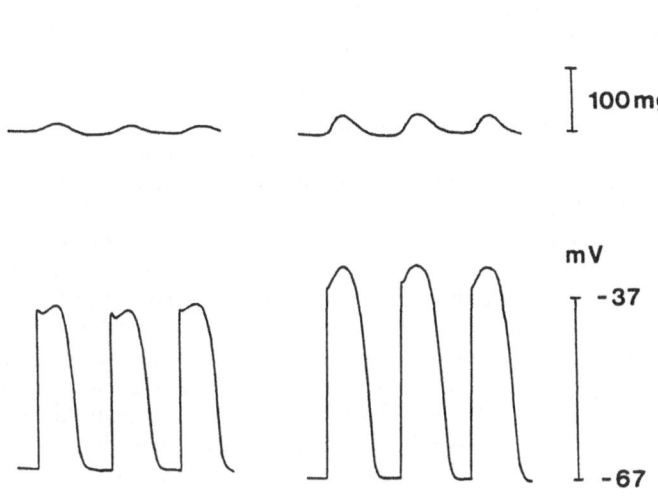

Figure 8.2 Simultaneous recording of mechanical (top trace, A and B) and intracellular electrical (bottom trace, A and B) activities of dog ileum circular muscle in Krebs' solution (A) and after treatment with 10^{-5} M indomethacin (B) (from Sanders, K.M. (1984). *Am. J. Physiol.*, **246**, G361, with permission)

muscle cells described above, must make these prostanoids good candidates for the role. Furthermore, both PGE_2 and PGI_2 dose dependently inhibit the spontaneous movements of dog antral circular muscle strips *in vitro*[6,61].

In conclusion, the results summarized in this section suggest that an endogenous prostanoid or prostanoids formed within the stomach, intestine and colon have a physiological role to play in the control of motility. The exact nature of this role is open to debate. Since gastrointestinal tissue has the capacity to synthesize prostanoids which contract or relax the two muscle layers, their effect *in vivo* will clearly depend upon the relative amounts of contractile and relaxant prostanoids present. *In vitro* experiments suggest that PGE_2 and PGI_2 are quantitatively the most important metabolites of arachidonic acid formed in the gut. If these prostanoids are also formed in significant concentration in the gut *in vivo* then their effect would be to promote motility of longitudinal muscle cells whilst relaxing the circular layer. Clearly, this combination of activity would have the effect of augmenting peristalsis and accelerating the passage of solids and fluids through the alimentary canal.

Effect of other spasmogens: role of prostanoids

Eicosanoids may also have a role to play in controlling the contractile response of the gut to other substances. For example, ATP-induced contraction of the isolated guinea-pig ileum is prevented by prior incubation with indomethacin suggesting that spasmogenic prostanoids may mediate the contractile effect of the purine[80]. Similarly, the rebound contraction of the intestine which follows the relaxation due to stimulation of non-adrenergic, non-cholinergic (NANC) nerves is also blocked by indomethacin, again implying a purine-induced biosynthesis of relaxant prostanoids[81].

The spasmogenic effect of pentagastrin on longitudinal muscle of human colon is suppressed by indomethacin treatment[76] whereas the response on circular muscle of the dog antrum is potentiated[62]. Presumably, pentagastrin stimulates the production of contractile prostanoids from longitudinal muscle and relaxant prostanoids from the circular muscle layer. At which point in the arachidonic acid cascade this stimulation takes place is not known.

Finally, the contractile effect of bradykinin on such commonly used gastrointestinal smooth muscle preparations as the guinea-pig ileum, chick rectum and rat fundus strip may also be reduced by indomethacin or aspirin pretreatment suggesting the mediation of contractile prostanoids. In this case, evidence from other non-gastrointestinal tissues (e.g. lung and kidney) suggests that bradykinin augments prostanoid formation by activating phospholipase A_2 and thereby increasing the de-esterification of arachidonic acid.

PATHOPHYSIOLOGICAL ROLES OF EICOSANOIDS

Diarrhoea

Eicosanoids may play a part in the aetiology of diarrhoea in two ways:

(1) By inhibiting the absorption of sodium ions and water in the small intestine, thereby increasing the volume of fluid in the intestine, and
(2) By promoting intestinal motility.

The major diarrhoeagenic action of eicosanoids is likely to be their effect on fluid transport into and out of the intestine (i.e. predominantly a 'secretory' diarrhoea). Elevated motility, caused either directly by the eicosanoid or indirectly by the presence of a large volume of fluid in the intestine, is probably only of secondary importance since hypermotility itself cannot liquefy the intestinal contents. The effect of eicosanoids on gut motility *in vivo* and *in vitro* have been dealt with in previous sections. The following discussion deals with the effect of eicosanoids on intestinal secretion.

It has been known for over a decade that injection of E and F prostanoids intravenously, intra-arterially or directly into the lumen of the small intestine in dogs or man produces an accumulation of fluid within the lumen[82]. This effect is similar to that produced by cholera toxin and vasoactive intestinal polypeptide each of which stimulates adenylate cyclase activity and increases cAMP levels in the intestinal mucosa. Prostanoids of the E and F series also inhibit absorption of sodium ions (and hence water) in the rabbit[83], rat[84] and human[85] intestine, almost certainly by similar action on mucosal cAMP production. The process whereby prostanoids induce intestinal fluid accumula-ation is referred to as 'enteropooling' and an assay to measure the diarrhoeagenic activity of eicosanoids (the enteropooling assay') has been developed in fasting rats[86]. According to this method, the rank order of diarrhoeagenic potency amongst E and F series prostanoids and their analogues is 16,16-dimethyl PGE_2 > 15-methyl PGE_2 > PGE_2 > 15-methyl $PGF_{2\alpha}$ > $PGF_{2\alpha}$ > $PGF_{2\beta}$. $PGF_{2\alpha}$ has less than 5% of the activity of PGE_2. The methylated prostaglandin analogues are more active than their naturally occurring counterparts most likely because they are broken down less rapidly in the circulation.

In contrast to E and F prostanoids, prostacyclin and its chemical analogues do not produce watery diarrhoea when administered to man or experimental animals[87]. Furthermore, PGI_2 has been found to inhibit the enteropooling effect of other prostanoids including $PGF_{2\alpha}$ in the rat[88]. These observations are supported by the finding that PGI_2 does not affect sodium ion transport in the rat jejunum, either *in vivo* or *in vitro*[89]. This so-called 'anti-enteropooling' effect of PGI_2, which is shared by PGD_2, may conceivably be exploited clinically as a treatment for those forms of diarrhoea in which prostanoids are implicated as discussed below.

The first experimental evidence that linked some forms of diarrhoea with overproduction of prostanoids in the gut was the finding of elevated plasma levels of PGE in patients experiencing the diarrhoea of medullary carcinoma of the thyroid and carcinoid syndrome[90].

High levels of PGE_2, estimated by a sensitive and selective radioimmunoassay, have also been detected in intestinal fluid of patients with irritable bowel syndrome[85] and in cultures of rectal mucosal biopsies from patients with ulcerative colitis[91]. Furthermore, experimentally induced diarrhoea, following intravenous injection of *E. coli* endotoxin to rabbits, produces greatly increased release of PGE from incubated intestinal segments[92], while treatment of rats with *Salmonella minnesota* increases intestinal fluid PGE_2 and 6-oxo-$PGF_{1\alpha}$ levels[93]. In intact animals both types of bacteria produce profuse, watery diarrhoea.

Other forms of diarrhoea which may involve eicosanoids include that associated with X-irradiation. Mennie and Daley[94] observed that diarrhoea in patients receiving radiation therapy for cancer of the cervix was resistant to conventional treatment but alleviated by aspirin. Later experiments suggested that exposure to X-irradiation may significantly elevate blood and organ prostanoid concentrations by destroying the 15-PGDH (15-hydroxyprostaglandin dehydrogenase) enzyme which normally catabolizes classical prostaglandins[95].

Indomethacin similarly inhibits the diarrhoea of dysmenorrhoea. In this case, treatment with the cyclo-oxygenase inhibitor was effective in 83% of subjects compared with those receiving placebo (46% relief) and also had the added benefit of reducing the incidence and severity of other gastrointestinal symptoms (e.g. nausea and vomiting) of this condition[96].

Paralytic ileus

In the same way that overproduction of intestinal prostanoids may precipitate or exacerbate diarrhoea, it is likely that a deficiency of these substances in the gut may produce hypomotility. One clinical condition characterized by gastrointestinal hypomotility in which prostanoids may be involved is post-operative ileus. This condition is one of delayed gastrointestinal propulsion and may occur in patients after abdominal surgery even in those whose recovery is otherwise uncomplicated. The cause(s) of post-operative ileus is not known but may be the result of stimulation of sympathetic nerves to the gut or suppression of cholinergic nervous activity or both. If not successfully treated the condition may progress to paralytic ileus.

Since E and F prostanoids contract longitudinal muscle of the intestines *in vivo* and PGE_1 and PGE_2 reduce noradrenaline efflux from sympathetic nerves, they would appear to be possible candidates for the clinical treatment of post-operative ileus. Laparotomized rats show reduced gastric emptying and slowed intestinal transit for up to 2 days after surgery. Administration of PGE_2, $PGF_{2\alpha}$ or 16,16-dimethyl $PGF_{2\alpha}$ to these animals restored normal gastric emptying[97]. Successful experiments of this type in animals will hopefully lead to an evaluation of eicosanoids in man for the treatment of this condition.

REFERENCES

1. Kurzrok, R. and Lieb, C. (1930). Biochemical studies of human semen: action of semen on the human uterus. *Proc. Soc. Exp. Biol. Med.*, **28**, 268–272
2. Bennett, A. and Fleshler, B. (1970). Prostaglandins and the gastrointestinal tract. *Gastroenterology*, **59**, 790–800
3. Bennett, A. (1976). Prostaglandins and the alimentary tract. In Karim, S.M.M. (ed.) *Prostaglandins: Physiological, Pharmacological and Pathological Aspects*, pp. 247–276. (Lancaster: MTP Press)
4. Robert, A. (1977). Prostaglandins and the digestive system. In Ramwell, P.W. (ed.) *The Prostaglandins*, pp. 225–266. (New York: Raven Press)
5. Moore, P.K. (1985) *Prostanoids: Pharmacological, Physiological and Clinical Relevance.* (Cambridge University Press)
6. Sanders, K.M. (1984). Role of prostaglandins in regulating gastric motility. *Am. J. Physiol.*, **247**, G117–G126
7. Moncada, S., Ferreira, S.H. and Vane, J.R. (1978). Bioassay of prostaglandins and biologically active substances derived from arachidonic acid. *Adv. Prostgl. Thromboxane Res.*, **5**, 211–236
8. von Euler, U.S. (1966). Introductory survey. *Mem. Soc. Endocrinol.*, **14**, 3–7
9. Bennett, A. and Posner, J. (1971). Studies on prostaglandin antagonists. *Br. J. Pharmacol.*, **42**, 584–594
10. Ishizawa, M. (1981). Effects of prostaglandins on the smooth muscle of the guinea pig stomach. *Arch. Int. Pharmacodyn. Ther.*, **253**, 80–89
11. Weeks, J.R., Schultz, J.R. and Brown, W.E. (1968). Evaluation of smooth muscle bioassays for prostaglandins E_2 and $F_{2\alpha}$. *J. Appl. Physiol.*, **25**, 783–785
12. Bennett, A., Eley, K.G. and Scholes, G.B. (1968). Effect of prostaglandins $F_{1\alpha}$ and $F_{2\alpha}$ on intestinal motility in the guinea pig and rat. *Br. J. Pharmacol.*, **34**, 639–647
13. Ferreira, S.H., Hermann, A. and Vane, J.R. (1972). Prostaglandin generation maintains the smooth muscle tone of the rabbit isolated jejunum. *Br. J. Pharmacol.*, **44**, 328–330
14. Turker, R.K. and Omer, R. (1971). Effect of prostaglandin E_1 on intestinal motility in the cat. *Arch. Int. Pharmacodyn. Ther.*, **253**, 80–89
15. Vanasin, B., Greenhough, W. and Schuster, M.M. (1970). Effect of prostaglandins on electric and motor activity of isolated colonic muscle. *Gastroenterology*, **58**, 1004
16. Vane, J.R. (1969). The release and fate of vasoactive hormones in the circulation. *Br. J. Pharmacol.*, **35**, 209–242

17. Omini, C., Moncada, S. and Vane, J.R. (1977). The effects of prostacyclin on tissues which detect prostaglandins. *Prostaglandins*, **14**, 25–31
18. Hamberg, M., Svensson, J. and Samuelsson, B. (1975). Thromboxanes: a new group of biologically active compounds derived from prostaglandin endoperoxides. *Proc. Natl. Acad. Sci.*, **72**, 2994–2998
19. Coleman, R.A., Humphrey, P.P.A., Kennedy, I., Levy, G.P. and Lumley, P. (1981). Comparison of the actions of U-46619, a prostaglandin H_2 analogue, with those of prostaglandin H_2 and thromboxane A_2 on some isolated smooth muscle preparations. *Br. J. Pharmacol.*, **73**, 773–778
20. Main, I.H.M. (1973). Prostaglandins and the gastrointestinal tract. In Cuthbert, M.F. (ed.) *The Prostaglandins*, pp. 287–323. (London: Heinemann Press)
21. Crutchley, D.J. and Piper, P.J. (1975). Comparative bioassay of prostaglandin E_1 and its pulmonary metabolites. *Br. J. Pharmacol.*, **54**, 397–399
22. Hoult, J.R.S. and Moore, P.K. (1979). Pathways of prostaglandin $F_{2\alpha}$ metabolism in mammalian kidneys. *Br. J. Pharmacol.*, **60**, 627–632
23. Moore, P.K. and Griffiths, R.J. (1983). 6-Keto prostaglandin E_1. *Prostaglandins*, **26**, 509–517
24. Bennett, A., Murray, J.G. and Wyllie, J.H. (1968). Occurrence of prostaglandin E_2 in the human stomach, and a study of its effects on human isolated gastric muscle. *Br. J. Pharmacol.*, **32**, 339–349
25. Bennett, A., Hensby, C.N., Sanger, G.J. and Stamford, I.M. (1981). Metabolites of arachidonic acid formed by human gastrointestinal tissues and their actions on the muscle layers. *Br. J. Pharmacol.*, **74**, 435–444
26. Bennett, A. and Stockley, H.L. (1977). The contribution of prostaglandins in the muscle of human isolated small intestine to neurogenic responses. *Br. J. Pharmacol.*, **61**, 573–578
27. Osaki, S., Omuro, S., Toyosaka, A., Kuwata, K., Miyamoto, T. and Okamoto, E. (1973). Effect of prostaglandin E on the smooth muscle of the human digestive tract. *Jpn. J. Smooth Muscle Res.*, **9**, 237–238
28. Horton, E.W. (1963). Action of prostaglandin E_1 on tissues which respond to bradykinin. *Nature*, **200**, 892–893
29. Khairallah, P.P., Page, I.H. and Turker, R.K. (1967). Some properties of prostaglandin E_1 action on muscle. *Arch. Int. Pharmacodyn. Ther.*, **169**, 328–341
30. Piper, P.J. (1983). Pharmacology of leukotrienes. *Br. Med. Bull.*, **39**, 255-259
31. Piper, P.J., Letts, L.G., Samhoun, M.N., Tippins, J.R. and Palmer, M.A. (1982). Actions of leukotrienes on vascular, airway and gastrointestinal smooth muscle. *Adv. Prostagl. Thromb. Leuk. Res.*, **6**, 169–181
32. Whittle, B.J.R., Mugridge, K.G. and Moncada, S. (1979). Use of the rabbit transverse stomach strip to identify and assay prostacyclin, PGA_2, PGD_2 and other prostaglandins. *Eur. J. Pharmacol.*, **53**, 167–172
33. Ishizawa, M. (1981). Effects of prostacyclin (PGI_2) on the smooth muscles of the guinea pig stomach. *Arch. Int. Pharmacodyn. Ther.*, **253**, 80–89
34. Sanger, G.J. and Bennett, A. (1976). Prostanoid agonists and antagonists: differentiation of prostanoid receptors in the gut. In Berti, F. and Velo, G. (eds.) *The Prostaglandin System*, pp. 372–391. (New York: Raven Press)
35. Ishizawa, M. and Minowa, T. (1982). Effects of PGD_2 and $PGF_{2\alpha}$ on longitudinal and circular muscle of the guinea pig isolated proximal colon. *Prostaglandins*, **24**, 843–851
36. Rattan, S., Hersh, T. and Goyal, R.K. (1972). Effect of prostaglandin $F_{2\alpha}$ and gastrin pentapeptide on the lower oesophageal sphincter. *Proc. Soc. Exp. Biol. Med.*, **141**, 573–575
37. Goyal, R.K. and Rattan, S. (1973). Mechanism of the lower oesophageal sphincter relaxation. Action of prostaglandin E_1 and theophylline. *J. Clin. Invest.*, **52**, 337–341
38. Dilawari, J.B., Newman, A., Poleo, J. and Misiewicz, J.J. (1973). The effect of prostaglandins and of anti-inflammatory drugs on the oesophagus and the cardiac sphincter in man. *Gut*, **14**, 822–826
39. Kruidinier, J., Tao, P. and Wilson, D.E. (1978). The role of prostaglandins in lower oesophageal sphincter pressure in man. *Clin. Res.*, **26**, 663
40. Bergstrom, S., Duner, H., von Euler, U.S., Pernow, B. and Sjovall, J. (1959). Observations on the effects of infusion of prostaglandin E_1 in man. *Acta Physiol. Scand.*, **45**, 145–151
41. Horton, E.W., Main, I.H.M., Thompson, C.J. and Wright, P.M. (1968). Effect of orally

administered prostaglandin E_1 on gastric secretion and gastrointestinal motility in man. *Gut*, **9**, 655–670

42. Bergstrom, S., Eliasson, R., von Euler, U.S. and Sjovall, J. (1959). Some biological effects of two crystalline prostaglandin factors. *Acta Physiol. Scand.*, **45**, 133–144
43. Carlson, L.A., Ekelund, L.G. and Oro, L. (1968). Clinical and metabolic effects of different doses of prostaglandin E in man. *Acta Med. Scand.*, **183**, 423–429
44. Bailey, C.D.H., Newman, C., Elinas, S.P. and Anderson, G.G. (1975). Use of prostaglandin E_2 vaginal suppositories in intrauterine foetal death and missed abortion. *Obstet. Gynaecol.*, **45**, 110–115
45. Kent, D.R. and Goldstein, A.L. (1976). Prostaglandin E_2 induction of labour for foetal demise. *Obstet. Gynaecol.*, **48**, 475–482
46. Karim, S.M.M. and Ratnam, S. (1976). Termination of abnormal intrauterine pregnancies with intramuscular administration of dihomo-15-methyl prostaglandin $F_{2\alpha}$. *Br. J. Obstet. Gynaecol.*, **83**, 885–889
47. Misiewicz, J.J., Waller, S.L., Kiley, N. and Horton, E.W. (1969). Effect of oral prostaglandin E_1 on intestinal transit in man. *Lancet*, **1**, 648
48. Newman, A., DeMoraes-Filho, J.P.P., Philippakos, D. and Misiewicz, J.J. (1975). The effect of intravenous infusions of prostaglandins E_2 and $F_{2\alpha}$ on human gastric function. *Gut*, **16**, 42–49
49. Hunt, R.H., Dilawari, J.B. and Misiewicz, J.J. (1975). The effect of intravenous prostaglandin $F_{2\alpha}$ and E_2 on the motility of the sigmoid colon. *Gut*, **16**, 47–52
50. Nylander, B. and Mattsson, O. (1975). Effect of 16,16-dimethyl PGE_2 on gastric emptying and intestinal transit of a barium meal in man. *Scand. J. Gastroenterol.*, **10**, 289–297
51. Wilson, D.E., Quertermus, J. and Raiser, M. (1976). Inhibition of stimulated gastric secretion by an orally administered prostaglandin capsule: A study in normal men. *Ann. Intern. Med.*, **84**, 688–691
52. Nompleggi, D., Myers, L. and Castell, D.O. (1980). Effect of a prostaglandin E_2 analogue on gastric emptying and secretion in rhesus monkeys. *J. Pharm. Exp. Ther.*, **212**, 491–495
53. Nylander, B. and Anderson, S. (1975). Effect of two methylated prostaglandin E_2 analogues on gastro-duodenal pressure in man. *Scand. J. Gastroenterol.*, **10**, 91–99
54. Shea-Donohue, P.T., Myers, L., Castell, D.O. and Dubois, A. (1980). Effect of prostacyclin on gastric secretion and emptying in rhesus monkeys. *Gastroenterology*, **78**, 1476–1479
55. Horton, E.W. (1979). Prostaglandins and smooth muscle. *Br. Med. Bull.*, **35**, 295–300
56. Horton, E.W. (1965). Biological activities of pure prostaglandins. *Experientia*, **21**, 113–118
57. Bennett, A., Eley, K.G. and Scholes, G.B. (1968). Effects of prostaglandins E_2 and E_1 on human, guinea pig and rat isolated small intestine. *Br. J. Pharmacol.*, **34**, 630–638
58. Kennedy, I., Coleman, R.A., Humphrey, P.P.A., Levy, G.P. and Lumley, P. (1982). Studies on the characterization of prostanoid receptors: a proposed classification. *Prostaglandins*, **24**, 667–689
59. Bennett, A. and Posner, J. (1971). Studies on prostaglandin antagonists. *Br. J. Pharmacol.*, **42**, 584–594
60. Coleman, P., Kennedy, I. and Sheldrick, R.C.G. (1985). AH 6809 – a prostanoid EP_1 receptor blocking drug. *Br. J. Pharmacol.*, **85**, 273P
61. Sanders, K.M. (1984). Evidence that prostaglandins are local regulatory agents in canine ileal circular muscle. *Am. J. Physiol.*, **246**, G361–371
62. Sanders, K.M. and Szurszewski, J.H. (1981). Does endogenous prostaglandin affect gastric antral motility. *Am. J. Physiol.*, **241**, G191–195
63. Mishima, K. and Kurijama, H. (1976). Effect of prostaglandins on electrical and mechanical activities of the guinea pig stomach. *Jpn. J. Physiol.*, **26**, 537–548
64. Kelly, K.A., Code, C.F. and Elvenack, L.R. (1969). Pattern of canine gastric electrical activity. *Am. J. Physiol.*, **217**, 461–470
65. Milenov, K. and Golenhofen, K. (1982). Contractile response of longitudinal and circular smooth muscle of the canine stomach to prostaglandins E_2 and $F_{2\alpha}$. *Prostagl. Leuk. Med.*, **8**, 287–300
66. Sanders, K.M. and Jones, C.D. (1982). Regulation of the muscles responsible for gastric emptying by endogenous prostaglandins. *Dig. Dis. Sci.*, **27**, 665
67. Pace-Asciak, C. and Rangaraj, G. (1977). Distribution of prostaglandin biosynthetic pathways in several rat tissues. *Biochim. Biophys. Acta*, **486**, 579–582

68. Ali, M. and McDonald, J.W.D. (1980). Synthesis of thromboxane B_2 and 6-keto prostaglandin $F_{1\alpha}$ by bovine gastric mucosal and muscle microsomes. *Prostaglandins*, **20**, 245–254
69. LeDuc, L.E. and Needleman, P. (1979). Regional localisation of thromboxane and prostacyclin synthesis in dog stomach and intestinal tract. *J. Pharm. Exp. Ther.*, **211**, 181–188
70. Sanders, K.M. and Northrup, T.E. (1983). Prostaglandin synthesis by microsomes of circular and longitudinal gastrointestinal muscles. *Am. J. Physiol.*, **244**, G442–448
71. Hall, W.J., O'Neill, P. and Sheehan, J.D. (1975). The role of prostaglandins in cholinergic neuro-transmission in the guinea pig. *Eur. J. Pharmacol.*, **34**, 39–47
72. Bennett, A., Eley, K.G. and Stockley, H.L. (1975). Modulation by prostaglandins of contractions in guinea pig ileum. *Prostaglandins*, **9**, 377–384
73. Yamaguchi, T., Hitzig, B. and Coburn, R.F. (1976). Endogenous prostaglandin in guinea pig taenia coli. *Am. J. Physiol.*, **230**, 149–157
74. Stockley, H.L. and Bennett, A. (1976). Modulation of activity by prostaglandins in human gastrointestinal muscle. In Vantrappen, G. (ed.) *Fifth International Symposium on gastrointestinal motility.* pp. 31–36. (Belgium: Typoff Press)
75. Bennett, A. and Stockley, H.L. (1977). The contribution of prostaglandins in the muscle of human isolated small intestine to neurogenic responses. *Br. J. Pharmacol.*, **61**, 573–578
76. Bruch, H.P., Schmidt, E. and Laven, R. (1978). The role of prostaglandins in peristalsis of the human colon. *Acta Hepato-Gastroenterol.*, **25**, 303–307
77. Nitta, H. and Ishizawa, M. (1980). Endogenous prostaglandins and spontaneous contractions in the circular muscle of the guinea pig stomach. *Jpn. J. Physiol.*, **30**, 815–826
78. Thor, P., Konturek, J.W. and Anderson, J.H. (1985). Role of prostaglandins in the control of intestinal motility. *Am. J. Physiol.*, **248**, 935–939
79. Sanders, K.M. (1978). Endogenous prostaglandin E and contractile activity of isolated ileal smooth muscle. *Am. J. Physiol.*, **234**, E209–212
80. Kamikawa, Y., Serizawa, K. and Shimo, Y. (1977). Some possibilities for prostaglandin mediation in the contractile response to ADP of the guinea pig digestive tract. *Eur. J. Pharm.*, **45**, 199–203
81. Burnstock, G., Cockes, T., Paddle, B. and Staszowska-Barczak, J. (1975). Evidence that prostaglandin is responsible for the rebound contraction following stimulation of non-adrenergic, non-cholinergic (purinergic) inhibitor nerves. *Eur. J. Pharmacol.*, **31**, 360–362
82. Greenough, W.B., Pierce, N.F., Al Awqati, Q. and Carpenter, C.C.J. (1969). Stimulation of gut electrolyte secretion by prostaglandins, theophylline and cholera exotoxin. *J. Clin. Invest.*, **48**, 32
83. Al Awqati, Q. and Greenhough, W.B. (1972). Prostaglandins inhibit intestinal sodium transport. *Nature*, **238**, 26–27
84. Declusin, R., Wall, M. and Whalen, G. (1974). Effect of prostaglandin E_2 on sodium and chloride transport in rat jejunum. *Clin. Res.*, **22**, 635
85. Bukhave, K. and Rask-Madsen, J. (1980). Saturation kinetics applied to *in vitro* effects of low prostaglandin E_2 and prostaglandin $F_{2\alpha}$ concentrations on ion transport across human jejunal mucosa. *Gastroenterology*, **78**, 32–42
86. Robert, A., Nezamis, J.E., Hancher, A.J., Lancaster, C. and Klepper, M.S. (1976). The enteropooling assay to test for diarrhoea due to prostaglandins. *Fed. Proc.*, **35**, 457
87. Whittle, B.J.R. and Boughton-Smith, N.K. (1979). 16-Phenoxy prostacyclin analogue – potent, selective anti-ulcer compound. In Vane, J.R. and Bergstrom, S. (eds.) *Prostacyclin,* pp. 159–171. (New York: Raven Press)
88. Robert, A., Hanchar, A.J., Lancaster, C. and Nezamis, J.E. (1979). Prostacyclin inhibits enteropooling and diarrhoea. In Vane, J.R. and Bergstrom, S. (eds.) *Prostacyclin,* pp. 147–157. (New York: Raven Press)
89. Hardcastle, J., Hardcastle, P.T. and Redfern, J.S. (1980). The effect of prostacyclin on intestinal ion transport in the rat. *Life Sci.*, **26**, 123–131
90. Jaffe, B.M. and Condon, S. (1976). Prostaglandins E and F in endocrine diarrhoeagenic syndromes. *Ann. Surg.*, **184**, 516–523
91. Ligumsky, M., Karmeli, F., Sharon, P., Zor, U., Cohen, F. and Rachmilewitz, D. (1981). Enhanced thromboxane A_2 and prostacyclin production by cultured rectal mucosa in ulcerative colitis and its inhibition by steroids and sulphasalazine. *Gastroenterology*, **81**, 444–449
92. Herman, A.G. and Vane, J.R. (1976). The effect of indomethacin on endotoxin-induced

production of prostaglandins in the isolated rabbit jejunum. *Adv. Prostagl. Thromboxane Res.*, **2**, 557–560

93. Peskar, B.M., Weiler, H., Kroner, E.E. and Peskar, B.A. (1981). Release of prostaglandins from small intestinal tissue in human and rat *in vitro* and the effect of endotoxin in rat *in vivo. Prostaglandins*, **21** (Suppl.), 9–14
94. Mennie, A.T. and Daley, V. (1973). Aspirin in radiation induced diarrhoea. Lancet, **1**, 1131
95. Eisen, V. and Walker, D.I. (1976). Effect of ionising radiation on prostaglandin-like activity in tissues. *Br. J. Pharmacol.*, **57**, 527–532
96. Kaupilla, A. and Ylikorkala, O. (1977). Indomethacin and tolfenamic acid in primary dysmenorrhoea. *Eur. J. Obstet. Gynaecol. Reprod. Biol.*, **7**, 59
97. Ruwart, M.J., Klepper, M.S. and Rush, B.D. (1980). Prostaglandin stimulation of gastrointestinal tract in post-operative ileus rats. *Prostaglandins*, **19**, 415–426

9
Effect of eicosanoids on gastrointestinal blood flow and microcirculation

G. Pihan and S. Szabo

INTRODUCTION

Eicosanoids, a term proposed by Corey et al.[1], encompasses a diverse group of mediators having in common polyunsaturated fatty acids of 20 carbons as precursors and potent biological actions[2–5]. The group encompasses the prostanoids[6–8], the thromboxanes[9], the leukotrienes[10,11], the 5-, 12- and 15-hydroxy and hydroperoxy fatty acids[12,13] and two newly described family of compounds: the lipoxins[14,15] and products derived from the metabolism of arachidonic acid by cytochrome P450[16]. All these compounds, except for the new families, are produced by either resident or circulating cells or both in the gastrointestinal tract[17–31] where they exert a variety of effects[32–34].

Eicosanoid effects on gastrointestinal blood flow have been extensively investigated (for previous reviews see references 35 and 36). Due to their protean effects and the multiplicity of their interactions[37], the exact physiological role of any given eicosanoid on the gastrointestinal circulation has to be defined individually.

Moreover, their well-recognized paracrine rather than endocrine mode of action[38] further complicates the interpretation of experimental results since their systemic or local administration may not reproduce with fidelity the mode in which they are normally delivered to their targets.

This chapter reviews the rather extensive data on the effects of eicosanoids on gastrointestinal vasculature and blood flow *in vivo* and *in vitro*. A special section at the end summarizes what we currently know about their role in certain pathological conditions.

EICOSANOIDS AND GASTRIC BLOOD FLOW

Eicosanoids can alter gastric flow either directly, by virtue of their action on the smooth muscle of the gastric vasculature, or indirectly, by modulating vascular noradrenergic transmission[39,40], the actions of other vasoactive substances[39,40], gastric acid secretion[41-43], gastric motility[44,45], and by producing systemic haemodynamic changes. Haemodynamic changes, particularly hypotension, have a profound effect on blood flow to the stomach[46]. This last consideration ought to be borne in mind when evaluating the effects of eicosanoids on gastrointestinal blood flow, since they can exert marked haemodynamic effects at very low systemic concentrations that are often achieved even when administered locally in the gastrointestinal tract.

Prostaglandins

Prostaglandins E_2, E_1 and analogues
In the non-stimulated stomach, prostaglandins (PG) E_1, E_2 and 16,16-dimethyl-PGE_2 have been shown to increase[47-57], or less often slightly decrease[58-60], or have no effect[61,62], on gastric blood flow. This overwhelming accumulation of experimental evidence, despite differences in animal species studied[47,49,55], route of administration of prostaglandins[47,48,50,52-55] and the techniques of assessing blood flow[47-49,53], indicates that PGs of the E series, under most circumstances, are gastric vasodilators. Studies in which mucosal blood flow has been measured simultaneously with total blood flow (fractional distribution of microspheres)[49,51] indicate that blood flow increases in the same proportion in both the mucosal and the non-mucosal (submucosal-muscle) compartments after topical mucosal administration of 16,16-dimethyl PGE_2. In vivo microscopy has revealed that PGE_2 dilates submucosal arterioles[63] and, together with PGE_1 and 16,16-dimethyl PGE_2, increase red blood cell velocity in superficial mucosal capillaries (an index of mucosal blood flow) when applied topically but decrease it when given intravenously (i.v.)[57]. This suggests that the occasional reports of decreased mucosal blood flow after local application of PGE_2 or analogues[58,60] may have been due to systemic absorption.

PGE_1, 16,16-dimethyl PGE_2 and ($\pm$)-15-deoxy-16-α,β-hydroxy-16-methyl PGE_1 methyl ester (SC-29333) have also been shown to lessen the decrease in gastric mucosal blood flow induced by haemorrhagic shock[64-66].

In the histamine- or pentagastrin-stimulated stomach, on the other hand, the increased mucosal blood flow is roughly parallel to the increase in acid secretion[42,43]. PGE_1, PGE_2 and analogues often decrease gastric mucosal blood flow (measured by clearance or microspheres) in dogs[49,51,55,59,61,67-73], rats[48,74,75], pigs[76] and cats[77], and markedly reduce acid secretion. In these studies, the ratio of mucosal blood flow to acid secretion (R) was either not changed[59,61] or increased[48,67-69,74], indicating that the changes in mucosal blood flow were, in all likelihood, secondary to the potent gastric antisecretory effects of the PGs studies[78,79] and mediated through the withdrawal of the stimulatory action on blood flow exerted by high gastric secretory rates. When administered by close intra-arterial (i.a.) injection into the vascular supply of the gastric mucosa in dogs, PGE_2 increased blood flow in both the resting and the histamine- or pentagastrin-stimulated stomach[50,80,81]. This result suggests that after local intravascular administration, the direct vasodilatory effects of these prostaglandins override the indirect effect mediated through gastric acid secretion inhibition. Alternatively, the lesser degree of systemic effects caused by i.a. injection might allow PGs to fully express their local vasodilatory actions without the intervening effect of systemic hypotension that naturally tend to reduce gastric blood flow. This view is supported by the findings of Francis and Smy who determined that low doses of PGE_1 and E_2, given i.a., increased, whereas given i.v. decreased, the ratio of mucosal blood flow to acid secretion[77].

Prostaglandin $F_{2\alpha}$
The few available studies on the effect of $PGF_{2\alpha}$ indicate that either it does not affect[55] or decreases[52,54] resting total gastric or mucosal blood flow when infused into the coeliac artery or its branches in anaesthetized dogs. $PGF_{2\alpha}$ is also a vasoconstrictor, yet less potent than norepinephrine in the isolated perfused stomach of rats and rabbits[82]. All these studies indicate that $PGF_{2\alpha}$ is predominantly a vasoconstrictor of the gastric circulation.

Prostaglandin A_1 and A_2
PGA_1 and A_2 have qualitatively and, to a certain extent, quantitatively similar effects, compared with PGs of the E series on resting gastric blood flow of dogs[47] and rats[48], and as PGE_2, they also reduce gastric mucosal blood flow in the pentagastrin- or histamine-stimulated stomach of the rat[48].

Prostacyclin
Considerably more information exists about the effects of PGI_2 on the gastric circulation than those of prostaglandins F and A. PGI_2, whether infused i.v.[59,83-86] or i.a., into the gastric circulation[50,52,53,80] always increases resting total gastric blood flow[50,52,59,80] and mucosal blood flow[53,83,86]. PGI_2 has been shown to be roughly equipotent with PGE_2 in vasodilating the resting stomach of the dog when administered by close i.a. infusion[52,80]. Administered i.v., however, PGI_2 is probably more potent than PGE_2[59]. The reasons for this difference are not known but might rest in the lower susceptibility of PGI_2 than PGE_2 to metabolic inactivation in the pulmonary circulation[87]. PGI_2 can also prevent the decrease in blood flow induced by concentrated ethanol in dogs[88,89] or a combination of vasopressin infusion and intragastric autogenous bile in pigs[90] and cause vasodilation in the isolated perfused stomach of the rat and rabbit[82,91].

Since PGI_2 possesses many desirable pharmacological properties yet its instability at neutral pH precludes sustained action, stable analogues have been developed[92]. Carbacyclin, 6β-PGI_1, and a 16-phenoxy derivative of PGI_2, all three PGI_2 analogues, have been shown to qualitatively exert the same effects as PGI_2, yet to be less potent gastric vasodilators[52]. In the canine histamine- or pentagastrin-stimulated stomach[93,94], PGI_2 given i.v. reduced mucosal blood flow (aminopyrine clearance)[59,93,95] without changing R but increased mucosal blood flow (despite secretory inhibition) when given by close i.a. infusion[86,50,73]. These apparently discordant effects of PGI_2 on the stimulated stomach are reminiscent of those of PGE_2 under similar conditions (see above), and again suggest that systemic effects of the autacoid might counteract and obscure the purely local actions.

Endoperoxides

U-46619 is a stable endoperoxide analogue, and, injected by close i.a. infusion in relatively high doses, reduces stimulated gastric mucosal blood flow to a greater extent than acid secretion ($\downarrow$R) in the dog[96]. More recent studies, also in the dog, have confirmed and extended these observations by demonstrating that U-44619 and U-44069 (another closely related analogue) decreased gastric mucosal blood flow equipotently[52]. In contrast to the analogues which are not further metabolized, PGH_2 itself was a weak vasodilator[52]. These results were interpreted as indicating that the action of the natural endoperoxides is predominantly vasoconstrictor. In the gastric circulation, however, PGH_2 is probably rapidly converted into a vasodilator product, more likely PGI_2[52]. This assumption is supported by the demonstration of a PGH_2-induced relaxation which can be converted to a contraction in isolated mesenteric vessels in which prostacyclin synthetase had been previously blocked with 15-HPAA[97]. In the blood perfused mesenteric circulation of the dog, however, 15-HPAA was unable to modify the vasodilatory action of PGH_2[98]. This lack of effect of hydroperoxides was ascribed to their rapid reduction in the circulation, precluding their inhibitory effect on prostaglandin synthetase[98]. The establishment of the definite mode of action of PGH_2 on the gastric circulation awaits the development of specific and more stable inhibitors of prostacyclin synthetase.

U-46619, administered at low doses, has also been shown to decrease mucosal blood flow in the stimulated stomach without reducing R. Thus, at low doses, the decrease in blood flow produced by U-46619 seems to be largely due to its inhibitory action on gastric acid secretion[96]. Caution needs to be exercised in the interpretation of results obtained with U-46619, however, since this compound has a pharmacological profile similar to those of thromboxanes and currently it is grouped under 'thromboxane mimetics'.

Thromboxanes

Since thromboxane A_2 (TxA_2) is extremely labile, the investigation of its action on the gastric circulation has relied mostly on indirect approaches. Whittle et al.[99] infused arachidonic acid (AA) into a delay coil (30 s) connected to an artery supplying a flap of gastric mucosa in the dog. In doses of 25–200 μg, AA induced a dose-dependent decrease in blood flow (rise in perfusion pressure). Since vasoconstriction caused by AA could be abolished by pretreatment with indomethacin or 1-benzyl-imidazole (a thromboxane syn-thetase inhibitor), it was concluded that a metabolite of AA, most likely TxA_2, was responsible for the vasoconstriction observed[99]. In a related study, AA, administered into the gastric circulation only through a 30 s (but not a 3 s) delay coil, was shown to induce vasoconstriction, again suggesting that the actions of AA were mediated through its conversion into a vasoconstrictor metabolite upon exposure to blood[52]. Similar results have been obtained by Moroni et al.[100] using the approach pioneered by Whittle. In addition, it was demonstrated that a putative thromboxane antagonist, the tripeptide ZAMI-420, could also inhibit AA-induced gastric vasoconstriction[100].

In a recent report, it has been shown that the stable endoperoxide analogue, U-46619, which is also a thromboxane mimetic, induced constriction of both arterioles and venules and sluggish blood flow in the gastric submucosal circulation[101].

Cyclo-oxygenase inhibitors

Indomethacin and aspirin have been shown to decrease gastric mucosal blood flow in the dog in both the resting[102,103] and stimulated[91] stomach and in the resting gastric mucosa of the rat[103–105], rabbits[106], and cats[107]. Indomethacin in the dog reduced basal blood flow by 45% and pentagastrin-stimulated blood flow by 43%. Aspirin was slightly less active than indomethacin[102]. As expected, the increase in blood flow induced by pentagastrin and the reduction induced by indomethacin were confined to the gastric mucosa, and, despite greater pentagastrin stimulation of blood flow in the fundus compared with the antrum or cardia, indomethacin decreased blood flow in all regions to a similar degree[102]. Based on similar results, Kauffman et al.[103] have postulated that endogenous prostaglandins may play a significant role in regulating basal gastric mucosal blood flow.

Lipoxygenase products

Very little is currently known about the effect of lipoxygenase products of arachidonic acid on the gastric circulation. In isolated perfused stomachs of the rat and rabbits, hydroperoxides produce vasodilation with a rank order of potency of the form 12-HPETE > 11-HPETE > 5-HPETE > 15-HPETE[82,91]. Additionally, 15-HPETE could abolish the vasodilation induced by arachidonic acid or PGH_2. This effect was presumably mediated by an inhibition of PGI_2 synthesis. LTC_4, but not LTD_4, applied topically to the submucosal vascular plexus of the rat induced marked vasoconstriction especially in venules[100], and, after i.v. injection, LTC_4, LTD_4 and LTE_4 caused a generalized increase in vascular permeability that was less marked in digestive organs than in others[108]. Since lipoxygenase products, particularly those of 5-lipoxygenase, seem to participate in a variety of pathological processes, the elucidation of their actions on the gastric circulation, both in physiological and pathological conditions, might prove rewarding in the future.

Arachidonic acid

Arachidonic acid (AA), given topically or i.a., has been shown to reduce mucosal blood flow in the stimulated stomach of the dog[109] and rats[110]. In both instances, the inhibitory effect of AA on blood flow and acid secretion could be substantially attenuated by administration of indomethacin[109,110], indicating that metabolites of the cyclo-oxygenase pathway, and not AA itself, meditated the observed effects. In subsequent studies, Whittle and Kauffman[52,99] have demonstrated that AA can induce both an increase or a decrease of gastric blood flow, apparently depending on whether AA is converted primarily to TxA_2 or to PGE_2 and PGI_2 before reaching the gastric resistance vessels. This was demonstrated by injecting AA into the gastric circulation through a 30 s delay coil; AA increased perfusion pressure whereas the same injection into a shorter delay coil (3 s) reduced perfusion pressure. Since the vasoconstriction caused by AA injected through the 30 s delay coil could be abolished by 1-benzylimidazole, it was concluded that the effect was mediated by TxA_2 generation.

EICOSANOIDS AND INTESTINAL BLOOD FLOW

The control of intestinal circulation is multifactorial. As in the stomach, local vascular myogenic[111-112], metabolic[113-115], neural[116,117] and functional factors, such as absorption[118-120], secretion[118] and motility[121,122], all play a role. In addition, extraintestinal factors, of which systemic haemodynamic changes are the most important, can influence blood flow and its distribution in the gut[123,124]. Since most of these regulatory mechanisms are sensitive to eicosanoids, it is not surprising that the effects of these compounds on intestinal blood flow are complex and varied, and many times depend on the experimental conditions, the species selected and the functional state of the intestinal segment investigated.

Prostaglandins

Prostaglandins E_2, E_1 and analogues

Prostaglandins of the E series as a group can be regarded as intestinal vasodilators. PGE_2 has been shown to increase superior mesenteric blood flow in dogs[125-129], cats[130-132] and pigs[133] under both spontaneous[125-129, 133] and controlled[130-132] blood flow conditions. Increased intestinal blood flow induced by PGE_2 was observed regardless of the route of administration of the prostaglandin or of systemic blood pressure changes: PGE_2 given into the superior mesenteric artery[126,133] induced little or no change in blood pressure whereas it produced a substantial drop after injection into the left ventricle[128] and after i.v. introduction[125]. However in all circumstances, mesenteric blood flow increased. Administered topically (mucosal side), PGE_2 increased blood flow in autoperfused jejunal segments of dogs[134].

In the isolated perfused rat mesenteric vascular bed, however, PGE_2 induced little or no effect[135] on basal perfusion pressure. This finding can be largely attributed to the low basal perfusion pressure exhibited by these preparations[136].

Authors who compared the potency of PGE_2 as a vasodilator, administered by close i.a. injection in different vascular beds, have reported that PGE_2 is a more potent vasodilator in the mesenteric bed than the renal vascular bed[126] yet less potent in the mesenteric than in the femoral circulation[127].

In related studies, in which PGE_2 was administered into the left ventricle and blood flow was measured simultaneously in several territories, it was observed that PGE_2 was a more potent vasodilator in the mesenteric circulation than on the renal, femoral or carotid systems[125,128]. Compared with other prostaglandins, PGE_2 had a similar vasodilatory potency than PGI_2 in the canine[129] and feline[132] mesenteric circulations. PGE_2, in addition to its direct effect on the intestinal circulation, also exerts indirect actions. At doses that have little or no effect on basal perfusion pressure, PGE_2 has been shown to markedly potentiate responses to noradrenaline and nerve stimulation in the isolated perfused superior mesenteric artery of the rat[135-137] but to have the opposite effect in rabbits[137]. These observations led Malik to propose that differing responses to PGE_2 could be explained on the basis of species differences[137]. Later, however, it was learned that PGE_2 in the blood perfused rat mesentery exerted an effect opposite to those seen by Malik, that is an attenuation of pressor responses to norepinephrine and nerve stimulation[138]. This reponse is qualitatively similar to that observed in most species, including human isolated arteries[139], and has been independently confirmed[140]. Thus, it can be concluded that, in all species, prostaglandins *in vivo* probably diminish the pressor effects of sympathetic stimulation or norepinephrine infusions.

PGE_1 is also a potent vasodilator of the intact mesenteric circulation. PGE_1 has been shown to increase mesenteric blood flow in dogs[125,128,141-143], cats[144] and humans[145-148] and jejunal blood flow in rats[149]. Comparison of potency of PGE_1 in several regional circulations reveals that PGE_1 administered into the left ventricle or intravenously is a more potent vasodilator in the mesenteric circulation than in others[125-128]. In fact, in one study, its hypotensive action could be attributed almost solely to mesenteric vasodilatation[128]. In the same study[128], in which PGE_1 was given into the left ventricle, mesenteric vascular resistance decreased by 70% yet renal vascular resistance decreased only by 50%; with close i.a. injection, however, it has been shown that the absolute vasodilatory potency of PGE_1 was similar in the mesenteric and carotid circulations of the dog[150]. Compared with other prostaglandins, PGE_1 is roughly equipotent with PGI_2 in the mesenteric circulation of anaesthetized dogs[128-150]. Although these studies agree in essence, additional investigations, such as those of Covino *et al.*[125], are needed to ascertain the exact rank order of potency of prostaglandins in different vascular beds and the relative potency of different prostaglandins in the mesenteric bed.

PGE_2 and PGE_1 also exert indirect effects in the mesenteric circulation: in the autoperfused feline intestine, it markedly inhibits vasoconstrictor responses to sympathetic nerve stimulation, norepinephrine and angiotensin II,[144] and in the rat perfused mesenteric artery, at low doses, it potentiates and at high doses inhibits pressor responses induced by norepinephrine[136]. In view of the results obtained by Jackson and Campbell[138] in the blood perfused rat mesenteric vascular bed with PGE_2 (see above), it would be interesting to determine whether PGE_1 will still exert the biphasic dose-related response observed *in vitro* or would only be inhibitory, regardless of dose, as shown for PGE_2.[138]

$PGF_{2\alpha}$

$PGF_{2\alpha}$, unlike E type prostaglandins, is an intestinal vasoconstrictor in most species. $PGF_{2\alpha}$, administered i.a., decreases mesenteric blood flow in dogs[141,142,126,151], pigs[133], humans[148], and baboons[151]. It also decreases blood flow in situ in isolated segments of ileum[152] and jejunum of the dog[134], whether administered i.a.[152] or topically (mucosal side)[134]. It also decreases blood flow in the isolated perfused rat mesenteric vascular bed[136]. In the rat isolated jejunal loop, however, it was reported to have no effect on blood flow when given topically, even in high doses[149].

PGA_1 and PGA_2

Early work indicated that PGA was a potent peripheral vasodilator, inducing a dose-related decrease in systemic vascular resistance and increasing cardiac output and heart rate in the conscious dog[153]. This systemic haemodynamic response was accompanied by a more marked decrease in vascular resistance and increase in blood flow in the mesenteric circulation than in the renal or iliac vascular beds[153]. In a related study, both PGA_1 and A_2 given i.v. increased blood flow in the superior mesenteric artery by 71–108% at doses that increased carotid blood flow by only 49–54% and had no effect on renal or femoral blood flow[125]. In a more recent study[150], in which the vasodilatory action of several prostaglandins were compared in the femoral, carotid and mesenteric vascular territories, these observations have been largely confirmed[150]. In addition, it has been suggested that, on a comparative basis, PGA_2 is less potent that either PGI_2 or PGE_2 as an intestinal vasodilator[150].

PGD_2

Reports about the effects of PGD_2 on canine intestinal blood flow are in conflict. PGD_2 has been reported both to decrease[126,129] and to increase[152,154] intestinal blood flow in the dog. In spite of methodological differences between these studies, such as assessment of blood flow in the entire mesenteric bed[126,129] versus an isolated autoperfused ileal segment[152,154], the reasons for these discordant observations are not apparent. In the cat, however, vascular intestinal responses to PGD_2 have been more uniform, and PGD_2 has always been shown to induce vasodilation[130,155] with only an occasional initial vasoconstrictor component[155]. As for other prostaglandins, PGD_2 has also been shown to have an inhibitory action on vascular sympathetic neurotransmission[132,155], substantially attenuating responses induced by most sympathetic stimuli.

Prostacyclin

Since the first description of the biological effects of PGI_2 in cascade superfused isolated vessels was made by Moncada et al.[8], it has become clear that PGI_2 is the vasodilator prostaglandin par excellence[156]. The mesenteric circulation in this regard is not an exception and, in fact is one of the territories most sensitive to PGI_2 vasodilator actions. PGI_2 dose-dependently increased blood flow in the canine superior mesenteric vascular bed[126–129,150,154]. It also increased portal venous flow in the pig[157], an action that is in keeping with its potent vasodilatory action on the mesenteric circulation. A stable analogue of PGI_2, 13,14-dehydroprostacyclin methyl ester, is also a potent mesenteric vasodilator in cats[132]. Under conditions of controlled blood flow, PGI_2 has been shown to dose-dependently decrease perfusion pressure in the feline mesenteric circulation[158]. The vasodilatory action of PGI_2 is not limited, however, to physiological conditions, but has also been observed under pathological circumstances, such as in the ischaemic intestine of the dog[154,159] and, albeit of lower magnitude, in the reperfusing intestine of the dog after a period of total superior mesenteric artery occlusion[160].

In comparative studies, PGI_2 has been shown to be equipotent[126,129] or more potent[128] than PGE_2 and equipotent to PGE_1[150] as a vasodilator of the canine mesenteric vascular bed. On the other hand, studies which have compared the potency of PGI_2 in several peripheral vessels indicate that PGI_2 is a more potent vasodilator in the mesenteric than in the renal[129,126], carotid or femoral[150] circulations. One study, however, reported that PGI_2 was about equipotent in both the mesenteric and femoral beds[127].

PGI_2 is highly unstable in aqueous solution and rapidly degrades nonenzymatically to form 6-keto-$PGF_{1\alpha}$[161], a compound which has been shown to be almost devoid of biological activity. In the mesenteric circulation, 6-keto-$PGE_{1\alpha}$ had little or no direct or indirect effect on blood flow[129]. PGI_2, however, also has other available metabolic degradation pathways. In blood vessels, it is enzymatically converted into 6,15-diketo-$PGF_{1\alpha}$, an action mediated by 15-OH prostaglandin dehydrogenase[162], and, in the liver it is converted to 6-keto-PGE_1 by the action of 9-OH prostaglandin dehydrogenase[163]. This last metabolite has been shown to retain substantial PGI_2-like biological activity, and, in fact, it increased blood flow in the territory of the superior mesenteric artery of dogs[128] and decreased perfusion pressure in the constant-flow perfused feline mesenteric vascular bed[144], with potencies comparable to those of PGI_2[128] or PGE_1[144].

PGI_2 also exerts indirect actions, primarily through modulating sympathetic neurotransmission as shown by its ability to inhibit vasoconstriction induced by nerve stimulation on norepinephrine in the feline intestine[161]. Interestingly, 6-keto-PGE_1, a vasoactive metabolite of PGI_2, also seems to share this action[146].

Endoperoxides

The analysis of the vascular actions of endoperoxides is complicated by their rapid conversion into other vasoactive metabolites of the arachidonate cascade (PGI_2, PGE_2, TxA_2), making it difficult to attribute the effect observed to the endoperoxides unambiguously. Although endoproxide conversion into TxA_2 can be selectively and effectively inhibited[164], blockade of their transformation into prostaglandins and prostacyclin *in vivo* has been difficult to achieve. Nevertheless, PGH_2, given by close i.a. injection into the inferior mesenteric artery, has been shown to increase blood flow in the dog[127,129,165-167]. The potency of PGH_2 as a vasodilator was shown to be equal to[127] or less than[129] that of PGI_2 under comparable conditions, leading to the suggestion that the effects of PGH_2 could be due largely to its bioconversion into PGI_2[127,166] or PGE_2[167]. One way of overcoming the difficulty posed by the instability of PGH_2 is to analyse the vascular responses induced by stable endoperoxide analogues which are not further metabolized into other active metabolites. Several compounds in this category have been synthesized, of which the epoximethano endoperoxide analogues, U-44069 and U-46619, are the most studied. U-46619 induces mesenteric vasoconstriction in the dog[127,167]. Recently, however, some doubts have been cast about the appropriateness of classifying U-46619 as an endoperoxide analogue since its biological profile resembles more closely that of thromboxanes (see above) For this reason, there is a rising tendency to group them under the designation 'thromboxane mimetics'.

Thromboxanes

Owing to the instability of TxA_2, few studies have been carried out to determine its effects on intestinal blood flow. In an early study, TxA_2 was shown to exert a potent vasoconstrictive effect on the mesenteric circulation of the dog[127] and to be less potent in the femoral bed[127,165]. The rise in perfusion pressure caused by TxA_2 was exacerbated by indomethacin pretreatment. This effect of indomethacin was attributed to inhibition of endogenous PGI_2 synthesis[127,165]. In addition to these direct and still not fully characterized effects of TxA_2, it has been shown that inhibition of thromboxane generation by dazoxiben or other thromboxane synthetase inhibitors leads to inhibition of vascular responsiveness to sympathetic nerve stimulation and angiotensin II in the blood perfused rat mesenteric vascular bed[140,168]. Since indomethacin could prevent the effect of thromboxane synthetase inhibitors on vascular responsiveness, the results are interpreted as indicating that the effect of thromboxane synthetase inhibitors was mediated through reorientation of AA cascade towards the production of metabolites such as PGE_2 and I_2 which are known to decrease vascular responsiveness to adrenergic stimuli (see above).

Cyclo-oxygenase inhibitors

Indomethacin reduces blood flow in the mesenteric vascular bed of dogs[127,169,170] and in the jejunum[150], and increases splanchnic vascular resistance in humans[146]. It also has been shown to reduce[170] or abolish[127] mesenteric vasodilatation induced by arachidonic acid and to have no effect on responses to nerve stimulation or norepinephrine in the dog[140], but in the rat it prevents the attenuation of reaction to sympathetic stimuli induced by chronic treatment with UK38,485, a thromboxane synthetase inhibitor[168]. Ibuprofen, however, in doses that inhibit arachidonate-induced mesenteric vasodilatation to the same extent that indomethacin does, caused no vasoconstriction[170]. Similar results with meclofenamate had been obtained earlier, although the completeness of cyclo-oxygenase blockade was not assessed in that study[169].

Additionally, indomethacin has been shown to have no effect on blood flow in the kidney[170].

Collectively, this evidence might be taken to indicate that inhibition of cyclo-oxygenase does not necessarily change mesenteric blood flow, and, therefore, the effects of indomethacin are not related to prostaglandin-synthesis inhibition. Whether this is true of false will be determined only after studies correlating the magnitude of blood flow changes with the extent of cyclo-oxygenase inhibition when other cyclo-oxygenase inhibitors become available.

Lipoxygenase products

The vascular action of lipoxygenase products, particularly leukotrienes (LT), in the intestinal circulation have received limited attention. Studies in the canine mesenteric vascular bed have shown LTC_4, LTD_4 and, to a lesser extent, LTE_4 to be potent vasoconstrictors[171,172]. Similar results were obtained in the feline mesenteric vascular bed perfused at constant flow[173]. Leukotrienes were more potent vasoconstrictors than norepinephrine in the dog[170] and equipotent with norepinephrine in the cat[173]. Since vasoconstriction induced by leukotrienes was not altered by indomethacin in the dog[171,172], or by meclofenamate in the cat[173], it was concluded that it was not mediated by cyclo-oxygenase metabolites. Furthermore, since FPL-55712 could inhibit the vasoconstriction induced by LTC_4 and LTD_4 in the dog[171], it is likely that the responses were mediated through LT receptors. Interestingly, the mesenteric vascular bed was much more sensitive to the pressor effect of leukotrienes than the renal circulation[171,172].

EICOSANOIDS AND ISOLATED GASTROINTESTINAL VASCULAR SMOOTH MUSCLE

The variable effects of eicosanoids on gastrointestinal blood flow reflect the complexity of their interactions with vascular effectors. In the intact circulation, two types of effects can be recognized in general: those that are exerted by direct interaction with vascular smooth muscle cells and those that are mediated by interaction with non-smooth muscle cells (endothelium, neurons, blood cells, etc.) and thus are essentially indirect. The response of a vascular territory *in vivo* to a particular eicosanoid thus depends on the relative contributions of these two general mechanisms.

Direct effects

Direct effects of eicosanoids on blood vessels are usually studied in isolated vascular strips in which generally the indirect effects do not participate to a great extent. Research in this area favours the view that the indirect effect of eicosanoids on vascular smooth muscle is mediated via receptors[174-179] rather than other actions such as a direct ionophoretic action, changes in membrane fluidity, or interaction with intracellular enzymes[174]. In spite of the progress made so far in clarifying and localizing eicosanoids receptors, it is not possible at present to ascertain the number and subclasses of such receptors, their distribution and the nature of their second messengers[175-178].

PGE_2 exerts variable effects on isolated gastrointestinal blood vessels. At concentrations up to $5.6 \times 10^{-6} mol L^{-1}$, PGE_2 relaxes the isolated canine mesenteric arteries and veins of dogs[179,180] and rabbits[181]. In small canine mesenteric arteries (outside diameter < 1 mm), however, PGE_2 increases vessel tone (ED_{50} $4 \times 10^{-7} mol L^{-1}$) without inducing relaxation at any given concentration[182]. In human isolated mesenteric arteries, low concentrations of PGE_2 ($0.7-3.6 \times 10^{-9} mol L^{-1}$) decreased, whereas higher concentrations (5.7×10^{-8} $mol L^{-1}$) increased basal tone[139]. PGE_1 has been found to be a potent vasodilator in the isolated mesenteric artery of the dog[182] but to have no effect on neonatal lamb mesenteric arteries[183,184].

$PGF_{2\alpha}$ is, in most circumstances, a vasoconstrictor. It contracts large[185] and small[182] isolated mesenteric arteries of the dog in a concentration range of $10^{-7}-10^{-6} mol L^{-1}$. In the same preparation in the rat, it induces contractions with a potency comparable to that of norepinephrine[186].

PGD_2 has little or no effect on resting tension of isolated dog mesenteric artery[187]. Coronary, renal and femoral arteries, however, respond to PGD_2 ($10^{-7}-10^{-5}$ $mol L^{-1}$) with contractions[187]. In the mesenteric artery precontracted with $PGF_{2\alpha}$ or norepinephrine, PGD_2 induces a marked relaxation[187].

Prostacyclin has been known to be a potent vasodilator since its discovery[8,97]. The potent vasorelaxing effect of PGI_2 on gastrointestinal blood vessels has been confirmed many times[180–182]. PGI_2 also relaxes the coeliac artery precontracted by electrical stimulation or norepinephrine in rabbits[188,189], dogs[190] and neonatal lambs[184].

Endoperoxides exert variable effects on gastrointestinal blood vessels. PGG_2 and PGH_2 relaxed coeliac and mesenteric arterial strips of rabbits, albeit with a fifth of the potency of PGE_2[191]. U-46619 and other related endoperoxide analogues are, however, potent vasoconstrictors in rabbit mesenteric artery strips[192].

TxA_2 has been shown to induce long-lasting contractions in both coeliac and superior mesenteric artery strips of rabbits assayed in the cascade superfusion system[191], as well as in mesenteric arteries of several other species[193,194]. In fact, carbocyclic TxA_2 (a stable analogue of TxA_2) at low concentrations ($10^{-10} - 10^{-9} mol L^{-1}$) induced contractions in all arteries tested[193]. The ED_{50} in mesenteric strips from dogs and monkeys was $\sim 4 \times 10^{-9} mol L^{-1}$. LTC_4 and D_4 are inactive in the isolated superior mesenteric artery of rabbits (up to $10^{-7} mol L^{-1}$)[195] but dose-dependently relax the mesenteric artery of the dog[196]. Interestingly, LTD_4-induced relaxation was observed only on those preparations in which care was taken to avoid damaging the intimal surface, suggesting that the endothelium mediated this response.

Indirect effects

Most indirect actions of eicosanoids on isolated vessels can be largely attributed to modification of vascular noradrenergic transmission or that of other vasoactive systems[197]. Recently, it has been realized that the endothelium can also modulate or mediate responses to vasoactive agents[198–200], and that eicosanoids may participate in these responses[201–203].

Although the complexity of these interactions precludes their full treatment in this review, some generalizations can be made. The effect of prostaglandins on noradrenergic transmission is highly variable between species and even within a single species among different vascular territories[197]. Most prostaglandins potentiate noradrenergic transmission in the perfused vascular bed of the rat[204-207] and in the isolated mesenteric artery of the dog[208-209], but inhibit them in mesenteric arteries of rabbits[188,204], neonatal lambs[183], and humans[182]. The demonstration by Jackson and Campbell[138] of inhibition of noradrenergic responses in the blood perfused mesenteric bed of the rat has raised the possibility that, in the intact circulation, PGs inhibit vascular noradrenergic responses in all species.

EICOSANOIDS, BLOOD FLOW AND GASTROINTESTINAL MUCOSAL DAMAGE

Vascular injury may accompany acute mucosal damage. In the absence of microvascular injury, the surface epithelium repairs rapidly (e.g. within hours) by cell migration restoring both morphological and physiological parameters traditionally associated with mucosal integrity[210-213]. This phenomenom has been termed 'epithelial restitution'[214] and seems to represent a first line of defence in epithelial injury of mild to moderate intensity[214]. Severe epithelial damage is invariably associated with extensive injury to the mucosal microcirculation resulting in haemorrhage and ischaemia (Figure 9.1). Severely damaged epithelium does not repair by restitution but instead by a process involving cell division that takes days or weeks to complete[215].

From the discussion above, it follows that the presence or absence of vascular injury is a critical factor in mucosal injury because it determines two radically different time frames for repair and restoration of functional integrity (Figure 9.1).

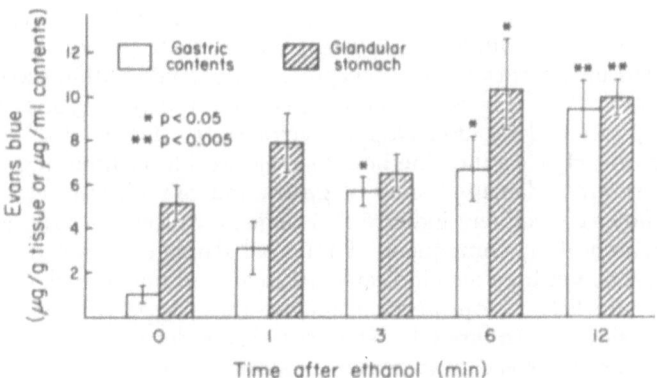

Figure 9.1 The time course of extravasation of Evan's blue (injected i.v.) into the glandular stomach tissue and gastric lumen of the rat after i.g. administration of 1 ml of 75% ethanol. (Reproduced with permission from Szabo *et al.* (1985). *Gastroenterology*, **88**, 228–236)

Ever since Virchow *et al* implicated ischaemia as a causative factor in ulceration[216], the aetiological importance of vascular changes in mucosal damage has been controversial[217]. We will describe below the different circumstances in which vascular injury is encountered in acute mucosal damage and outline both the importance of vascular changes and the perceived role of eicosanoids in ameliorating or exacerbating such vascular damage. The discussion will focus entirely on the gastric mucosa, since only limited data are available for the rest of the gut mucosa.

Mucosal damage caused by concentrated ethanol, HCl and NaOH

Experimental intragastric administration of 100% ethanol, strong acids and alkali, hypertonic NaCl or hot liquids induce severe mucosal damage with rapid development[218-220], involving the gastric glands and the mucosal microcirculation[215,218-222]. These lesions heal slowly by cell division[215]. Pretreatment with small doses of prostaglandins prevents mucosal damage to structures located deeper than the monolayer of surface mucous cells[218-225]. This property of PGs has been termed cytoprotection by Robert *et al.*[223,224]. As defined originally, cytoprotection excludes, as a mechanism of action, inhibition of gastric acid secretion, since PGs devoid of antisecretory action, or at doses that do not inhibit acid secretion, were able to elicit protection in the rat[223].

In spite of extensive research in the last decade, the mechanism(s) of cytoprotection has remained elusive (for review, see references 226–229). Recently, it has become apparent from work in our[60, 218–220, 230] and other[221,225,231–233] laboratories that damaging agents rapidly produce extensive microcirculatory changes both structurally[218–221,225] and functionally[60,230–233] preceding the development of intramucosal haemorrhage[218–220]. Seconds after ethanol, there is a massive and rapid increase in vascular permeability to albumin (Evan's blue extravasation) (Figure 9.1) and extensive labelling of mucosal microvessels with monastral blue (a marker of vascular injury) (Figure 9.2). These changes could be substantially attenuated by PG pretreatment[218–220]. Furthermore, $16,16$-dmPGE$_2$ ($10 \mu g \, kg^{-1}$) was able to prevent the microcirculatory stasis in superficial mucosal capillaries observed within seconds after topical ethanol[60,230,231] (Figure 9.3) and the ensuing mucosal hypoperfusion as continuously assessed by laser-Doppler velocimetry (Figure 9.4)[60,230]. Leung *et al.*, using the H$_2$ clearance method to measure blood flow, found absent blood flow in gross damaged areas of gastric mucosa 1 h after ethanol[58].

These studies collectively indicate that damage to the mucosal microcirculation is an important component of mucosal damage caused by necrosis-inducing agents, yet they also indicate that increased mucosal blood flow per se does not mediate cytoprotection against these type of agents as once thought[88,89], since $16,16$-dmPGE$_2$, at doses that induce mucosal protection, slightly decreased, instead of increasing, mucosal blood flow.

An all important issue that has remained unsolved in these studies is whether PGs protect the mucosal microcirculation directly or whether they do so as a consequence of preserving epithelial integrity in the first place.

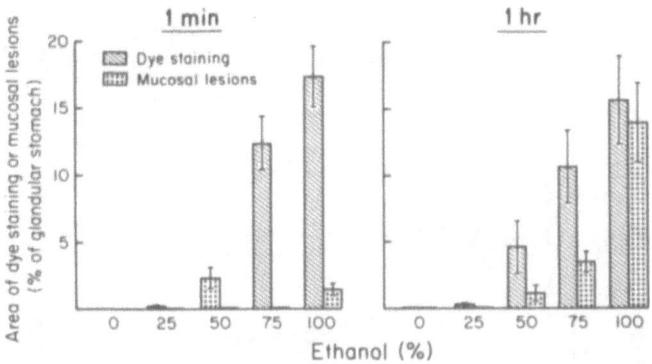

Figure 9.2 The area of vascular injury as revealed by monastral blue deposition 1 min or 1 h after various doses of ethanol. (Modified from Szabo *et al.* (1985). *Gastroenterology*, **88**, 228–236)

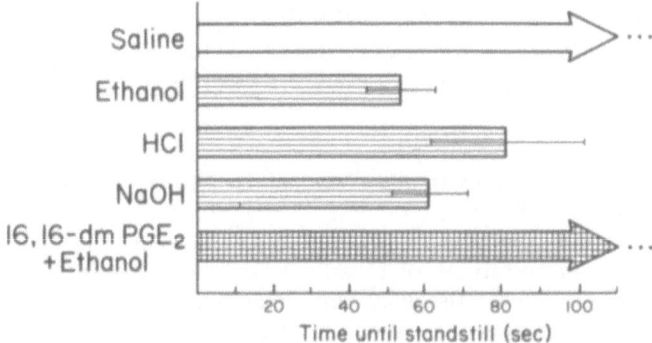

Figure 9.3 *In vivo* microscopy of microcirculation (passage of erythrocytes in subepithelial capillaries) in a chambered area of the glandular stomach in an anaesthetized rat after topical application of 100% ethanol, $0.6\,mol\,L^{-1}$ HCl or $0.2\,mol\,L^{-1}$ NaOH. In the last column, exposure to ethanol was preceded by 16, 16-dmPGE$_2$ ($10\,\mu g\,kg^{-1}$ i.g.)

Fragmentary evidence suggests that PGs protect the microcirculation directly. For instance, neither the morphological[212,222,225] nor the functional[215,222] indices of surface epithelial injury observed after ethanol are prevented by PGs, making it unlikely that the prevention of vascular injury is secondary to epithelial preservation. Moreover, the intramucosal concentration of ethanol[234] has been shown to be similar in animals pretreated with prostaglandins and those left untreated, suggesting that the microcirculation was in contact with as much ethanol in untreated damaged mucosa, as it was in PG-pretreated mucosa, in which vascular lesions were prevented. This strongly suggests that vascular protection is a direct action of PGs on blood vessels. Further studies in this direction, however, are needed since the immediate perivascular concentration of ethanol is unknown and might be lower in PG-treated mucosa than in control mucosa. A related unsolved issue is whether PGs can increase cellular resistance to noxious agents, as claimed by Robert[228], and

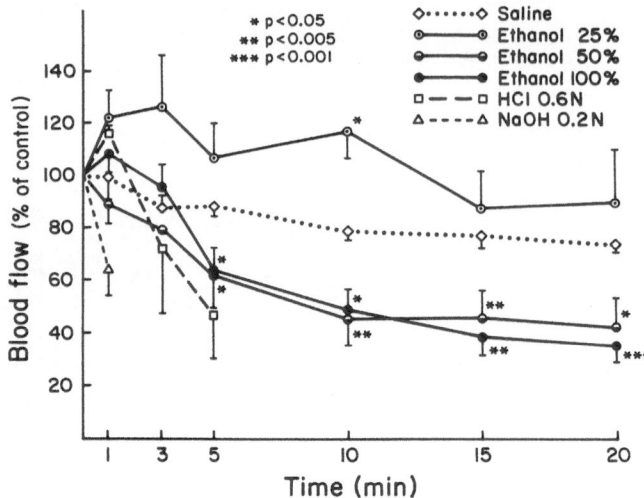

Figure 9.4 Laser-Doppler velocimetry of mucosal blood flow measured under experimental conditions described in Figure 9.3. 25% and 50% ethanol were also used. (Reprinted with permission from Pihan *et al.* (1986). *Gastroenterology*, **91**, 1415–1426.)

whether this includes the vascular endothelium. Studies addressing this issue using isolated epithelial cells have been largely inconclusive. Recent work in our laboratory indicates that 16,16-dmPGE$_2$ can decrease the direct cytotoxic effect of low concentrations of ethanol in cultured endothelial cells in the presence of plasma in the tissue culture medium (Szabo *et al.*, in preparation). This effect could explain the maintenance of mucosal blood flow associated with mucosal protection as found by Guth *et al.*[58,231,232] and our laboratory[60,230]. Further studies are required, however, before concluding that these are the mechanisms by which PGs prevent gastric mucosal lesions after damaging agents.

Recently, emerging evidence indicates that leukotrienes may play a role in acute mucosal damage induced by chemicals. LTC$_4$ and D$_4$ potentiated ethanol-induced mucosal injury[235] by a mechanism apparently dependent on vascular factors since close i.a. infusion of LTs in the rat stomach induced extensive vascular injury (as revealed by monastral blue labelling) yet minor or no epithelial damage was observed[235] (Figure 9.5). Furthermore, dietary treatment with eicosapentaenoic acid, a substrate which competes with arachidonic acid in the lipoxygenase pathway resulting in LTs of lowered

Figure 9.5 End face view of gastric mucosa after the fixed stomach was cleared in glycerol. The rats were injected with monastral blue (3 mg (100 g)$^{-1}$ i.v.) 3 min before starting the intra-arterial infusion. (A) Control rat infused with saline ($\times$ 28). (B) Rat infused with LTD$_4$ (1 nmol (100g)$^{-1}$ min^{-1}). Notice the labelling of collecting venules in B (arrows) ($\times$ 28). (C) Same rat with microscopic focus on labelling of submucosal venules and veins (arrows) and congested blood vessels in muscularis propria or serosa (*) ($\times$ 28)

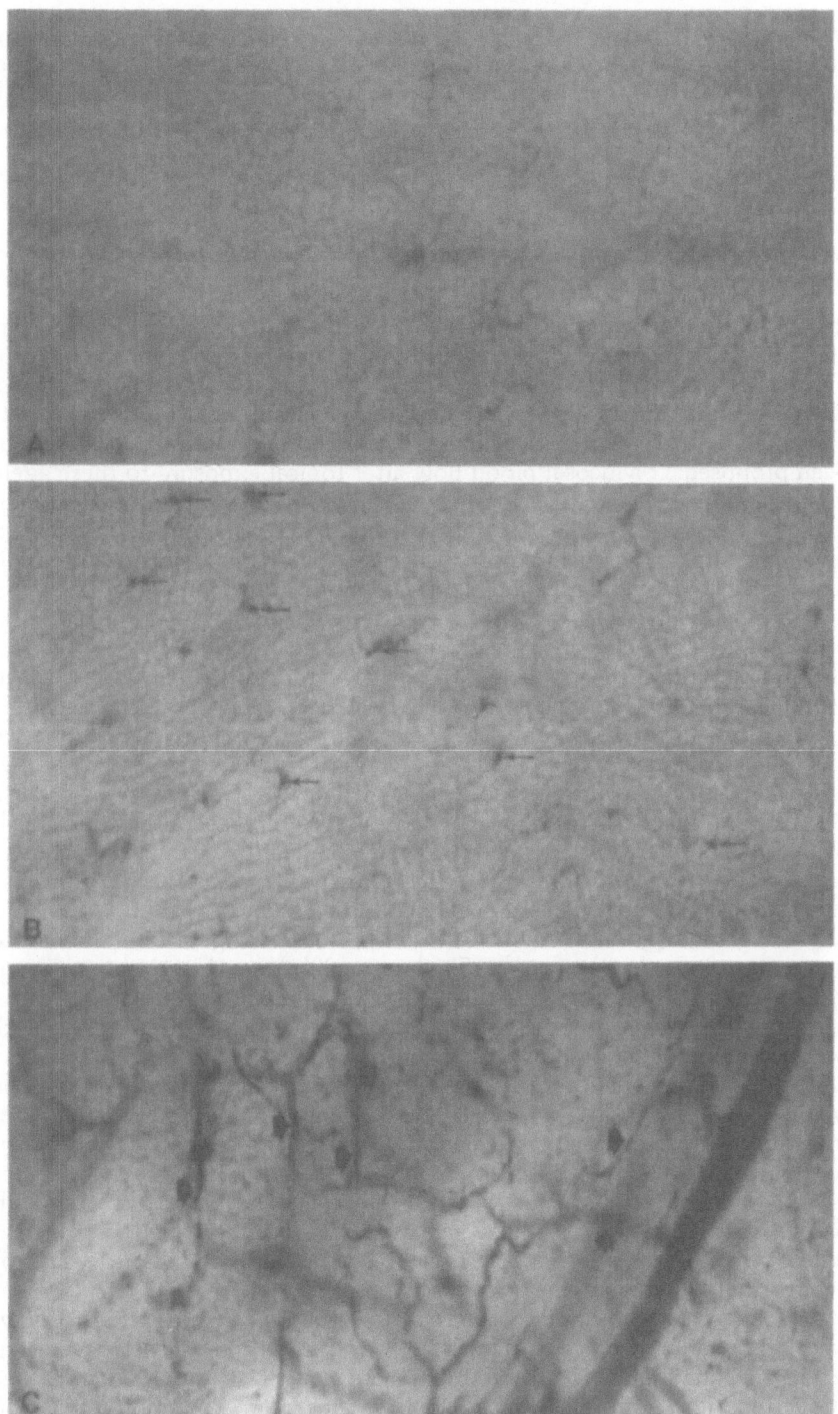

inflammatory potency, decreases both acute haemorrhagic mucosal damage and microvascular injury induced by several damaging agents[216]. This evidence, together with the demonstration of increased leukotriene levels in the gastric mucosa exposed to ethanol[237], suggests that LT may contribute to microvascular injury in acute mucosal damage.

Mucosal damage induced by aspirin, indomethacin, bile acids and other barrier breakers

It is currently believed that mucosal damage induced by indomethacin, aspirin and bile salts results from back-diffusion of lumenal H^+ into the gastric mucosa as originally proposed by Davenport et al.[238-240]. The mechanism whereby these agents induce H^+ back-diffusion are largely unknown but a combination of direct surface mucosal injury and decreased PG synthesis has been proposed[241]. Mucosal blood flow after topical exposure to these agents invariably increases, often in direct proportion to the severity of gross mucosal injury[242-245]. The exact relationship between mucosal blood flow and lesion development, however, has not been easy to establish since most studies have correlated mucosal blood flow and lesion development in a mucosal area in which lesions cover just a small fraction of the area. Recent studies using the H_2 gas clearance technique, which is capable of assessing focal changes in blood flow, have indicated that, after both topical bile acid and aspirin, blood flow decreases or does not show compensatory increase in areas which subsequently develop lesions[246-247] (Figure 9.6), suggesting that mucosal ischaemia is indeed an important factor in the development of these lesions and that increased blood flow is an important defensive mechanism. Reduction of mucosal blood flow by the infusion of vasoconstrictors[245] or by haemorrhagic shock[248] aggravates, whereas vasodilators, such as isoproterenol, reduce mucosal lesions induced by bile salts[248,249]. Indomethacin and aspirin, two agents that reduce mucosal blood flow presumably through inhibition of prostaglandin synthesis, aggravate, whereas PGs mitigate, bile-acid induced mucosal lesions in the rat[105]. Similar results have been obtained with indomethacin in the dog[152], and PGI_2 in the miniature swine[90] after topical exposure to bile. Two mechanisms have been postulated to explain the beneficial effect of blood flow: (1) maintenace of normal mucosal ATP levels[251] and optimal oxygenation resulting in maintenance of the proliferative zone of the gastric mucosa[225,252]; and (2) dissipation of back-diffusion[253,254]. Both mechanisms have experimental support. On the basis of these findings, it has been proposed that cytoprotection by prostaglandins against 'barrier breakers' is due to increased blood flow. This hypothesis needs further testing by determining whether PGs that reduce mucosal blood flow or do not increase mucosal blood flow in areas that develop lesions, also lack protective actions against these agents, as the hypothesis predicts.

Among other eicosanoids, thromboxanes have been suggested to play a role in bile-induced mucosal damage[99,255,256]. Since both mucosal lesions and ischaemia could be reduced by thromboxane synthetase inhibition, it has been suggested that thromboxanes may contribute to lesion formation by inducing

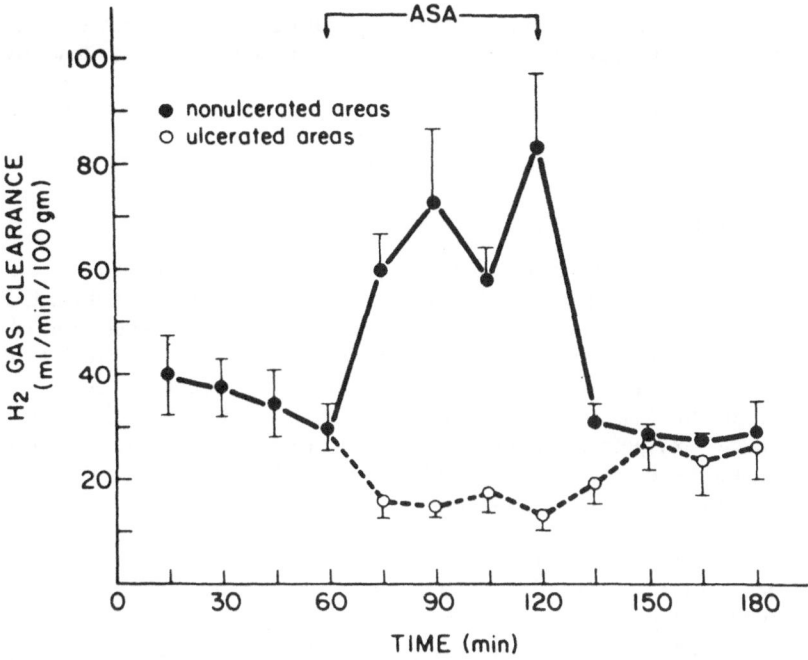

Figure 9.6 Gastric mucosal blood flow measured by hydrogen gas clearance after topical application of aspirin. (Reprinted with permission from Ashley, S.E. *et al.* (1985). *Am. J. Surg.*, **149**, 53–58)

ischaemia[99,255,256]. Similar results have been obtained with the thromboxane mimetic, U-46619[257].

Mucosal damage induced by stress and circulatory shock

There is an intimate relationship between the development of stress ulceration and circulatory shock. Nearly all investigators agree that mucosal ischaemia is one of the most important factors in the development of acute stress ulceration[258,261]. Mucosal ischaemia per se, however, does not cause grossly evident mucosal lesions unless severe or followed by reperfusion[262]. Therefore, mucosal ischaemia seems to play a permissive role, i.e. it is needed for lesions to develop, yet, by itself, is not sufficient to cause lesions. The explanation of this apparent paradox is found in studies simultaneously measuring H^+ back-diffusion and mucosal ischaemia. These studies have found that the presence of either factor alone does not lead to lesion development yet their combination always does[46,245]. It follows that maintenance of blood flow would preclude lesion development and this has been demonstrated experimentally[246].

Several PGs have been shown to prevent stress-induced lesions[64–66,90,263]. Under these conditions, PGs lessen mucosal hypoperfusion but not H^+ back-diffusion. Therefore, lessening of mucosal hypoperfusion is, in all likelihood, the most important mechanism of PG-induced mucosal protection during stress.

There is some fragmentary evidence implicating thromboxanes as contributors to mucosal hypoperfusion during water-immersion stress[264]and hypothermic restraint stress[265].

However, whether thromboxanes have a wider role in conditions leading to mucosal ischaemia is not currently known.

SUMMARY

Evidence accrued during the past few years indicates an important role for eicosanoids in the regulation of blood flow in the gastrointestinal tract, both under physiological and pathological conditions. With the exception of the F series, prostaglandins as a group have been shown to be vasodilators in the gastrointestinal circulation, whereas thromboxanes and leukotrienes, under most circumstances, are vasoconstrictors. The reduction in blood flow observed after cyclo-oxygenase inhibition indicates that, under basal conditions, prostaglandins exert a tonic vasodilatory effect on gastrointestinal blood vessels, and thus the local prostaglandin levels may have a regulatory role in blood flow.

It has also been learned recently that the interactions of eicosanoids with vascular targets are complex and involve a variety of mechanisms that can be broadly categorized into direct and indirect effects.

The role of altered blood flow regulation by eicosanoids in pathological conditions of the gut, particularly of upper gastrointestinal tract, is also emerging. In acute gastric mucosal protection, for example, blood flow maintenance by prostaglandins seems to be an important mechanism. Further insights into the actions of eicosanoids on gastrointestinal blood flow will hopefully lead to new and effective therapeutic agents.

REFERENCES

1. Corey, E.J., Hiwa, H., Falck, J.R., Mioskowski, C., Arai, Y. and Marfat, A. (1987). Recent studies on the chemical synthesis of eicosanoids. In Samuelsson, B., Ramwell, R.W. and Paoletti, R. (eds.). *Advances in Prostaglandin and Thromboxane Research*. Vol. 6, pp. 19–25. (New York: Raven Press)
2. Moncada, S. (ed.). (1983). Prostacyclin, thromboxane and leukotrienes. *Br. Med. Bull.*, **39**, 209–289
3. Samuelsson, B., Goldyne, M., Granström, E., Hamberg, M., Hammarstrom, S. and Malmsten, C. (1978). Prostaglandin and thromboxanes. *Ann. Rev. Biochem.*, **47**, 997–1029
4. Moncada, S. and Vane, J.R. (1979). Pharmacology and endogenous roles of prostaglandin endoperoxides, thromboxane A_2, and prostacyclin. *Pharmacol. Rev.*, **30**, 293–331
5. Samuelsson, B. and Hammarström, S. (1982). Leukotrienes: A novel group of biologically active compounds. *Vitam. Horm.*, **39**, 1–30
6. Von Euler, U.S. (1937). On the specific vasodilating and plain muscle stimulating substance from accessory genital glands on man and certain animals (prostaglandin and vesiglandin). *J. Physiol.*, **88**, 213–234
7. Bergström, S. and Sjövall, J. (1960). The isolation of prostaglandin F from sheep prostate glands. *Acta Chem. Scand.*, **14**, 1693–1701
8. Moncada, S., Gryglewski, R.J., Bunting, S. and Vane, J.R. (1976). An enzyme isolated from arteries transforms prostaglandin endoperoxide to an unstable substance that inhibits platelet aggregation. *Nature (London)*, **263**, 663–665

9. Hamberg, M., Svensson, J. and Samuelsson, B. (1975). Thromboxanes: A new group of biologically active compounds derived from prostaglandin endoperoxides. Proc. Natl. Acad. Sci. USA, 72, 2994–2998

10. Feldberg, W. and Kellaway, C.H. (1938). Liberation of histamine and formation of lysolecithin-like substances by cobra venom. J. Physiol. (Lond.), 94, 187–226

11. Murphy, R.C., Hammarström, S. and Samuelsson, B. (1979). Leukotriene C: A slow reacting substance from murine mastocytoma cells. Proc. Natl. Acad. Sci. USA, 76, 4275–4279

12. Samuelsson, B. (1983). Leukotrienes: Mediators of immediate hypersensitivity reactions and inflammation. Science, 220, 568–575

13. Needleman, P., Turk, J., Jakschick, B.A., Morrison, A.R. and Lefkowith, J.B. (1986). Arachidonic acid metabolism. Ann. Rev. Biochem., 55, 69–102

14. Serhan, C.N., Hamberg, M. and Samuelsson, B. (1984). Lipoxins: Novel series of biologically active compounds formed from arachidonic acid in human leukocytes. Proc. Natl. Acad. Sci. USA, 81, 5335–5339

15. Serhan, C.N., Hamberg, M. and Samuelsson, B. (1986). Novel mechanisms in arachidonic acid cascade: formation of lipoxins. In Russo-Marie F., Mencia-Huerta J.M. and Chignard M. (eds). Advance in Inflammation Research, Vol. 10, pp. 117–128. (New York: Raven Press)

16. Schwartzman, M., Ferreri, N.R., Carroll, M.A., Songu-Mize, E. and McGiff, J.C. (1985). Renal cytochrome P450-related arachidonate metabolite inhibits $(Na^+ + K^+)$ ATPase. Nature (London) 314, 620–622

17. Bennett, A., Friedman, C.A. and Vane, J.R. (1967). Release of prostaglandin E_1 from the rat stomach. Nature (London) 216, 873–876

18. Bennett, A., Stamford, I.F. and Stockley, H.L. (1977). Estimation and characterization of prostaglandins in the human gastrointestinal tract. J. Pharmacol., 61, 579–586

19. Ahlquist, D.A., Duenes, J.A., Madson, T.H., Romero, J.C., Dozois, R.R. and Malagelada, J-R. (1982). Prostaglandin generation from gastroduodenal mucosa: Regional and species difference. Prostaglandins, 24, 115–125

20. Ligumsky, M., Karmeli, F., Sharon, P., Zor, V., Cohen, F. and Rachmilewitz, D. (1981). Enhanced thromboxane A_2 and prostaglandin production by cultured rectal mucosa in ulcerative colitis and its inhibition by steriods and sulphasalazine. Gastroenterology, 81, 444–449

21. Aly, A., Johansson, C., Slezak, P. and Green, K. (1984). Bioconversion of arachidonic acid in the human gastrointestinal tract. Biochem. Med., 31, 319–331

22. Peskar, B.M., Seyberth, H.W. and Peskar, B.A. (1980). Synthesis and metabolism of endogenous prostaglandins by human gastric mucosa. In Samuelsson, B., Ramwell, P.W. and Paoletti, R. (eds.). Advances in Prostaglandins and Thromboxane Research, Vol. 8, pp. 1511–1514. (New York: Raven Press)

23. LeDrec, L.E. and Needleman, P. (1979). Regional localization of prostacyclin and thromboxane synthesis in dog stomach and intestinal tract. J. Pharmacol. Exp. Ther., 211, 181–188.

24. Wölblong, R.H., Aehringhaus, V., Peskar, B.A., Morgenroth, K. and Peskar, B.M. (1983). Release of slow-reacting substance of anaphylaxis and leukotriene C4-like immunoreactivity from guinea pig colonic tissue. Prostaglandins, 25, 809–822

25. Boughton-Smith, N.K., Hawkey, C.J. and Whittle, B.J.R. (1983). Biosynthesis of lipoxygenase and cyclo-oxygenase products from [^{14}C]-arachidonic acid by human colonic mucosa. Gut, 24, 1176–1182

26. Zifroni, A., Treves, A.J., Sacher, D.B. and Rachmilewitz, D. (1983). Prostanoid synthesis by cultured intestinal epithelial and mononuclear cells in inflammatory bowel disease. Gut, 24, 659–664

27. Postius, S., Ruoff, H-J. and Szelenyi, I. (1985). Prostaglandin formation by isolated gastric parietal and nonparietal cells of the rat. Br. J. Pharmacol., 84, 871–877

28. Bonney, R.J., Wightman, P.D., Dahlgren, M.E., Davies, P., Kuehl, F.A., Jr. and Humes, J.L. (1978). Regulation of prostaglandin synthesis and of selective release of lysosomal hydrolases by mouse peritoneal macrophages. Biochem. J., 179, 433–442

29. Bonney, R.J., Opas, E.E. and Humes, J.L. (1985). Lipoxygenase pathways of macrophages. Fed. Proc., 44, 2933–2936

30. Steinhoff, M.M., Lee, L.H. and Jakschik, B.A. (1980). Enzymatic formation of prostaglandin D_2 by rat basophilic leukemia cells and normal rat mast cells. Biochim. Biophys. Acta, 618, 28–34
31. Lewis, P.A., Wasserman, S.I., Goetzl, E.J. and Austen, K.F. (1974). The release of four mediators of immediate hypersensitivity from human leukemic basophils. J. Exp. Med., 140, 1133–1146
32. Robert, A. and Ruwart, M.J. (1982). Effects of prostaglandins on the digestive system. In Lee, J.B. (ed.). Prostaglandins, pp. 113–176. (New York: Elsevier)
33. Robert, A. (1981). Prostaglandins and the gastrointestinal tract. (1981). In Johnson, L.R. (Chief ed.). Physiology of the Gastrointestinal Tract, pp. 1407–1434. (New York: Raven Press)
34. Robert, A. (1977). Prostaglandins and the digestive system. In Ramwell. P.W., (ed.). The Prostaglandins. pp. 225–266. Vol. III, (New York: Plenum Press)
35. Gallavan, R.H. and Jacobson, E.D. (1982). Minireview: Prostaglandins and the splanchnic circulation. Proc. Soc. Exp. Biol. Med., 170, 391–397
36. Whittle, B.J.R. and Vane, J.R. (1983). Prostacyclin, thromboxanes, and prostaglandins. Actions and roles in the gastrointestinal tract. In Glass, G.B.J. and Sherlock, P. (eds.). Progress in Gastroenterology, Vol. IV, pp. 3–30. (New York: Grune & Stratton)
37. Williams, T.J. (1983). Interactions between prostaglandins, leukotrienes and other mediators of inflammation. Br. Med. Bull., 39, 239–242
38. Armstrong, J.M., Dusting, G.J., Moncada, S. and Vane, J.R. (1978). Cardiovascular actions of prostacyclin (PGI_2) a metabolite of arachidonic acid which is synthesized by blood vessels. Circ. Res., 43, (Suppl. 1), 112–119
39. Malik, K.V. (1978). Prostaglandins—modulation of adrenergic nervous system. Fed. Proc., 37, 203–207
40. Messina, E.J., Weiner, R. and Kaley, G. (1976). Prostaglandins and local circulatory control. Fed. Proc., 35, 2367–2375
41. Guth, P.H. (1982). Stomach blood flow and acid secretion. Ann. Rev. Physiol., 44, 3–12
42. Kaufman, G.L. Jr. (1982). Blood flow and gastric secretion. Fed Proc., 41, 2080–2083
43. Perry, M.A., Haedicke, G.J., Bulkley, G.B., Kvietys, P.R. and Granger, D.N. (1983). Relationship between acid secretion and blood flow in the canine stomach: Role of oxygen consumpution. Gastroenterology, 85, 529–534
44. Chou, C.C. and Gallavan, R.H. (1982). Blood flow and intestinal motility. Fed. Proc., 41, 2090–2095
45. Chou, C.C. (1982). Relationship between intestinal blood flow and motility. Ann. Rev. Physiol., 44, 29–42
46. Leung, F.W., Itoh, M., Hirabayashi, K. and Guth, P.H. (1985). Role of blood flow in gastric and duodenal mucosal injury in the rat. Gastroenterology, 88, 281–289
47. Nakano, J. and Prancan, A.V. (1972). Effect of prostaglandin E_1 and A_1 on the gastric mucosal circulation in dogs. Proc. Soc. Exp. Biol. Med., 139, 1151–1154
48. Main, I.H.M. and Whittle, B.J.R. (1973). The effects of E and A prostaglandins on gastric mucosal blood flow and acid secretion in the rat. Br. J. Pharmacol., 49, 428–436
49. Cheung, L.Y. (1980). Topical effects of 16, 16-dimethyl prostaglandin E_2 on gastric blood flow in dogs. Am. J. Physiol., 238, G514–G519
50. Walus, K.M., Gustaw, P. and Konturek, S.J. (1980). Differential effects of prostaglandins and arachidonic acid on gastric circulation and oxygen consumption. Prostaglandins, 20, 1089–1102
51. Chung. L.Y. and Lowry, S.F. (1981). Local effects of 16, 16-dimethyl prostaglandin E_2 on gastric blood flow and acid secretion. Surgery, 90, 291–298
52. Kauffman, G.L. and Whittle, B.J.R. (1982). Gastric vascular actions of prostanoids and the dual effect of arachidonic acid. Am. J. Physiol., 242, G582–G587
53. Gerberg, J.G. and Nies, A.S. (1982). Canine gastric mucosal vasodilation with prostaglandins and histamine analogs. Dig. Dis. Sci., 27, 870–874
54. Inatomi, N. and Maki, Y. (1983). Effect of prostaglandins on mucosal blood flow and aspirin-reduced damage in the canine stomach. Jpn. J. Pharmacol., 33, 1263–1270
55. Balint, G.A., Sagi, I., Dobronte, Z. and Varro, V. (1984). Effect of different prostaglandin analogs on gastric acid secretion and mucosal blood flow in the dog: Action on the stimulated and resting mucosa. Acta Med. Hung., 41, 149–155

56. Holm-Rutili, L. and Obrink, K.J. (1984). Effects of prostaglandin E_1 on gastric mucosal microcirculation and spontaneous acid secretion in the rat. In Allen, A., Flemstrom, G., Garner, A., Silen W. and Turnberg, L.A. *Mechanisms of Mucosal Protection in the Upper Gastrointestinal tract*. pp 279–283, (New York: Raven Press)

57. Holm-Rutili, L. (1986). Effects of prostaglandin E_1, E_2 and 16, 16-dimethyl-E_2 on gastric acid output in the rat. *Acta Physiol. Scand.*, **127**, 313–321

58. Leung, F.W., Robert A. and Guth, P.H. (1985). Gastric mucosal blood flow in rats after administration of 16, 16-dimethyl prostaglandin E_2 at a cytoprotective dose. *Gastroenterology*, **88**, 1948–1953

59. Konturek, S.J., Robert A., Hanchar, A.J. and Nezamis, J.E. (1980). Comparison of prostacyclin and prostaglandin E_2 on gastric secretion, gastrin release and mucosal blood flow in dogs. *Dig. Dis. Sci.*, **25**, 673–679

60. Pihan, G., Majzoubi, D., Haudenschild, C., Trier, J.S. and Szabo, S. (1986). Early microcirculatory stasis in acute gastric mucosal injury in the rat and prevention by 16, 16-dimethyl prostaglandin E_2 or sodium thiosulfate. *Gastroenterology*, **91**, 1415–1426

61. Miller, T.A., Henagan, J.M. and Robert, A. (1980). Effect of 16, 16-dimethyl PGE_2 on resting and histamine-stimulated gastric mucosal blood flow. *Dig. Dis, Sci.*, **25**, 561–567

62. Moody, F.G., McGreevy, J. and Zalewski, C. (1979). Role of gastric blood flow in the pathogenesis of erosions and ulcers. In *Peptic Ulcer Disease and Update*, pp. 135–150 (New York: BMI Publications)

63. Guth, P.H. and Moller, T.L. (1982). The role of endogenous prostanoids in the response of the rat gastric microcirculation to vasoactive agents. *Microvasc. Res.*, **23**, 336–346

64. Gaskill, H.V., Sirinek, K.R. and Levine, B.A. (1984). 16, 16-dimethyl prostaglandin E_2 reverses focal mucosal ischemia associated in the stress ulcers. *J. Surg. Res.*, **37**, 83–88

65. Gaskill, H.V., Sirinek, K.R. and Levine, B.A. (1980). PGE_1 protects gastric mucosal blood flow during hypovolemic shock. *Surg. Forum*, **31**, 123–124

66. Larsen, K.R., Jensen, N.F., Davis, E.L., Jensen, J.C. and Moody, F.G. (1981). The cytoprotective effects of $(\pm)$-15-deoxy-16-1α1β-hydroxy-16-methyl PGE_1 methyl ester (SC-29333) versus aspirin-shock gastric ulcerogenesis in the dog. *Prostaglandins*, **21**, (Suppl.), 119–124

67. Jacobson, E.D. (1970). Comparison of prostaglandins E_1 and norepinephrine in gastric mucosal circulation. *Proc. Soc. Exp. Biol. Med.*, **133**, 516–519

68. Colton, D.G., Driskill, D.R., Phillips, E.L., Poy, P. and Dajani, E.Z. (1978). Effect of SC-29333, an inhibitor of gastric secretion, on canine gastric mucosal blood flow and serum gastrin levels. *Arch. Int. Pharmacodyn.*, **236**, 86–95

69. Wilson, D.E. and Levine, R.A. (1972). The effect of prostaglandin E_1 on canine gastric acid secretion and gastric mucosal blood flow. *Dig. Dis.* **17**, 527–532

70. Wilson, D.E. and Levine, R.A. (1969). Decreased canine gastric mucosal blood flow induced by prostaglandin E_1: A mechanism for its inhibitory effect on gastric secretion. *Gastroenterology*, **56**, 1268

71. Konturek, S.J., Walus, K. and Pawlik, W. (1978). Comparison of prostaglandin I_2 and E_2 on gastric acid secretion and mucosal blood flow. *Gastroenterology*, **74**, 1130

72. Cheung, L.Y. and Lowry, S.F. (1976). Effect of prostaglandin E_2 (PGE_2) and 16, 16-dimethyl PGE_2 ($DMPGE_2$) on gastric acid secretion and blood flow. *Gastroenterology*, **70**, 870

73. Walus, K.M., Pawlik, W. and Konturek, S.J. (1980). Prostacyclin-induced gastric mucosal vasodilation and inhibition of acid secretion in the dog. *Proc. Soc. Exp. Biol. Med.*, **163**, 228–232

74. Main, I.H.M. and Whittle, B.J.R. (1972). Effects of prostaglandin E_2 on rat gastric mucosal blood flow as determined by ^{14}C-aniline clearance. *Br. J. Pharmacol.*, **44**, 331P

75. Main, I.H.M. and Whittle, B.J.R. (1975). Potency and selectivity of methyl analogs of prostaglandin E_2 on rat gastrointestinal function. *Br. J. Pharmacol.*, **54**, 309–317

76. Zamora, G., Reddy, V.K., Johnson, P. and Gallagher, L. (1981). Effect of histamine and prostaglandin E_2 on gastric blood flow in swine. *Am. J. Vet. Res.*, **42**, 956–959

77. Francis H.P. and Smy. J.R. (1978). Comparison of intravenous and close arterial infusions of prostaglandins E_1 and E_2 on gastric acid secretion and mucosal blood flow in anaesthetized cats. *J. Physiol. (Lond.)*. **285**, 38P

78. Robert, A., Nezamis, J.E. and Phillips, J.P. (1967). Inhibition of gastric secretion by prostaglandin. *Am. J. Dig. Dis.*, **12**, 1073–1076
79. Robert, A. (1977). The inhibitory effects of prostaglandins on gastric secretion: their possible role in the treatment of gastric hypersecretion and peptic ulceration. In Jerzy Glass G.B. (ed.) *Progress in Gastroenterology*, Vol. III, pp. 777–801. (New York: Grune and Stratton)
80. Gerkens, J.F., Gerberg, J.G., Shand, D.G. and Branch, R.A. (1978). Effect of PGI_2, PGE_2 and 6-keto $PGF_1\alpha$ on canine gastric blood flow and acid secretion *Prostaglandins*, **16**, 815–822
81. Cheung, L.Y. and Lowry, S.F. (1978). Effect of intra-arterial infusion of prostaglandin E_1 on gastric secretion and blood flow. *Surgery*, **83**, 699–703
82. Salvati, P. and Whittle, B.J.R. (1981). Investigation of the vascular actions of arachidonate, lipoxygenase and cyclooxygenase products on the isolated perfused stomach of the rat and rabbit. *Prostaglandins*, **2**, 141–156
83. Whittle, B.J.R., Boughton-Smith, N.K., Moncada, S. and Vane, J.R. (1978). Actions of prostacyclin (PGI_2) and its product, 6-oxo-PGI_{12} on the rat gastric mucosa in vivo and in vitro. *Prostaglandins*, **15**, 955–967
84. Gaskill, H.V., Sirinek, K.R. and Levine, B.A. Prostacyclin increases gastric mucosal blood flow via cyclic AMP. *J. Surg. Res.*, **33**, 140–145
85. Gaskill, H.V., Sirinek, K.R. and Levine, B.A. (1984). Prostacyclin selectivity enhances blood flow in areas of the GI tract prone to stress ulceration. *J. Trauma*, **24**, 397–400
86. Einzing, S., Rao, G.H.R. and White, J.G. (1980). Differential sensitivity of regional vascular beds in the dog to low-dose prostacyclin infusion. *Can. J. Physiol. Pharmacol.*, **58**, 940–946
87. Gryglewski, R.J. (1982). Prostacyclin, prostaglandins, thromboxanes, and platelet function. In Lee. J.B. (ed.) *Prostaglandins*, pp. 303–350 (New York: Elsevier North Holland)
88. S.J. Konturek, Bowman, J., Lancaster, C., Hanchar, A.J. and Robert, A. (1979). Cytoprotection of the canine gastric mucosa by prostacyclin: possible mediation by increased mucosal blood flow. *Gastroenterology*, **76**, 1173a
89. S.J. Konturek and Robert, A. (1982). Cytoprotection of canine gastric mucosa by prostacyclin: possible mediation by increased mucosal blood flow. *Digestion*, **25**, 155–163
90. Gaskill, H.V., Sirinek, K.R. and Levine, B.A. (1982)., Prostacyclin-mediated gastric cytoprotection is dependent on mucosal blood flow. *Surgery*, **92**, 220–224
91. Salvati, P. and Whittle, B.J.R. (1981). The vasoactive effects of some arachidonate lipoxygenase and cyclo-oxygenase products on the isolated perfused stomach of rabbit and rat. *Br. J. Pharmacol.*, **73**, 256P–257P
92. Nickolson, R.C., Town, M.H. and Vorbrüggen, H. (1985). Prostacyclin analogs. *Med. Res. Rev.*, **5**, 1–53
93. Kauffman, G.L. Jr., Whittle, B.J.R., Aures, D., Vam, J.R. and Grossman, M.I. (1979). Effects of prostacyclin and a stable analog, 6β–PGI_1, on gastric acid secretion, mucosal blood flow, and blood pressure in conscious dogs. *Gastroenterology*, **77**, 1301–1306
94. Kauffman, G.L., Whittle, B.J.R., Aurus, D. and Grossman, M.I. (1980). Gastric antisecretory and cardiovascular actions of a stable 16-phenoxy prostacyclin analog in the dog. In Samuelsson, B., Ramwell, P.W. and Paoletti, R. (eds.) *Advances in Prostaglandin and Thromboxane Research*, Vol. 8, pp. 1521–1524. (New York: Raven Press)
95. Konturek, S.J., Lancaster, C., Hanchar, A.J., Nejamis, J.E. and Robert, A. (1979). The influence of prostacyclin on gastric mucosal blood flow in resting and stimulated canine stomach. *Gastroenterology*, **76**, 1173b
96. Tao, P., Scruggs, W. and Wilson, D.E. (1979). The effects of a prostaglandin endoperoxide analogue on canine gastric acid and mucus secretion. *Dig. Dis. Sci.*, **24**, 449–454
97. Bunting, S., Gryglewski, R., Moncada, S. and Vane, J.R. (1976). Arterial walls generate from prostaglandin endoperoxides a substance (prostaglandin X) which relaxes strips of mesenteric acid coeliac arteries and inhibits platelet aggregation. *Prostaglandins*, **12**, 897–913
98. Dusting, G.J., Moncada, S. and Vane, J.R. (1978). Vascular actions of arachidonic acid and its metabolites in perfused mesenteric and femoral beds of the dog. *Eur. J. Pharmacol.*, **49**, 65–72

99. Whittle, B.J.R., Kauffman, G.L. and Moncada, S. (1981). Vasoconstriction with thromboxanes A_2 induces ulceration in the gastric mucosa. *Nature (London)*, **292**, 472—474

100. Moroni, D., Gervasi, G.B., Patella, P., Visentin, L., Masselli, M.A. and Bergamaschi, M. (1983). The tripeptide ZAMI-420 inhibits thromboxane-induced gastric vasoconstriction and ischemia. *Int. J. Tiss. Reac.*, **5**, 249—252

101. Whittle, B.J.R., Oren-Wolman, N. and Guth, P.H. (1985). Gastric vasoconstrictor actions of leukotriene C_4, $PGF_{2\alpha}$ and thromboxane mimetic U-46619 on rat submucosal microcirculation in vivo. *Am. J. Physiol.*, **248**, G580—G586

102. Gerkens, J.F., Shand, D.G., Flexner, Ch., Nies, A.S., Oates, J.A. and Data, J.L. (1977). Effect of indomethacin and aspirin on gastric blood flow and acid secretion. *J. Pharmacol. Exp. Ther.*, **203**, 646—652

103. Kauffman, G.L. Jr., Aures, D. and Grossman, M.I. (1980). Intravenous indomethacin and aspirin reduce basal gastric mucosal blood flow in dogs. *Am. J. Physiol.*, **238**, G131—G134

104. Main, I.H.M. and Whittle, B.J.R. (1973). Effects of indomethacin in rat gastric acid secretion and mucosal blood flow. *Br. J. Pharmacol.*, **47**, 666P

105. Whittle, B.J.R. (1977). Mechanisms underlaying gastric mucosal damage induced by indomethacin and bile-salts, and the action of prostaglandins. *Br. J. Pharmacol.*, **60**, 455—460

106. Bill. A. (1979). Effects of indomethacin on regional blood flow in conscious rabbits—A microsphere study. *Acta Physiol. Scand.*, **105**, 437—442

107. Skarstein, A. (1979). Effect of indomethacin on blood flow distribution in the stomach of cats with acute gastric ulcer. *Scand. J. Gastroenterol.*, **14**, 905—911

108. Hua, H.Y., Dahlen, S.E., Lundberg, J.M., Hammarstrom, S. and Hedqvist, P. (1985). Leukotrienes C_4, D_4 and E_4 cause widespread and extensive plasma extravasation in the guinea pig. *Naunyn-Schmeidebergs Arch. Pharmacol.*, **330**, 136—141

109. Konturek, S.J., Mikos, E., Pawlik, W. and Walus, K. (1979). Direct inhibition of gastric secretion and mucosal blood flow by arachidonic acid. *J. Physiol. (Lond.)*, **286**, 15—28

110. Frame, M.H. and Main, I.H.M. (1980). Effects of arachidonic acid on rat gastric acid secretion in response to different secretagogues: inhibition of these effects by indomethacin. *Br. J. Pharmacol.*, **69**, 171—178

111. Johnson, P.C. (1980). Autoregulation of intestinal blood flow. *Am. J. Physiol.*, **199**, 311—318

112. Johnson, P.C. (1984). Myogenic and venous-arteriolar responses in intestinal circulation. In Shepherd, A.P. and Granger, D.N. (eds.) *Physiology of the Intestinal Circulation.* pp. 49—60. (New York: Raven Press)

113. Granger, H.J. and Shepherd, A.P. Jr. (1973). Intrinsic microvascular control of tissue oxygen delivery. *Microvasc. Res.*, **5**, 49—72

114. Texter, E.C. Jr., Merrill, S., Schwartz, M., Van Derstrappen, G. and Haddy, F.S. Relationship of blood flow to pressure in the intestinal bed of the dog. *Am. J. Physiol.*, **202**, 253—256

115. Shepherd, A.P. and Granger, D.N. (1984). Metabolic regulation of the intestinal circulation. In Shepherd, A.P. and Granger, D.N. (eds.) *Physiology of the Intestinal Circulation*, pp. 33—47. (New York: Raven Press)

116. Folkow, B., Lewis, D.H., Lundgren, O., Mellander, S. and Wallentin, I. (1964). The effect of graded vasoconstrictor fibre stimulation on the intestinal resistance and capacitance vessels. *Acta Physiol. Scand.*, **61**, 458—466

117. Greenway, C.V. (1984). Neural control and autoregulatory escape. In Shepherd, A.P. and Granger, D.N. (eds.) *Physiology of the Intestinal Circulation.* pp. 61—71. (New York: Raven Press)

118. Fara, J.W., (1984). Post prandial mesenteric hyperemia. In Shepherd, A.P. and Granger, D.N. (eds.) *Physiology of the Intestinal Circulation*, pp. 99—106. (New York: Raven Press)

119. Chou, C.C. and Kvietys, P.R. (1981). Physiological and pharmacological alterations in gastrointestinal blood flow. In Granger, D.N. and Bulkley, G.B. (eds.) *Measurement of Blood Flow, Application to the Splanchnic Circulation*, pp. 475—509. (Baltimore: Williams and Wilkins)

120. Shepherd, A.P. (1982). Local control of intestinal oxygenation and blood flow. *Ann. Rev. Physiol.*, **44**, 13—27

121. Chou, C.C. (1982). Relationship between intestinal blood flow and motility. *Ann. Rev. Physiol.*, **44**, 29–42
122. Foncadaro, J.D. (1984). Intestinal blood flow and motility. In Shepherd, A.P. and Granger, D.N. (eds.) *Physiology of the Intestinal Circulation*, pp. 107–120 (New York: Raven Press)
123. Haglund, V. (1973). The vascular reactions in the small intestine of the cat during haemorrhage. *Acta Physiol. Scand.*, **89**, 129–141
124. Haglund, V. (1973). The small intestine in hypotension and hemorrhage. An experimental cardiovascular study in the cat. *Acta Physiol. Scand.*, **387** (Suppl.), 1–37
125. Covino, B.G., Lee, J.B. and McMorrow. (1968). Circulatory effects of renal prostaglandins. *Circulation*, **38**, (Suppl. 6), 60
126. Chapnick, B.M., Feingen, L.P., Hyman, A. and Kadowitz, P.J. (1978). Differential effects of prostaglandins in the mesenteric vascular bed. *Am. J. Physiol.*, **235**, H326–H332
127. Dusting, G.J., Moncada, S. and Vane, J.R. (1978). Vascular action of arachidonic acid and its metabolites in perfused mesenteric and femoral beds of the dog. *Eur. J. Pharmacol.*, **48**, 65–72
128. Feingen, L.P., Chapnick, B.M., Hyman, A.L., King, L., Marascaldo, B. and Kadowitz, P.J. (1980). Peripheral vasodilator effects of prostaglandins: Comparison of 6-keto-prostaglandin E_1 with prostacyclin and escape from prostaglandin E_2 in the mesenteric vascular bed. *J. Pharmacol. Exp. Ther.*, **214**, 528–534
129. Cahpnick, B.M., Feingen, L.P., Hyman, A.L. and Kadowitz, P.J. (1978). Vasodilator effects of prostacyclin in the canine intestine. *Fed. Proc.*, **37**, 732
130. Lippton, H.L., Camin, S. and Kadowitz, P.J. (1980). Comparative effects of PGD_2 and PGE_2 on vasoconstrictor responses in the feline vascular bed. *Prostagl. Med.*, **5**, 297–305
131. Lippton, H.L., Paustian, P.W., Sporl, L. and Kadowitz, P.J. (1980). Comparative effects of PGD_2 and PGE_2 in the regional circulation of the cat. *Prostagl. Med.*, **5**, 365–373
132. Paustian, P.W., Chapnick, B.M., Feingen, L.P., Hyman, A.L. and Kadowitz, P.J. (1977). Effects of 13, 14-dehydroprostacyclin methyl ester on the feline intestinal vascular bed. *Prostaglandins* **14**, 1141–1152
133. Houvenaghel, A. and Wechsung, E. (1977). Influence of prostaglandins on blood flow through the superior mesenteric artery in the pig. *Arch. Int. Pharmacodyn.*, **230**, 332–334
134. Balint, G.A., Kiss, Zs. F., Varkonyi, T., Wittman, T. and Varro, V. (1979). Effects of prostaglandin E_2 and $F_{2\alpha}$ on the absorption and portal transport of sugar and on the local intestinal circulation. *Prostaglandins*, **18**, 265–268
135. Kondo, K., Misumi, J., Okuno, T., Nakamura, R., Saruta, T. and Kato, E. (1978). Effect of prostaglandin E_2 on vascular reactivity to norepinephrine in isolated rat mesenteric artery, hind limb and splenic artery. *Prostagl. Med.*, **2**, 67–72
136. Manku, M.S., Mtabaji, J.P. and Horrobin, D.F. (1977). Effects of prostaglandins on baseline pressure and responses to noradrenaline in a perfused rat mesenteric artery preparation: PGE_1 as an antagonist of PGE_2. *Prostaglandins*, **13**, 701–709
137. Malik, K.U., Ryan, P. and McGiff, J.C. (1976). Modification by prostaglandins E_1 and E_2, indomethacin and arachidonic acid of the vasoconstrictor responses of the isolated perfused rabbit and rat mesenteric arteries to adrenergic stimuli. *Circ. Res.*, **39**, 163–168
138. Jackson, E.K. and Campbell, W.B. (1980). The in situ blood perfused rat mesentery: A model for assessing modulation of adrenergic neurotransmission. *Eur. J. Pharmacol.*, **66**, 217–224
139. Hadhazy, P., Nagy, L., Juhasz, F., Malomvolgyi, B. and Magyark. (1983). Effects of indomethacin and prostaglandin I_2 and E_2 on the tone of human isolated mesenteric arteries. *Eur. J. Pharmacol.*, **91**, 477–484
140. Dennis, M.F., Richard, L.I., DeGaris, M. and Dusting, G.J. (1985). Inhibition of vasoconstrictor mechanisms by dazoxiben in the rat mesenteric vasculature. *Eur. J. Pharmacol.*, **110**, 351–356
141. Shehadeh, Z., Price, W.E. and Jacobson, E.D. (1969). Effects of vasoactive agents on intestinal blood flow and motility in the dog. *Am. J. Physiol.*, **216**, 386–392
142. Pawlik, W., Shepherd, A.P. and Jacobson, E.D. (1975). Effects of vasoactive agents on intestinal oxygen consumption and blood flow in dogs. *J. Clin. Invest.*, **56**, 488–490

143. Granger, D.N., Shackleford, J.S. and Taylor, A.E. (1979). PGE$_1$-induced intestinal secretion: mechanism of enhanced transmucosal protein efflux. Am. J. Physiol., **236**, E788–E796

144. Lippton, H.L., Chapnick, B.M., Hyman, A.L. and Kadowitz, P.J. (1980). Inhibition of vasoconstrictor responses by 6-keto-PGE$_1$ in the feline mesenteric vascular bed. Prostaglandin, **19**, 299–310

145. Davis, L.J., Anderson, J.H., Wallace, S., Gianturco, C. and Jacobson, E.D. (1975). The use of prostaglandin E$_1$ to enhance the angiographic visualization of the splanchnic circulation. Radiology, **114**, 281–286

146. Nowak, J. and Wenmalm, A. (1978). Influence of indomethacin and of prostaglandin E$_1$ on total and regional blood flow in man. Acta Physiol. Scand., **102**, 484–491

147. Clark, R.A., Colley, D.P., Jacobson, E.D., Herman, R., Tyler, G. and Stahl, D. (1980). Superior mesenteric angiography and blood flow measurement following intra-arterial injection of prostaglandin E$_1$ Radiology, **134**, 327–333

148. Adachi, H., Sugihara, H., Nakagawa, H. et al. (1984). Effect of prostaglandin E$_1$ on fractional distribution of cardiac output and organ blood flow in man: a simultaneous and non-invasive determination using double dose thallium-201 scintigraphy. Cardiovasc. Res., **18**, 657–662

149. Beubler, E. and Juan, H. (1977). The function of prostaglandins in transmucosal water movement and blood flow in the rat jejunum. N-S Arch. Pharmacol., **299**, 89–94

150. Lumley, P., Humphrey, P.P.A., Kennedy, I. and Coleman, R.A. (1982). Comparison of the potencies of some prostaglandins as vasodilators in three vascular beds of the anesthetized dog. Eur. J. Pharmacol., **81**, 421–430

151. Fara, J.W., Barth, K.H., White, R.I. and Bynum, T.E. (1979). Mesenteric effects of prostaglandins F$_{2\alpha}$ and B$_2$ Radiology, **133**, 317–320

152. Walus, K.M., Fondacaro, J.D. and Jacobson, E.D. (1980). Hemodynamic and metabolic changes during stimulation of ileal motility. Dig. Dis. Sci., **26**, 1069–1077

153. Higgins, C.B., Vatner, S.V. and Braunwald, E. (1973). Regional hemodynamic effects of prostaglandin A$_1$ in the conscious dog. Am. Heart J., **85**, 349–357

154. Fondacaro, J.D., Walus, K.M., Schwaiger, M. and Jacobson, E.D. (1981). Vasodilation of the normal and ischemic canine mesenteric circulation. Gastroenterology, **80**, 1542–1549

155. Paustian, P.W., Gottlieb, A.J., Ritchie, E., Chapnick, B.M., Hyman, A.L. and Kadowitz, P.J. (1978). The effects of prostaglandin D$_2$ infusion on the feline intestinal vascular bed. Clin. Res., **26**, 10A

156. Moncada, S. and Vane, J.R. (1981). Prostacyclin: Its biosynthesis, actions and clinical potential. Phil. Trans. R. Soc. Lond., **B294**, 305–329

157. Traverso, L.W., O'Benar, J.D. and Buchalter, C.C. (1984). Prostacyclin increases portal venous flow. Prostaglandins, **28**, 679–693

158. Lippton, H.L., Chapnick, B.M., Hyman, A.L. and Kadowitz, P.J. (1979). Inhibition of vasoconstrictor responses by prostacyclin (PGI) in the feline mesenteric vascular bed. Arch. Int. Pharmacodyn., **241**, 214–223

159. Seeling, R.F., Kerr, J.C., Hobson, R.W. and Machiedo, G.W. (1981). Prostacyclin (Epoprostenol). Its effect on canine splanchnic blood flow during haemorrhagic shock. Arch. Surg., **116**, 428–430

160. Shapiro, D.M., Cronenwelt, J.L., Lindenauer, S.M., Luce, J.L. and Stanley, J.C. (1984). Effect of glucagon and prostacyclin in acute occlusive and post-occlusive canine mesenteric ischemia. J. Surg. Res., **36**, 535–546

161. Cho, M.J. and Allen, M.A. (1978). Chemical stability of prostacyclin (PGI$_2$) in aqueous solutions. Prostaglandins, **15**, 943–954

162. Nong, PY-K., Sun, F.F. and McGiff, J.C. (1978). Metabolism of prostacyclin in blood vessels. J. Biol. Chem., **253**, 5555–5557

163. Pace-Asciak, C.R., Carrara, M.C. and Domzet, Z. (1977). Identification of the major urinary metabolites of 6-keto-prostaglandins F$_{1\alpha}$ (6K-PGF$_{1\alpha}$) in the rat. Biochem. Biophys. Res. Commun. **78**, 115–121

164. Randall, M.J., Parry, M.J., Hawkeswood, E., Gross, P.E. and Dickinson, R.P., (1981). UK-37,248, a novel, selective thromboxane synthetase inhibitor with platelet anti-aggregatory and anti-thrombotic activity. Thromb. Res., **23**, 145–162

165. Dusting, G.J., Moncada, S. and Vane, J.R. (1979). Prostaglandins, their intermediates

and precursors: cardiovascular actions and regulatory roles in normal and abnormal circulatory systems. *Progr. Cardiov. Dis.*, **21**, 405–430

166. Feingen, L.P., Chapnick, B.M., Gorman, R.R., Hyman, A.L. and Kadowitz, P.J. (1978). The effect of PGH$_2$ on blood flow in the canine renal and superior mesenteric vascular beds. *Prostaglandins*, **16**, 803–813

167. Chapnick, B.M., Feingen, L.P., Flemming, J.M., Hyman, A.L. and Kadowitz, P.J. (1977). Comparison of the effects of prostaglandin H$_2$ and an analog of prostaglandin H$_2$ on the intestinal vascular bed of the dog. *Pharmacologist*, **19**, 148

168. Jackson, E.K. (1985). Effects of thromboxane synthetaze inhibition on vascular responsiveness in the in vitro rat mesentery. *J. Clin. Invest.*, **76**, 2286–2295

169. Gaffney, G.R. and Williamson, H.E. (1979). Effect of indomethacin and meclofenamate on canine mesenteric and celiac blood flow. *Res. Commun. Chem. Pathol. Pharmacol.*, **75**, 165–168

170. Feingen, L.P., King, L.W., Ray, J., Beckett, W. and Kadowitz, P.J. (1981). Differential effects of ibuprofen and indomethacin in the regional circulation of the dog. *J. Pharmacol. Exp. Ther.* **219**, 679–684

171. Feingen, L.P. (1983). Differential effects of leukotrienes C$_4$, D$_4$ and E$_4$ in the canine renal and mesenteric vascular beds. *J. Pharmacol. Exp. Ther.*, **225**, 682–687

172. Chapnick, B.M. (1984). Divergent influences of leukotrienes C$_4$, D$_4$ and E$_4$ on mesenteric and renal blood flow. *Am. J. Physiol.*, **246**, H518–H524

173. Lippton, H.L., Armstead, W.M., Hyman, A.L. and Kadowitz, P.J. (1984). Vasoconstrictor effects of leukotrienes C$_4$ and D$_4$ in the feline mesenteric vascular bed. *Prostaglandins*, **27**, 233–243

174. Hall, A.K. and Behrman, H.R. (1982). Prostaglandins: biosynthesis metabolism, and mechanism of cellular action. In Lee, J.B. (ed.), *Prostaglandins*, pp. 1–38. (New York: Elsevier)

175. Coleman, R.A., Humphrey, P.P.A., Kennedy, I. and Lumley, P. (1984). Prostanoid receptors—the development of a working classification. *Trends Pharmaceut. Sci.*, **5**, 303–306

176. Aiken, J.W. (1984). Prostaglandins. *J. Cardiovasc. Pharmacol.*, **6**, 5413–5420

177. Kennedy, I., Coleman, R.A., Humphrey, P.P.A. and Lumley, P. (1983). Studies on the characterization of prostanoid receptors. In Samuelsson, B., Paoletti, R. and Ramwell, P., (eds.). *Advances in Prostaglandin, Thromboxane and Leukotriene Research*, Vol. II, pp. 327–332. (New York: Raven Press)

178. Lewis, R.A. and Austen, K.F. (1984). Molecular determinants for functional responses to the sulfidopeptide leukotrienes: metabolism and receptor subclasses. *J. Allergy Clin. Immunol.*, **74**, 369–372

179. Greenberg, S.P., Kadowitz, J., Long, J.P. and Wilson, W.R. (1976). Studies on the nature of a prostaglandin receptor in canine and rabbit vascular smooth muscle. *Circ. Res*, **39**, 66–76

180. Sterin-Borda, L., Franchi, A.M., Borda, E.S., DelCastillo, E., Gimeno, M.F. and Gimeno, A. (1984). Augmented thromboxane generation by mesenteric arteries from pancreatectomized diabetic dogs is coincident with the vascular tone enhancement evoked by sodium arachidonate and prostacyclin. *Eur. J. Pharmacol.*, **103**, 211–221

181. Ercan, Z.A. and Turker, R.K. (1985). The relaxing activity of iloprost and prostaglandin E$_2$ in the various isolated vascular smooth muscle of the rabbit. *Pharmacology*, **31**, 61–66

182. Hatano, Y., Yohli, J.D., Goldberg, L.I. and Fried, J. (1981). Relative contracting and relaxing potencies of a series of prostaglandins on isolated canine mesenteric artery strips. *Prostaglandins*, **21**, 515–529

183. Yabek, S.M. and Avner, B.P. (1979). Effect of prostaglandin E$_1$ and indomethacin on fetal and neonatal lamb mesenteric responses to norepinephrine. *Prostaglandins*, **17**, 227–233

184. Yabek, S.M. and Avner, B.P. (1980). Effects of prostacyclin (PGI$_2$) and indomethacin on neonatal lamb mesenteric and renal artery responses to electrical stimulation and norepinephrine. *Prostaglandins*, **19**, 23–30

185. Goldberg, L.I. (1975). Dopamine induced relaxation of isolated canine renal, mesenteric, and femoral arteries contracted by prostaglandin F$_{2\alpha}$ *Circ. Res.*, **37**, (Suppl. I), 197–1120

186. Godfraind T. and Miller, R.C. (1982). Actions of prostaglandin F$_{2\alpha}$ and noradrenaline

on calcium exchange and contraction in rat mesenteric arteries and their sensitivity to calcium entry blockers. *Br. J. Pharmacol.*, **75**, 229–236

187. Toda, N. (1982). Different responsiveness of a variety of isolated dog arteries to prostaglandin D₂. *Prostaglandins*, **23**, 99–112

188. Hadhazy, P., Malomvolgyi, B. and Magyer, K. (1984). Differential contractile responsiveness of isolated rabbit arteries from different vascular beds to cyclooxygenase inhibitors and PGI₂. *Eur. J. Pharmacol.*, **98**, 323–330

189. Malomvolgyi, B., Hadhazy, P. and Nagyar, K. (1984). Effects of cyclooxygenase inhibitors and PGI₂ on the adrenergic contractions of isolated rabbit arteries. *Biomed. Biochim. Acta*, **43**, S277–S280

190. Koltay, M.Z., Hadhazy, P., Malomvolgyi, B., Wagner, M. and Pogatsa, G. (1984). Effect of cyclooxygenase inhibitors, prostaglandins F₂α and I₂ on isolated celiac and basilar arteries of alloxan-diabetic dogs. *Eur. J. Clin. Invest.*, **14**, 130–134

191. Bunting, S., Moncada, S. and Vane, J.R. (1976). The effect of prostaglandin endoperoxides and thromboxane A₂ on strips of rabbit celiac artery and certain other smooth muscle preparations. *Br. J. Pharmacol.*, **57**, 462P–463P

192. Banerjee, A.K., Tuflin, D.P. and Walker, J.L. (1985). Pharmacological effects of (±)-11-deoxy-16-phenoxy prostaglandin E₁ derivatives in the cardiovascular system. *Br. J. Pharmacol.*, **84**, 71–80

193. Toda, N. (1982). Mechanisms of action of carbocyclic thromboxane A₂ and its interaction with prostaglandin I₂ and verapamil in isolated arteries. *Circ. Res.*, **51**, 672–682

194. Yarmada, K., Kubo, K., Shuto, K. and Nakamuzo, N. (1984). Inhibition of thromboxane A₂-induced vasoconstriction by KF 4939, a new antiplatelet agent in rabbit mesenteric and dog coronary arteries. *Jpn. J. Pharmacol.* **36**, 283–290

195. Kito, G., Okuda, H., Ohkawa, SH., Terao, SH. and Kikuchi, K. (1981). Contractile activites of leukotrienes C₄ and D₄ on vascular strips from rabbits. *Life Sci.* **29**, 1325–1332

196. Secrest, R.J., Olsen, E.J. and Chapnick, B.M. (1985). Leukotriene D₄ relaxes canine renal and superior mesenteric arteries. *Circ. Res.*, **57**, 323–329

197. Malik, K.V. (1978). Prostaglandins-modulation of adrenergic nervous system. *Fed. Proc.*, **37**, 203–207

198. Furchgott, R.F. (1984). The role of endothelium in the responses of vascular smooth muscle to drugs. *Ann. Rev. Pharmacol. Toxicol.*, **24**, 175–197

199. Vanhoutte, P.M. and DeMey, J. (1983). Control of vascular smooth muscle function by the endothelial cells. *Gen. Pharmacol.*, **14**, 39–41

200. Chand, N. and Altura, B.M. (1981). Endothelial cells and relaxation of vascular smooth muscle cells: possible relevance to lipoxygenase and their significance in vascular disease. *Microcirculation*, **1**, 297–317

201. Gerritsen, M.E., Morgan, D.O., Parks, T.P., Printz, M.P. and Lederis, K.P. (1981). A proposed role for prostaglandins in the modulation of the relaxation response to urotensin I in isolated rat arteries. *Prostaglandins*, **22**, 873–892

202. Kaiser, L. and Sparks, H.V. Jr. (1986). Mediation of flow-dependent arterial dilation by endothelial cells. *Circ. Shock*, **18**, 109–114

203. Busse, R., Forstermann, V., Matsuda, H. and Pohl, V. (1984). The role of prostaglandins in the endothelium-mediated vasodilatory response to hypoxia. *Pflugers Arch.*, **401**, 77–83

204. Malik, K.V., Ryan, P. and McGiff, J.C. (1976). Modification by prostaglandins E₁ and E₂, indomethacin and arachidonic acid of the vasoconstrictor responses on the isolated perfused rabbit and rat mesenteric arteries to adrenergic stimuli. *Circ. Res.*, **39**, 163–172

205. Manku, M.S. and Horrobin, D.F. (1976). Indomethacin inhibits responses to all vasoconstrictors in the rat mesenteric vascular bed: restoration of responses by prostaglandin E₂. *Prostaglandins*, **12**, 369–376

206. Coupar, I.M. and McLennan, P.L. (1978). The influence of prostaglandins on noradrenaline-induced vasoconstriction in isolated perfused mesenteric blood vessels of the rat. *Br. J. Pharmacol.*, **62**, 51–59

207. Kondo, K., Okuno, T., Suzuki,. H. and Suruta, T. (1980). Effects of prostaglandins E₂ and I₂, and arachidonic acid on vascular reactivity to norepinephrine in isolated rat mesenteric artery, hind limb and splenic artery. *Prostagl. Med.*, **1**, 21–30

208. Greenberg, S. and Long, J.P. (1973). Enhancement of vascular smooth muscle responses to vasoactive stimuli by prostaglandin E_1 and E_2. Arch. Int. Pharmacodyn., 206, 94–104

209. Greenberg, S., Kadowitz, P.J. and Diecke, F.P.J. (1973). Effect of prostaglandin $F_{2\alpha}$ ($PGF_{2\alpha}$) on arterial and venous contractility and ^{45}Ca uptake. Arch. Int. Pharmacodyn., 205, 381–398

210. Morris, G.P. and Wallace, J.L. (1981). The roles of ethanol and of acid in the production of gastric erosions in rats. Virchow's Arch., B., 38, 23–28

211. Svanes, K., Ito, S., Takeuchi, K. and Silen, W. (1982). Restitution of the surface epithelium of the in vitro frog gastric mucosa after damage with hyperosmolar NaCl. Gastroenterology, 82, 1409–1427

212. Lacy, E.R. and Ito, S. (1984). Ethanol-induced insult to the superficial rat gastric epithelium: a study of damage and rapid repair. In Allen, A.D., Flemstrom, G., Garner, A., Silen, W. and Turnberg, L.A. (eds.) Mechanisms of Mucosal Protection in the Upper Gastrointestinal Tract, pp. 49–56. (New York: Raven Press)

213. Lacy, E.R. and Ito, S. (1984). Rapid epithelial institution of the rat gastric mucosa after ethanol injury. Lab. Invest., 51, 573–583

214. Silen, W. and Ito, S. (1985). Mechanisms for rapid re-epithelization of the gastric mucosal surface. Ann. Rev. Physiol., 47, 217–229

215. Ito, S. and Lacy, E.R. (1984). Characteristics of ethanol-induced lesions in rat gastric mucosa. In Allen, A.D., Flemstrom, G., Garner, A., Silen, W. and Turnberg, L.A. (eds.) Mechanisms of Mucosal Protection in the Upper Gastrointestinal Tract, pp. 57–62. (New York: Raven Press)

216. Virchow, R. (1953). Historisches, Kritisches unt positive zur lehre der unter leibsaffektionen. Virchow's Arch. F. Patyhol. Anat., 5, 632–650

217. Svanes, K., Varhang, J.E., Dzienis, H. and Gronbeck, J.E. (1984). Gastric mucosa blood flow related to acute mucosal damage. Scand. J. Gastroenterol., (Suppl. 105), 62–66

218. Szabo, S., Trier, J.S., Brown, A. and Maull, E.A. (1982). Increased vascular permeability appears early in ethanol-induced gastric injury and is reduced by prostaglandins or cysteamine. Gastroenterology, 82, 1191

219. Szabo, S. and Trier, J.S. (1984). Pathogenesis of acute gastric mucosal injury: sulfhydryls as a protector, adrenal cortex as a modulator, and vascular endothelium as a target. In Allen, A., Flemstrom. G., Garner, A., Silen, W. and Turnberg, L.A., (eds.) Mechanisms of Mucosal Protection in the Upper Gastrointestinal Tract. pp. 287–293 (New York: Raven Press)

220. Szabo, S., Trier, J.S., Brown, A. and Schnoor, J. (1985). Early vascular injury and increased vascular permeability in gastric mucosal injury caused by ethanol in the rat. Gastroenterology, 88, 228–236

221. Guth, P.H., Paulsen, G. and Nagata, H. (1984). Histologic and microcirculatory changes in alcohol-induced gastric lesions in the rat: effect of prostaglandin cytoprotection. Gastroenterology, 87, 1083–1090

222. Wallace, J.L., Morris, G.P., Krausse, E.J. and Greaves, S.E. (1982). Reduction by cytoprotective agents of ethanol-induced damage to the rat gastric mucosa: a correlated morphological and physiological study. Can. J. Physiol. Pharmacol., 60, 1686–1699

223. Robert, A., Nezamis, J.E., Lancaster, C. and Hanchar, A.J. (1979). Cytoprotection by prostaglandins in rats. Prevention of gastric necrosis produced by ethanol, HCl, NaOH, hypertonic NaCl, and thermal injury. Gastroenterology, 77, 433–443

224. Robert, A. (1979). Cytoprotection by prostaglandins. Gastroenterology, 77, 761–767

225. Tarnawski, A., Hollander, D., Stachura, J., Krause, W.J. and Gargeley, H. (1985). Prostaglandin protection of the gastric mucosa against alcohol injury—A dynamic time-related process. Role of the proliferative zone. Gastroenterology, 88, 334–352

226. Johansson, C. and Bergstrom, S. (1982). Prostaglandins and protection of the gastroduodenal mucosa. Scand. J. Gastroenterol., (Suppl. 77), 21–46

227. Miller, T.A. (1983). Protective effects of prostaglandins against gastric mucosal damage: current knowledge and proposed mechanisms. Am. J. Physiol., 245, G601–G623

228. Robert, A. (1984). On the mechanism of cytoprotection by prostaglandins. Ann. Clin. Res., 16, 335–338

229. Hawkey, C.J. and Ramptom, D.S. (1985). Prostaglandins and the gastrointestinal mucosa: Are they important in its function, diease, or treatment. Gastroenterology, 89, 1162–1188

230. Pihan, G., Majzoubi, D., Trier, J.S. and Szabo S. (1986). Microcirculatory stasis and mucosal hypoperfusion in acute gastric mucosal injury in the rat; prevention by a prostaglandin and thiosulfate. *Gastroenterology*, **90**, 1586

231. Ohya, Y. and Guth, P.H. (1985). Effect of ethanol on rat gastric microcirculation. *Gastroenterology*, **88**, 1522

232. Guth, P.H., Paulsen, G., Nagata, H., Leung, F., Robert, A. and Ohya, Y. Prostaglandin cytoprotection: role of microcirculatory changes. In Hayaishi, O. and Yamamoto, S. (eds.) *Advances in Prostaglandin, Thromboxane and Leukotriene Research*. Vol. 15, pp. 637–639. (New York: Raven Press)

233. Guth, P.H., Paulsen, G. and Nagata, H. (1984). Prostaglandin cytoprotection: effect on histologic and microcirculatory changes in alcohol-induced gastric mucosal injury. In Allen, A., Flemstrom, G., Garner, A., Silen, W. and Turnberg, L.A. (eds.), *Mechanisms of Mucosal Protection in the Upper Gastrointestinal Tract*, pp. 285–286 (New York: Raven Press)

234. Robert, A., Lancaster, C., Davis, J.P., Field, S.O., Wickrema Sinha, A.J. and Thornburgh, B.A. (1985). Cytoprotection by prostaglandin occurs in spite of penetration of absolute ethanol into the gastric mucosa. *Gastroenterology*, **88**, 328–333

235. Pihan, G. and Szabo, S. (1986). Leukotriene (LTD$_4$) enhances gastric mucosal lesions induced by ethanol or HCl. *Dig. Dis. Sci.*, **31**, (Suppl.), 57S

236. Rogers, C., Pihan, G. and Szabo, S. (1986). Role for leukotrienes in the pathogenesis of haemorrhagic mucosal lesions induced by ethanol or HCl in the rat. *Gastroenterology*, **90**, 1797

237. Peskar, B.M., Lange, K., Hoppe, U. and Peskar, B.A. (1986). Ethanol stimulates formation of leukotriene C$_4$ in rat gastric mucosa. *Prostaglandins*, **31**, 283–293

238. Davenport, H.W., Warner, H.A. and Code, C.F. (1964). Functional significance of gastric mucosal barrier to sodium. *Gastroenterology*, **47**, 142–152

239. Davenport, H.W. (1964). Gastric mucosal injury by fatty and acetylsalicylic acids. *Gastroenterology*, **46**, 245–253

240. Davenport, H.W. (1965). Damage to the gastric mucosa: effect of salicylates and acid stimulation. *Gastroenterology*, **49**, 189–196

241. Whitle, B.J.R. (1981). Prostaglandin-cyclooxygenase inhibition and its relationship to gastric damage. In Harmon, J.W. (ed.). *Basic Mechanisms of Gastrointestinal Mucosal Cell Injury and Protection*, pp. 197–210 (Baltimore: Williams and Wilkins)

242. Augur, N.A. (1970). Gastric mucosal blood flow following damage by ethanol, acetic acid, or aspirin. *Gastroenterology*, **58**, 311–320

243. Moody, F.G. and Durbin, R.P. (1965). Effects of glycine and other instillates on concentration of gastric acid. *Am. J. Physiol.*, **209**, 122–126

244. Cheung, L.Y., Moody, F.G. and Reese, R.S. (1975). Effect of aspirin, bile salt, and ethanol on canine gastric mucosal blood flow. *Surgery*, **77**, 786–792

245. Ritchie, W.P. (1975). Acute gastric mucosal damage induced by bile salts, acid and ischemia. *Gastroenterology*, **68**, 699–707

246. Ashley, S.W., Sonnenschein, L.A. and Cheung, L.Y. (1985). Focal gastric mucosal blood flow at the site of aspirin-induced ulceration. *Am. J. Surg.* **149**, 53–58

247. Yan, Z–Y., Ashley, S.W., Sonnenschein, L.A. and Cheung, L.Y. (1984). Changes in focal gastric mucosal blood flow associated with bile salt-induced injury. *Surg. Forum*, **35**, 189–191

248. Ritchie, W.P. and Shearburn, E.W. (1977). Influence of isoproterenol and cholestyramine on acute gastric mucosal ulcerogenesis. *Gastroenterology*, **73**, 62–65

249. McGreevy, J.M. and Moody, F.G. (1977). Protection of gastric mucosa against aspirin-induced erosions by enhanced blood flow. *Surg. Forum*, **28**, 357–359

250. Cloud, W.G. and Ritchie, W.P. Jr. (1982). Evidence for cytoprotection by endogenous prostaglandins on gastric mucosa treated with bile acids. *Surg. Forum*, **33**, 150–152

251. Menguy, R., Desbaillets, L. and Master, Y.F., (1974). Mechanisms of stress ulcer: influence of hypovolemic shock on energy metabolism in the gastric mucosa. *Gastroenterology*, **66**, 46–51

252. Szabo, S., Pihan, G. and Trier, J.S. (1986). Alterations in blood vessels during gastric injury and protection. *Scand. J. Gastroenterol.*, **21**, (Suppl. 125), 92–96

253. Kivilaakso, E., Fromm, D. and Silen, W. (1987). Relationship between ulceration and intraluminal pH of gastric mucosa during haemorrhagic shock. *Surgery*, **84**, 70–78

254. Cheung, L.Y. and Toenjes, A.A. (1980). Effect of intra-arterial infusion of bicarbonate on gastric intramural pH and ulceration. *Surg. Forum*, **31**, 117–118

255. Konturek, S.J., Brzozowski, T., Piastucki, I., Radicki, T. and Dembinska-Kiu, A. (1983). Role of prostaglandin and thromboxane biosynthesis in gastric necrosis produced by taurocholate and ethanol. *Dig. Dis. Sci.*, **28**, 154–160

256. Whittle, B.J.R. (1984). Cellular mediators in gastric damage: actions of thromboxane A_2 and its inhibitors. In Allen, A., Flemstrom, G., Garner, A., Silen, W. and Turnberg, L.A. (eds.) *Mechanisms of Mucosal Protection in the Upper Gastrointestinal Tract*, pp. 295–300. (New York: Raven Press)

257. Gervasi, G.B., Forsati, A., Caliari, S., Rapalli, L. and Bergamaschi, M. (1983). Prevention of experimentally induced gastric damage with the tripeptide Zami-420. A new thromboxane synthesis inhibitor. *Int. J. Tiss. Reac.*, **5**, 253–256

258. Kivilaakso, E. and Silen, W. (1978). Pathogenesis of experimental gastric mucosal injury. *N. Engl. J. Med.*, **301**, 364–369

259. Silen, W., Merhav, A. and Simson, J.N.L. (1981). The pathogenesis of stress ulcer disease. *World J. Surg.*, **5**, 165–174

260. Guth, P.H. (1982). Pathogenesis of gastric mucosal injury. *Ann. Rev. Med.*, **33**, 183–196

261. Kauffman, G.L. (1985). The gastric mucosal barrier. Component control. *Dig. Dis. Sci.*, **30**, (Suppl. 1), 69S–76S

262. Leung, F.W., Itoh, M., Hirabayashi, K. and Guth, P.H. (1985). Role of blood flow in gastric and duodenal mucosal injury in the rat. *Gastroenterology*, **88**, 281–289

263. Larsen, K.R., Niels, F.J., Davis, E.K., Jensen, J.C. and Moody, F.G. (1981). The cytoprotective effects of ($\pm$)-15-deoxy-16-α, hydroxy-16-methyl PGE_1 methyl ester (SC-29333) versus aspirin-shock gastric ulcerogenesis in the dog. *Prostaglandins*, **21**, (Suppl.), 119–124

264. Kitagawa, H., Kurahashi, K. and Fujiwara, M. (1984). Water immersion stress induces mucosal ischemia due to thromboxane A_2-like substance and ulcer formation in rats. *Jpn. J. Pharmacol.*, **35**, 478–483

265. Murakami, M., Kum Lam, S., Inada, M. and Miyake, T. (1985). Pathophysiology and pathogenesis of acute gastric mucosal lesions after hypothermic restraint stress in rats. *Gastroenterology*, **88**, 660–665

10
The gastroduodenal mucus barrier and the place of eicosanoids

A. Allen A. Garner, A.C. Hunter and J. P. Keogh

Mucus is ubiquitous throughout the gastrointestinal tract and is a major organic secretion in terms of output by weight and biosynthetic requirements. From the stomach to the colon the primary mucus secretion is a water insoluble gel which adheres to the mucosal surfaces. A soluble mucus is also produced which is mixed with luminal juices and can be removed from the mucosal surface by gentle washing. Salivary mucus is secreted only in the soluble phase and is present in the mouth as a viscous solution. To date the effects of eicosanoids on mucus secretions in the gastrointestinal tract have been almost entirely confined to the stomach and duodenum. It is here that the mucus:bicarbonate barrier is considered to be the first line in mucosal defence against autodigestion by the corrosive gastric juices. This chapter is specifically addressed to the effect of prostaglandins on the gastroduodenal mucus barrier and its relation to mucosal protection. For more general surveys of the biochemistry and physiology of mucus secretions the reader is referred to specialized reviews[1-4].

MUCUS IN SITU

Mucus in vivo can be identified in three phases: (i) presecreted mucus stored intracellularly in vesicles; (ii) the water insoluble mucus gel layer adherent to the mucosal surfaces and (iii) soluble mucus mixing with the luminal contents. Mucus is composed of large molecular weight glycoproteins or mucins which confer on the secretion its viscous and gel-forming properties. Admixed with secreted mucus are other gastrointestinal secretions (e.g. enzymes and secretory IgA), micro-organisms, sloughed off cells and ingested matter at various stages of digestion.

Presecreted mucus can be readily identified in histologically prepared sections stained for neutral mucins by the periodic acid Schiff stain or for acidic mucins by Alcian blue and high iron diamine. Mucus originates from a variety of cell types including surface epithelial and mucus neck cells of the stomach, Brunner's glands of the duodenum and goblet cells of the small and large intestines[5,6]. Electron microscopy studies[2,3,7] have shown intracellular mucus is stored in membrane bound secretory vesicles, which, on stimulation, move to and fuse with the apical plasma membrane before releasing their contents into the lumen. Scanning electron microscopy[8] has shown three mechanisms for mucus release from gastric surface epithelial cells: (i) a continuous exocytosis of a few granules at a time, (ii) explosive release of mucus by apical expulsion of older cells in the interfoveolar area, and (iii) the relatively rare event of cell exfoliation.

The adherent mucus gel can be observed *in situ* on unfixed mucosal sections as a clearly visible thin layer of translucent gel between the mucosal surface and luminal bathing solution. The mucus adherent to the gastric and duodenal mucosa is always seen to be continuous, varying in thickness from 50–450 μm, median 180 μm for human stomach and 10–300 μm, median 80 μm for rat stomach and duodenum[9]. Mucus appears as a layer between 10–250 μm thick overlying the villi in the ileum and as a discrete, continuous layer in the colon of rodents and man[10]. The layer of adherent mucus gel in the stomach is not solubilized over the pH range of 1–8 by bile or hypertonic solutions (2 mmol L^{-1} NaCl). It is a relatively rigid structure that is resistant to mechanical disruption and will only perceptibly flow over a relatively long time scale of about an hour[11]. Exposure to proteolytic enzymes (e.g. excess pepsin) or disulphide bond disrupting agents (e.g. *N*-acetylcysteine) will however result in disruption and dissolution of the adherent mucus layer over a period of an hour. This extracellular adherent mucus gel layer is either absent or very much reduced on mucosal sections that have been fixed and stained for histological observation. This is because the mucosal gel is 95% water and histological fixatives, such as ethanol and glutaraldehyde, cause it to dehydrate and shrink[12]. In contrast, the presecreted mucus contained within intracellular mucus vesicles remains after histological processing to give the mucus-secreting epithelia its characteristic neutral mucin and basophilic staining properties[5,6]. Extracellular mucus is visible on electron micrographs of the mucosa partly as sheets but frequently as threads over the mucosal surface[8,13]. If, however, it is stabilized first with antibody, mucus gel can be observed as a continuous layer by electron microscopy[14].

MUCUS STRUCTURE

Major technical problems have been associated with the isolation and characterization of mucus glycoproteins due to their large complex structure and association with other macromolecules particularly proteins and lipids[1,3,15]. However, the general structure of mucus glycoproteins (or mucin) from the gastrointestinal tract as well as other tracts of the body is well established as a distinct class of macromolecules. Mucus glycoproteins in general contain over 70% by weight carbohydrate (salivary mucins contain somewhat less, 50–70%, by weight carbohydrate) in the form of carbohydrate chains around a central protein core (Figure 10.1)[16,17]. The tertiary structure of mucus is often referred to as the 'bottle brush' where the bristles represent the sugar chains with the wire support representing the central protein core. The constituent sugars are N-acetylglucosamine, N-acetylgalactosamine, fucose, galactose and sialic acid. The size of the carbohydrate side chains varies according to the origin of the secretion, ranging from 2–5 sugars per chain in salivary mucus glycoproteins to up to 19 sugars per chain in colonic and gastric mucus glycoproteins[16,18–20]. The terminal sugars of the carbohydrate chains of human mucus glycoproteins have ABH antigenic activity while those of the pig[21] have A and H. Why mucus glycoproteins possess structures characteristic of the erythrocyte surface is unknown. Mucus glycoproteins are strongly negatively charged primarily because of the presence of carbohydrate bound ester sulphate and sialic acid residues. The content of sialic acid and ester sulphate varies from one mucus glycoprotein secretion to another and is the basis of the Alcian blue and high iron diamine mucin stains[5].

The protein core has an unusual amino acid composition with as much as 40% by weight being composed of the amino acids threonine, serine and proline. This reflects the high density of attachment sites for the carbohydrate side chains which occurs through an O-glycosidic linkage between N-acetylgalactosamine and serine or threonine[16–18]. The carbohydrate chains are tightly packed together along the protein core forming a protective sheath against proteolysis of 'the bristle section of the bottle brush'. However, there are parts of the protein core low in serine and threonine which are essentially non-glycosylated and therefore susceptible to proteolysis[22,23].

Proteolytic enzymes fragment larger molecular weight mucus glycoproteins into smaller glycosylated units of M_r between 3 and 7.5 × 10^5 in size[1,4,23]. These proteolytically digested mucus glycoproteins have lost between 30–50% of the protein core of the original glycoprotein without detectable loss of carbohydrate. The three amino acids associated with the glycosylated regions, threonine, serine and proline, are conserved and can constitute up to 78% by weight of the total protein after proteolytic digestion.

Glycoproteins isolated directly from mucus secretions are very large in size[1,4] ranging from M_r about 2 × 10^6 to 45 × 10^6. They consist of a polymeric structure of glycoprotein subunits joined together by disulphide bridges between the non-glycosylated regions of the protein core[1,24]. An example is the glycoprotein isolated from gastric mucus[25,26] (pig and human) which is of molecular weight 2 × 10^6. Following reduction with thiol agents or proteolysis[23,24], the glycoprotein consistently produces subunits of molecular weight approximately 5 × 10^5. From detailed structural studies, including chemical analysis, analytical ultracentrifugation and viscosity measurements, it is concluded that gastric mucus glycoprotein is a polymer consisting on average of four subunits joined together by disulphide bridges located in regions of the protein core that are non-glycosylated and hence susceptible to proteolytic attack[27]. Polymeric structures based on disulphide bridges and non-glycosylated protein cores have also been shown for other gastro-intestinal mucus glycoproteins, including human, pig and rat small intestinal mucus[28–30] pig colonic mucus[31] and human and pig biliary mucus[32]. An

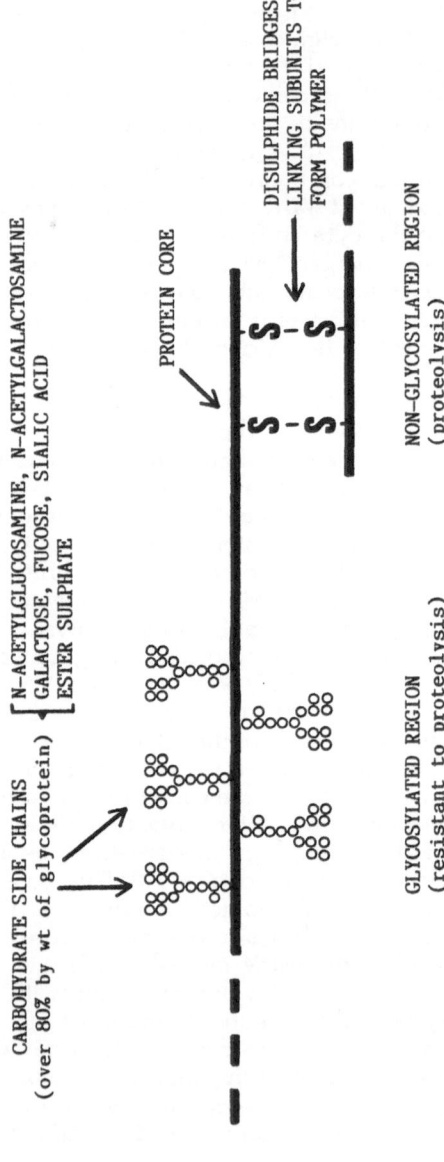

Figure 10.1 General structure of mucus glycoproteins

interesting structural observation is the release of a separate protein from pig and human gastric[26] and pig, rat and human small intestinal[28–30] mucus glycoproteins on reduction. These protein components range in size from M_r 70 000 to M_r 120 000 for gastric and small intestinal mucus respectively and in the latter case are glycosylated. All preparations of mucus glycoproteins viewed by electron microscopy appear as complex linear chains[33–35]. How the subunits are spacially arranged to form the polymeric mucus glycoprotein has still to be determined. Whether the very large glycoproteins isolated are non-covalent associations of smaller (e.g. 2×10^6) units as yet is also uncertain.

Rheological studies on isolated gastrointestinal mucus show it has mechanical properties characteristic of a weak viscoelastic gel. This type of gel structure has been shown for mucus secretions from all regions of the pig gastrointestinal tract, stomach to colon, as well as human gastric mucus[11,36]. Gels with the same characteristic mechanical properties as the native secretions can be reproduced from the isolated purified gastrointestinal mucus glycoproteins at concentrations equivalent to that of the native secretion. This demonstrates that mucus glycoproteins alone can account for the viscous and gel-forming properties of the native mucus secretion, although other components, proteins and nucleic acids, can affect its rheological properties. Adherent gastrointestinal mucus gel is insoluble and does not dissolve when exposed to solutions of high acidity (pH 1), high osmolality (2 mol L^{-1} NaCl), dilute ethanol (less than 40%, v/v), or bile collected directly from the gall bladder[11,36]. Mucus gels are, however, readily dissolved by a wide variety of proteases or by reduction of disulphide bridges with thiol agents, e.g. 2-mercaptoethanol, dithiothreitol or the mucolytic drug, N-acetylcysteine. The mucolytic effect of such procedures is due to cleavage of the covalent structure of the protein core of the polymeric glycoproteins to yield smaller sized glycoprotein units of lower viscosity and which are devoid of gel-forming properties[1,11,24]. The solubilization of mucus by proteolytic enzymes, e.g. luminal pepsins, have important implications *in vivo* where a dynamic balance exists between erosion of the adherent mucus gel by proteolysis augmented by mechanical sloughing and the secretion of new mucus by the epithelial cells (Figure 10.2).

Adherent mucus gel is considered to form a first line defence between the underlying gastroduodenal epithelium and the digestive juices present in the lumen. It is useful to categorize the protective role of adherent mucus in mucosal protection into two parts, depending on the nature of the damaging agent (Table 10.1)[37]. Firstly, protection against the endogenous aggressors (acid, pepsin and bile acids) and secondly, protection against exogenous damaging agents (e.g. alcohol and non-steroidal anti-inflammatory drugs). Natural defence mechanisms have presumably evolved against acid and pepsin and evidence points to an important role played by mucus. Adherent mucus alone does not appear to function as an effective barrier against mucosal damaging agents, such as ethanol and aspirin, which rapidly penetrate the mucus gel and damage the underlying epithelium. The response of the mucosa to such damage and the role of mucus in this process is discussed in the final section in relation to prostaglandins. The viscous, soluble, mucus present in the lumen is unlikely to protect against acid and pepsin in gastric juice

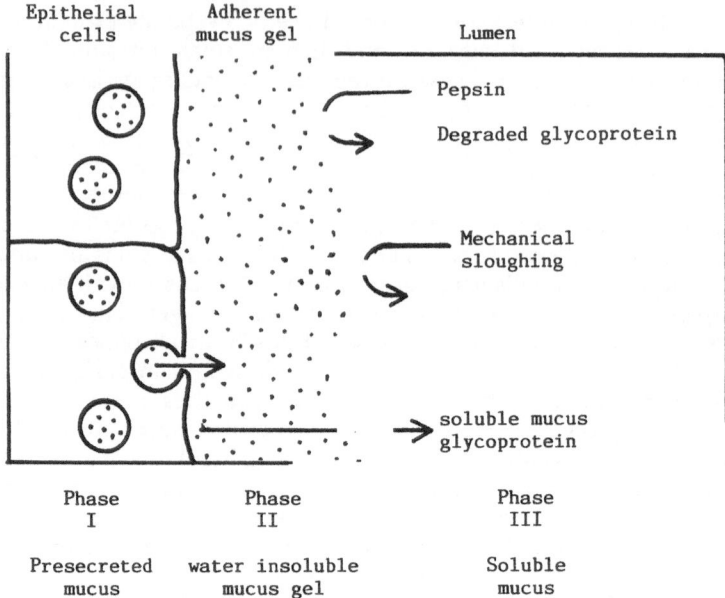

Figure 10.2   The three phases of mucus

Table 10.1   Role of mucus in gastroduodenal protection

Damaging factors	Protective action of mucus
Endogenous aggressors	
Acid	Stable unstirred layer: mixing barrier supporting surface neutralization by bicarbonate
Pepsin	Permeability barrier
Biliary reflux	Bile permeates through mucus to epithelium; mucus structure unchanged, continues to protect against acid and pepsin
Exogenous damaging agents	
Ethanol	Mucus permeated but remains: fibrin gel
Non-steroidal anti-inflammatory drugs	with mucus and necrotic cells protects
Hypertonic solutions	re-epithelializing cells: mucus may
Bile salts (high concentration)	act as template for fibrin formation
Severe damage resulting in lesions	—
Mechanical damage from abrasion	Lubricant (particularly soluble mucus)

Taken from Allen *et al.*, 1986[37].

although it will act as a lubricant preventing excessive depletion of the adherent mucus layer and damage to the mucosa from mechanical forces associated with digestion.

The foundations for the current concepts of the mucus:bicarbonate barrier were laid by Hollander[38] and Florey[39] The former proposed a dual barrier consisting of an alkaline mucus cover and an underlying, rapidly regenerating epithelial cell layer. The role of mucus was further developed by Heatley[40], who, recognizing that acid could rapidly permeate the mucus layer, proposed that surface neutralization occurred within this layer by bicarbonate secreted from the epithelium (Figure 10.3). Research over the last decade has now provided clear evidence for the existence of surface neutralization within the mucus layer adherent to both gastric and duodenal mucosal surfaces. Bicarbonate secretion by the gastric and duodenal mucosa has been demonstrated both *in vitro* and *in vivo* in a number of species, including man (see chapter by Aly and Flemström). Direct evidence for the surface neutralization of acid by bicarbonate has been provided by the demonstration of pH gradients across the mucus layer of both the gastric and duodenal mucosal surfaces[41–43]. Using H^+-sensitive microelectrodes, gradients have been shown to range from an acid pH in the lumen to a near neutral pH at the mucosal surface. In the duodenum, the maximum measured bicarbonate secretion is sufficient to account for the neutralization of acid down to the lowest pH values likely to occur in the duodenal bulb[44]. In the stomach, the measured bicarbonate release is not sufficient to neutralize acid below about pH 1.5–2, and, under conditions of high luminal acidity, the pH gradient is dissipated. As pH values below 1.5 are common in the gastric lumen, further neutralizing capacity must be provided[45]. The protective mechanisms which operate at

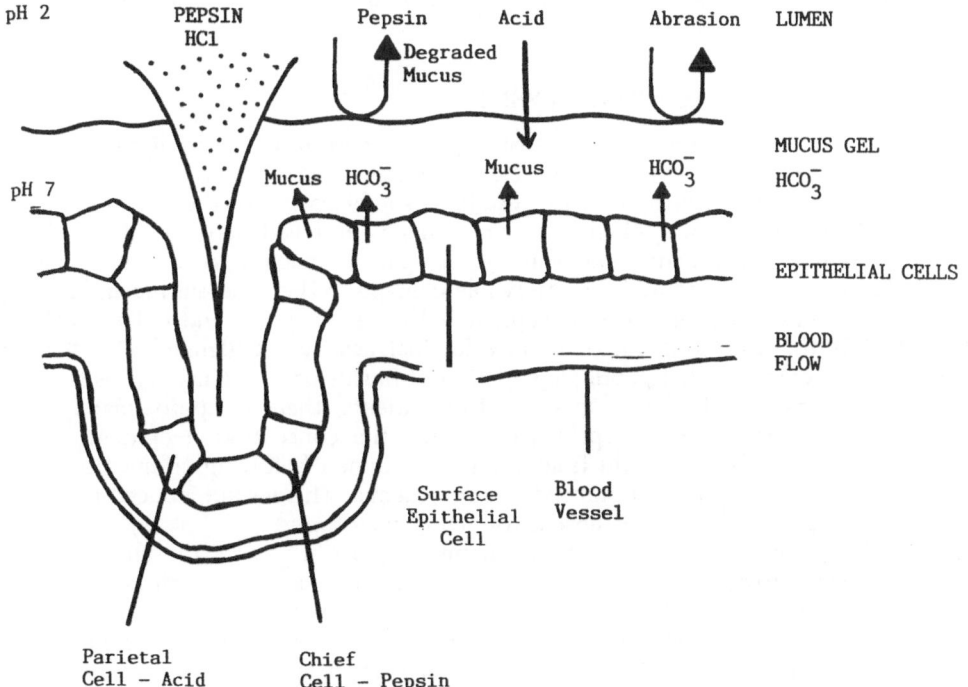

Figure 10.3 Mechanisms of gastroduodenal defence

the gastric epithelial surface or within the mucosa when the luminal pH falls below 1.5 remain to be elucidated. However, considerable neutralizing capacity is available from bicarbonate in the blood and interstitial fluid. If the epithelium is damaged and becomes leaky, then efflux of mucosal bicarbonate can maintain a neutral surface microenvironment enabling rapid re-epithelialization and recovery of mucosal barrier function[46].

The essential function of the adherent mucus layer in protection against acid is to provide a stable unstirred layer at the mucosal surface. In this way, mucus prevents the relatively small amount of secreted bicarbonate, which amounts to about 10% of the maximal acid secretion, from mixing with the bulk of the acid in the lumen[37,45]. The existence of this unstirred layer depends on the structure of the mucus, which consists of a matrix of non-covalently-bonded interlocking glycoprotein molecules. The matrix is about 5% by weight of the gel, the remaining 95% being solution held within the interstices of the gel network. This structure provides an excellent unstirred layer, which remains undisturbed by the mechanical forces involved in digestion. Although H^+ ions penetrate mucus gel more slowly (i.e. at about one quarter the rate) than through a truly unstirred layer of solution, the rate of penetration is extremely rapid and mucus must act primarily as a mixing barrier between bicarbonate and acid rather than as a diffusion barrier to H^+ ions. Furthermore, bicarbonate appears to be the only significant source of neutralizing capacity at the mucosal surface, because isolated mucus has very little buffering capacity, even when mixed with substantial amounts of mucosal cell debris.

PROTECTION AGAINST PEPSIN

The other aggressive factor in gastric juice is pepsin, which itself has ulcerogenic properties. For example, excess pepsin at pH 2.2 instilled into the stomach of an anaesthetized rat results in solubilization of the mucus layer, marked histological epithelial damage and gastric bleeding within 1 hour[37]. In control experiments, exposure of the gastric mucosa to pH 2.2 in the absence of pepsin caused no observable damage to the adherent mucus layer or the underlying epithelium. Thus, it is the pepsin *per se* and not the acid that is the damaging factor at low luminal acidity ($< 10 \, mmol \, L^{-1}$ HCl). Indirect evidence that peptic degradation of mucus occurs in man arises from the observation that in duodenal ulcer patients, there is approximately a three-fold rise in both pepsin activity and the concentration of degraded mucus glycoprotein products in the gastric lumen following stimulation of acid secretion by insulin-induced hypoglycaemia. This insulin-induced rise in both pepsin and mucus is absent following vagotomy[47].

The continuous cover of adherent mucus gel can protect the underlying epithelium from attack by luminal pepsin despite its solubilization as a result of proteolysis. Thus the mucus gel, while permeable to small ions and molecules, is not permeable to large protein molecules like pepsin[48]. Therefore, pepsin, will progressively dissolve the mucus layer at its luminal surface, but cannot diffuse through the matrix of the gel to reach the underlying epithelium. Since a continuous adherent layer of mucus is observed to cover the epithelium *in vivo*, new mucus secretion normally balances that lost by peptic erosion. In this way, mucus acts as an expendable but renewable permeability barrier, protecting the underlying epithelium against pepsin (Figure 10.3).

The properties of mucus which enable it to protect against acid and pepsin clearly depend on its ability to form a stable water-insoluble gel. The structure of the mucus gel layer adherent to the antral gastric mucosa has been shown to be impaired in gastric ulcer patients, and, to a lesser extent, in duodenal ulcer patients[49]. Quantitative analysis of adherent gastric mucus from antral mucosa resected from peptic ulcer patients has shown that there is significantly less polymerization of the glycoprotein. Detailed structural studies have shown that the mucus gel strength is directly related to the amount of polymerized glycoprotein[11]. Therefore, a weaker mucus layer, less resistant to erosion by mechanical forces and peptic digestion, covers the diseased gastric mucosa. Impairment of the protective mucus layer is not necessarily a primary factor in aetiology of peptic ulceration. Indeed, recent evidence suggests this weaker mucus barrier may be secondary to changes in the relative amounts of different forms of pepsin in the gastric juice[50].

Pepsin 3 is the major pepsin in man, pepsin 1 accounting for only 3.6% of the total activity in normal controls[51]. However, pepsin 1 accounts for 23% and 16.5% of the total pepsin activity in gastric and duodenal ulcer patients respectively. Recently it has been shown that pepsin 1, the ulcer-associated pepsin, dissolves mucus much more readily than pepsin 3, both at the optimum pH 2, when it has twice the activity, and in the higher pH range 4–5, when it has a six-fold greater activity. This increased mucolytic activity in gastric juice from peptic ulcer patients indicates the potential for increased breakdown of the mucus barrier under the higher pH conditions likely to be found in the duodenal bulb as well as in the stomach. Another factor which may cause a weakening of the mucus barrier in peptic ulcer patients is the associated increased shedding of epithelial cells, which is known to occur in the disease[52]. Such cell shedding will result in release of intracellular, lysosomal proteinases, which might also be expected to erode the mucus layer at the mucosal surface.

It is important to note that the gastric glands which produce acid and pepsin do not secrete mucus or bicarbonate. Acid concentrations resulting in a pH below 1 are attained in the lumen of the gastric glands during acid secretion, and, under these conditions, newly secreted pepsinogen will rapidly be converted autocatalytically into pepsin. Therefore, the apical membranes of the gastric glands must be resistant to their own secretions[53]. In contrast, the apical surface of the epithelial cells lining the gastric lumen appear to be sensitive to both acid and proteolysis. Excess acid or pepsin in the lumen is known to cause epithelial damage *in vivo*, but just how sensitive the apical membranes *per se* of the epithelial cells are to acid and pepsin will only be determined by future research.

EFFECTS OF EICOSANOIDS ON MUCUS SECRETION

When considering the effects of eicosanoids and other agents on gastrointestinal mucus dynamics it is important to consider its three phases: presecreted mucus in intracellular vesicles, insoluble mucus gel adherent to the mucosa, and freely mobile (largely soluble) luminal mucus (Figure 10.2). These phases are not related to each other quantitatively and all three forms of mucus should be assayed. For example, a major source of luminal mucus is derived from erosion of the adherent mucus gel by proteolysis due to endogenous secretions or bacteria as well as by shear forces. Hence, the content of luminal glycoprotein is not a measure of either secretion of the protective adherent mucus barrier or biosynthesis of the glycoprotein[1,54]. For an accurate picture of the physiological status of mucus, it is necessary to estimate quantitatively both biosynthesis and secretion, as well as to distinguish between the respective amounts present as adherent gel and as mucus in the lumen.

Several groups have demonstrated that different prostanoids increase the output of luminal mucus in the stomach in a variety of species (Table 10.2). Prostaglandins of the E series, both natural and synthetic analogues, have been most commonly used but A, F and H type prostaglandins have also been shown to increase luminal gastric mucus output. These studies reveal a two- to five-fold stimulation of glycoprotein output into the lumen compared with that of controls. The most potent agents appear to be the stable E type analogues and the endoperoxide PGH_2. Stimulation of soluble mucus output by PGs was independent of their inhibitory action on acid secretion[56,59]

Table 10.2 Luminal mucus glycoprotein output in response to prostaglandin administration

Species	Prostaglandin analogues and dose	Method of glycoprotein estimation	Reference
Man	15(R)-15-Me PGE_2 (80–400 µg, oral) 9-OH-19,20-bisnorprostanoic acid (400–3200 mg, oral)	Sialic acid	55
	PGE_2 (2 mg, oral)		56
	Rioprostil (PGE_1, oral)		57
Dog	PGH_2 (0.25 µg/kg, i.v.)	Sialic acid	58
Rat	PGE_2 (0.6 mg/kg, i.v. bolus; 1.3 mg/kg, oral) 15-Me PGE_2 (0.6 µg/kg, i.v. bolus; 0.13 mg/kg, oral) 16,16-dm PGE_2 (0.6 µg/kg i.v. bolus; 0.13 mg/kg, oral)	Alcian blue	59
	16,16-dm PGE_2 (5 µg/kg s.c., oral)	Hexosamines, sialic acid	60
	15-Me PGE_2, E_1, $F_{1\alpha}$, $F_{2\alpha}$, A_1, A_2 (0.1–4.0 mg/kg, oral)	Anthrone–total hexoses	61
	16,16-dm PGE_2 (25–50 µg/kg, oral)	Periodic acid–Schiffs	9,65
	$PGF_{2\beta}$ (0.5–2.0 mg/kg,oral)	Alcian blue. Sialic acid hexoses	62
	Enprostil (PGE_2) (19–250 µg/kg, p.o.)	Anthrone–total hexoses	63
	PGE_2 (200 µg/100g, s.c.)	Fucose	64
	PGE_2(1.5 mg/kg) 16,16-dm PGE_2 (0.18 mg/kg) U46619 (PGH_2) (1.5 mg/kg, intragastric)	Sialic acid	74

In each case, an increase was observed of 2- to 5-fold over the control without prostaglandin thereby reflecting a direct action on the epithelial surface cells. However, this rise in luminal mucus output could be associated with the ability of PGs to stimulate non-parietal secretions[45,65], since increased flow through the surface mucus layer can wash soluble mucus glycoprotein associated with the surface gel into the lumen. Such an explanation could also account for the increased output of luminal mucus glycoprotein into the gastric lumen of the rat after topical application of damaging agents which are known to increase mucosal permeability, e.g. absolute ethanol and non-steroidal anti-inflammatory drugs. In many cases, a substantial increase in luminal mucus viscosity is observed following prostaglandin administration indicative of polymeric glycoprotein. This points to the rise in luminal mucus originating by an increase in secretion rather than peptic erosion.

The magnitude of the increase in output of luminal mucus glycoprotein following PG administration (Table 10.2) varies between different studies and there are two reports, both in the rat, where no increase was recorded[67,69]. These differences may in part be attributable to the particular PG used, its dose and route of administration. However, the various methods and approaches used to estimate mucus glycoprotein in the luminal juice can also be a source of variable results. A wide variety of chemical methods have been used to estimate mucus glycoprotein in gastric juice. Simple colorimetric assays that have been most commonly employed to estimate mucus are: the anthrone estimation for neutral sugars, sialic acid estimation, the periodic acid Schiff reaction and the binding of Alcian blue to the negative charges of the mucus glycoprotein (Table 10.2). These methods are rapid but great care is necessary to ensure that they are measuring mucus glycoprotein alone and are not subject to interference from other macromolecular contaminants (e.g. protein and nucleic acid) as well as more specific interference from other glycosaminoglycans which arise from sources such as proteoglycans, connective tissue, serum glycoproteins and glycolipid cell debris[1].

The variability in results for estimating soluble mucus is demonstrated in a study which measured mucus glycoprotein in the rat stomach simultaneously using three different methods: Alcian blue binding, sialic acid content, and total hexose by anthrone estimation[62]. The increase in soluble mucus glycoprotein output following administration of $PGF_{2\beta}$ (2.0 mg kg^{-1}) was two-fold when measured by Alcian blue binding and almost three-fold by hexose content, while the sialic acid content was unchanged. The amount of insoluble mucus, estimated from mucosal scrapings, also increased over two-fold following $PGF_{2\beta}$ when measured by Alcian blue binding or as total hexose, but increased only 40% when measured by sialic acid content. Using an Alcian blue binding method, an increase was reported in the soluble mucus output in rat gastric contents, but not in the binding of dye to the adherent gel, after intravenous or topical administration of PGE_2 and methylated analogues[59]. Sialic acid is found in the terminal position on carbohydrate chains of mucus glycoprotein and can vary in content for given glycoprotein preparations according to the secretory status. For satisfactory chemical estimation of mucus it is desirable to first partially purify the glycoprotein from other components that interfere with these assays[1].

EFFECT OF EICOSANOIDS ON THE ADHERENT MUCUS GEL

When considering the effects of eicosanoids on the mucus barrier it is changes in the adherent mucus gel that are relevant rather than the soluble mucus which mixes freely with the gastric juices. This adherent mucus gel in theory can be estimated by gently scraping it from the surface of the mucosa, but in practice this is almost impossible to achieve without removing epithelium or else inducing release of presecreted mucus. A satisfactory method for measuring changes in adherent mucus in different physiological and pharmacological states is to measure changes in the adherent mucus thickness[9,12,65]. This can be done by observing the adherent mucus on thick (1.6 mm) unfixed transverse sections of gastrointestinal mucosa. On such sections, the adherent mucus layer is readily distinguished as a thin layer of translucent gel optically distinct from the mucosa and bathing solution. The thickness of this mucus layer, taken as the distance between the soluble mucus interface and the mucus:mucosa interface, can be directly measured with an eye piece graticule. Wide variations (up to 10-fold) in the thickness of the mucus layer are observed across a single gastric or duodenal mucosal section. To obtain values of average mucus thickness, and enable comparisons of different treatment groups, a minimum of 6 animals per treatment group are necessary. An alternative method for estimating mucus thickness is to use a slit lamp and pachymeter[67]. This indirect method gives values for mucus thickness about twice those measured by direct observation of unfixed mucosal sections. A probable explanation for this overestimation is that the pachymeter value also incorporates a layer of unstirred solution exterior to the adherent mucus gel[70]. Such an explanation probably also accounts for the fact that dimensions of the measured pH gradients at the gastroduodenal mucosal surface can exceed observed mucus thickness by up to 10-fold.

Intragastric instillation of 16,16-dimethyl PGE_2 or misoprostol both increase significantly adherent gastric mucus gel thickness up to 3-fold in the rat (Table 10.3). With topical 16,16-dimethyl PGE_2, the maximal response was obtained after 2 h when mean gastric mucus thickness was 139 μm, an increase of 74% over the control[65]. This increase was rapid, with 70% of maximal response achieved within 5 min of dosing. Such a rapid increase in mucus thickness is consistent with the release of preformed mucus[8]. Comparison of the distribution of individual readings for the control and PG-treated animals showed that the increase in mucus thickness was not restricted to the areas where the gel was thinnest. An increase in mean gastric mucus gel thickness was observed in the frog (*Rana pipiens*) following topical 16,16-dimethyl PGE_2 via an orogastric tube 2 h previously[9]. Mean mucus thickness in the fasted frog was 47 μm after 0.15 mol L^{-1} NaCl and this increased to 73 μm after PG administration. Similarly, in chambered preparations of *Rana temporaria*, gastric mucosa mean mucus thickness was 72 $\pm$ 11 μm immediately after mounting, which increased to 192 $\pm$ 16 μm after exposure to bathing solution alone for 1 h, and to 267 $\pm$ 11 μm when 16,16-dimethyl PGE_2 was included in the nutrient solution[12]. Much of this increase in mucus thickness in chambered preparations of *Rana temporaria* gastric mucosa has been shown to be due to distension of the mucosa[68], although 16,16-dimethyl PGE_2 still gives a significant increase in thickness in addition to that due to mucosal distension.

Table 10.3 Adherent gastric mucus gel: increased thickness in response to prostaglandin administration

Species	Prostaglandin analogue and dose	Time course	Increase compared with control (%)	Reference
Rat *in vivo*	16,16-dm PGE$_2$ (25 μg/kg)	2 h	74	9
Rat *in vivo*	Misoprostil (1000 μg/kg)	1 h	236	66
Rat *in vivo*	16,16-dm PGE$_2$ (25 μg/kg)	2 h	139	67
Rana pipiens in vivo	16,16-dm PGE$_2$ (25 μg (animal))	2 h	29	9
Rana temporaria (mucosal sheets)	16,16-dm PGE$_2$ (10^{-5} mol/L)	1 h	40	68
Rana temporaria (stomach sacs)	16,16-dm PGE$_2$ (10^{-5} mol/L)	1 h	170	68

EFFECT OF EICOSANOIDS ON MUCUS BIOSYNTHESIS

The intracellular pathways for mucus glycoprotein biosynthesis have been extensively investigated[2,4,17,71]. The protein core of the mucus glycoprotein is synthesized by translation of mRNA in the rough endoplasmic reticulum. The carbohydrate chains are formed by direct transfer of nucleotide sugars to the nascent molecule, primarily in the Golgi complex. The first step in biosynthesis of the sugar chains is the transfer of N-acetylgalactosamine to either seryl or threonyl residues of the protein core. This is followed by a stepwise addition of single sugars one at a time to complete the carbohydrate chain. The glycosidases which catalyse these transfers are highly specific for the structure of their growing oligosaccharide chain substrate. Sialic acid and ester sulphate are added at a late stage and the glycoprotein is packed into secretory granlules which then move to the apical aspect of the cell prior to secretion. There must be a mechanism which keeps the mucus glycoprotein in a compact state prior to its secretion, since the dimensions of freshly secreted mucus gels far exceed those of the epithelia which produce them. Techniques which have been applied to measure mucus biosynthesis have utilized radiolabelled substrates such as ^{14}C- or ^{3}H-labelled amino acids and sugars, and $^{35}SO_4^{2-}$. Their incorporation has been measured either autoradiographically by determining the density of silver grains or by measurement of incorporation into isolated mucus preparations (Table 10.4). In such studies it is important to show that the measured radioactivity is unambiguously incorporated into mucus glycoprotein and not other macromolecules, e.g. proteins and connective tissue proteoglycans: this is seldom achieved.

The stimulation by prostaglandins of the incorporation of radioactive mucus glycoprotein precursors into trichloroaecetic acid (TCA) precipitable

Table 10.4 Rat gastric mucus biosynthesis: effect of prostaglandins

Species	Prostaglandin analogue and dose	Method of estimation	Reference
Rat in vivo	Rioprostil (PGE$_1$) (1.5 µg/kg, oral)	[^{3}H]gluosamine into mucosal tissue	57
Rat in vivo	16,16-dm PGE$_2$ PGE$_2$, U46619 (PGH$_2$) (10^{-4}–10^{-8} mol/L oral)	[^{3}H]glucosamine into trichloroacetic acid precipitates	73
Rat in vivo	16,16-dm PGE$_2$ (10 µg/kg, i.v.)	[^{3}H]galactose, [^{3}H]glucosamine incorporation assay by autoradiography	72
Rat in vitro	Arachidonic acid (5–50 µmol/L)	[^{3}H]glucosamine into cells in culture	74
Rat in vitro	PGE$_2$ (200 µmol/L)	[^{3}H]N- acetylglucosamine and [^{14}C]amino acids into isolated cells	64

In all cases a significant increase in incorporation was observed following prostaglandin administration

material or into whole cells has been demonstrated (Table 10.4). 16,16-Dimethyl PGE$_2$ and an endoperoxide analogue both stimulated strips of rat gastric mucosa *in vitro* to incorporate [^{3}H]glucosamine into TCA precipitable protein[74]. These effects were observed at eicosanoid levels below the antisecretory dose. PGE$_2$ stimulated the incorporation by cultured rat non-parietal cells of [^{3}H]glucosamine into TCA precipitable protein[64]. Vascularly perfused rat stomachs incorporated [^{3}H]glucosamine almost exclusively into mucus glycoprotein[72]. Radioactive mucus was identified by autoradiography but its identity was confirmed by analysis by equilibrium centrifugation in a caesium chloride gradient. In contrast, the incorporation of radioactive serine into mucus glycoprotein by perfused rat stomach was only 8% of the total radioactivity incorporated. Much of the radioactivity incorporated was into pepsinogen and this was not stimulated by 16,16-dimethyl PGE$_2$.

MUCOSAL PROTECTION AND INJURY

Gastroduodenal mucosal protective mechanisms are several and include the mucus:bicarbonate barrier, re-epithelialization and mucosal blood flow (Figure 10.3)[75,76]. As already discussed, adherent mucus and epithelial bicarbonate secretion are the initial barrier against the natural aggressors, acid and pepsin. The ability of prostaglandins to stimulate both mucus and bicarbonate secretions by the gastric and duodenal mucosa (see also chapter by Aly and Flemström) would be expected to enhance such protection. A thicker adherent mucus cover would provide a better unstirred layer for surface neutralization and a more effective barrier against penetration by pepsin and proteolytic digestion of the underlying epithelium. In the stomach, where the mucus:bicarbonate barrier is insufficient at luminal pH 1.5 and below, other mechanisms are necessary to dispose of H^+ ions which may diffuse into the mucosa. Under these circumstances, mucosa acid–base balance is maintained in both the interstitial and intracellular compartments as a consequence of perfusion with HCO_3^- exchangers[77]. There is no evidence that prostaglandins influence these events at the cellular level although a thicker mucus barrier will contribute to maintaining stability and increased protection of the underlying epithelium.

The phenomenon of cytoprotection described in laboratory animals refers to an ability of prostaglandins to attenuate acute mucosal damage induced by exogenous agents such as aspirin and alcohol[78] (see chapter by Robert). These small molecular weight compounds permeate through the surface mucus gel extremely rapidly and a PG-induced thicker layer of glycoprotein will remain ineffective in terms of protection against such exogenous chemical aggressors[37]. Rather, the protective actions of prostaglandins against acute injury seem to operate at the vascular level and result from their ability to prevent vascular stasis[79]. Maintaining mucosal perfusion, thereby preventing ischaemia or reperfusion and injury is a critical factor in limiting acute mucosal damage. In the case of exogenous chemical injury, blood flow is also important as a means of mucosal clearance of the compound which would otherwise build up and induce the formation of mucosal erosion and haemorrhage.

An important phenomenon for limiting acute damage is the ability of the stomach to rapidly re-epithelialize areas of superficial cell loss by a process termed 'restitution'[47,80]. This property is distinct from both normal mucosal proliferation and chronic wound repair which involve cell division and occur over much longer time scales. Restitution follows superficial damage causing widespread shedding of necrotic interfoveolar epithelial cells and involves migration of viable mucus cells from the gastric pits across the basal lamina. Formation of tight junctions with complete restoration of epithelial continuity and barrier functions occurs in less than one hour of the surface being totally denuded of cells. Protection of the exposed basal lamina from luminal acid and pepsin is achieved by formation of an overlying, thick (1 mm), gelatinous layer of a fibrin-based gel with mucus and necrotic cells[81]. This thick, fibrin, gelatinous coat, with essentially unlimited neutralizing capacity from the plasma exudate, should be quite effective in protecting re-epithelialization from acid and pepsin in the lumen. The gelatinous coat has also been shown to have protective properties against ethanol, not shown by the adherent mucus layer. Thus, in contrast to the original adherent mucus barrier on the undamaged mucosa, this fibrin gelatinous coat protects the newly regenerated epithelium from further mucosal damage on re-exposure to ethanol[46]. If the gelatinous coat is removed from the surface (it can be easily removed), the epithelium is as sensitive to ethanol damage as the original epithelium, if not more so. As yet, there is no evidence for a role of prostaglandins in re-epithelialization or formation of the protective fibrin-based cover.

REFERENCES

1. Allen, A. (1981). Structure and function of gastrointestinal mucus. In Johnson, L.R. and associates (eds.) *Physiology of the Gastrointestinal Tract*, 1st Edn., pp. 617–639. (New York: Raven Press)

2. Neutra, M.R. and Forstner, J.F. (1986). Gastrointestinal mucus synthesis, secretion, function. In Field, M. and associates (eds.) *Physiology of the Gastrointestinal Tract*, 2nd Edn. (In press)
3. Ciba Foundation (1984). *Mucus and Mucosa. Ciba Foundation Symposium 109*. (London: Pitman)
4. Carlstedt, I., Sheehan, J.K., Corfield, A.P. and Gallagher, J.T. (1985). Mucous glycoproteins, a gel of a problem. *Essays Biochem.*, **20**, 40−76
5. Filipe, M.I. (1979). Mucins in the human gastrointestinal epithelium: A review. *Invest. Cell Pathol.*, **2**, 195−216
6. Culling, F.A. and Reid, P.E. (1984). Histochemistry of sialic acids. In Schauer (ed.) *Sialic Acids*, pp. 173−191. (Heidelberg: Springer Verlag)
7. Neutra, M.R. and Leblond, C.P. (1966). Synthesis of the carbohydrate of mucus in the Golgi complex as shown by electron microscope radioautography of goblet cells injected with glucose H^3. *J. Cell Biol.*, **30**, 119−136
8. Zalewsky, C.A. and Moody, F.G. (1979). Mechanisms of mucus release in exposed canine gastric mucosa. *Gastroenterology*, **77**, 719−729
9. Kerss, S., Allen, A. and Garner, A. (1982). A simple method for measuring thickness of the mucus gel layer adherent to rat, frog and human gastric mucosa: influence of feeding, prostaglandin, N-acetylcysteine and other agents. *Clin. Sci.*, **63**, 187−195
10. Sakata, T. and Englehart, W.V. (1981). Luminal mucin in the large intestine of mice, rats and guinea pigs. *Cell Tissue Res.*, **219**, 629−635
11. Bell, A., Sellers, L.A., Allen, A., Cunliffe, W.J., Morris, E.R. and Ross-Murphy, S.B. (1985). Properties of gastric and duodenal mucus: effect of proteolysis, disulfide reduction, bile acid, ethanol and hypertonicity on mucus gel structure. *Gastroenterology*, **88**, 269−280
12. McQueen, S., Allen, A. and Garner, A. (1984). Measurements of gastric and duodenal mucus gel thickness. In Allen, A., Flemström, G., Garner, A., Silen, W. and Turnberg, L.A. (eds.) *Mechanisms of Mucosal Protection in the Upper Gastrointestinal Tract*, pp. 215−221. (New York: Raven Press)
13. Morris, G.P. Harding, P.L. and Wallace, J.L. (1984). A functional model for extracellular gastric mucus in the rat. *Virchows Arch. (Cell Pathol.)*, **46**, 239−251
14. Walker, R.J., Brook, I., Costerton, J.W., MacVittie, T. and Myhal, M.L. (1985). Possible association of mucous blanket integrity with postirradiation colonisation resistance. *Rad. Res.*, **104**, 346−357
15. Creeth, J.M. (1978). Constituents of mucus and their separation. *Br. Med. Bull.*, **34**, 17−24
16. Gottschalk, A., Bhargava, A.S. and Murty, V.L.N. (1972). Submaxillary gland glycoproteins. In Gottschalk, A. (ed.) *Glycoproteins: their Composition, Structure and Function*, 2nd Edn., pp. 810−829. (Amsterdam: Elsevier)
17. Horowitz, M.I. and Pigman, W. (1977). *The Glycoconjugates*, Vol. 1. (New York: Academic Press)
18. Carlson, D.M. (1968). Structures and immunochemical properties of oligosaccharides isolated from pig submaxillary mucins. *J. Biol. Chem.*, **243**, (Suppl. 3), 616−626
19. Slomiany, B.L. and Meyer, K. (1972). Isolation and structural studies of sulphated glycoproteins of hog gastric mucosa. *J. Biol. Chem.*, **247**, 5062−5070
20. Podolsky, D.K. (1985). Oligosaccharide structures of human colonic mucin. *J. Biol. Chem.*, **260**, 8262−8271
21. Watkins, W.M. (1974). Genetic regulation of the structure of blood group specific glycoproteins. *Biochem. Soc. Symp.*, **0**, 125−146
22. Donald, A.S.R. (1973). The products of pronase digestion of purified blood group-specific glycoproteins. *Biochim. Biophys. Acta*, **37**, 420−436
23. Scawen, M. and Allen, A. (1977). The action of proteolytic enzymes on the glycoprotein from pig gastric mucus. *Biochem. J.*, **163**, 363−368
24. Snary, D., Allen, A. and Pain, R.H. (1970). Structural studies on gastric mucoproteins. Lowering of molecular weight after reduction with 2-mercaptoethanol. *Biochem. Biophys. Res. Commun.*, **40**, 844−851
25. Pearson, J.P., Allen, A. and Venables, C.W. (1981). Gastric mucus: isolation and polymeric structure of the undegraded glycoprotein: its breakdown by pepsin. *Gastroenterology*, **78**, 709−715
26. Pearson, J.P., Allen, A. and Parry, S. (1981). A 70,000-molecular weight protein, isolated

from purified pig gastric mucus glycoprotein by reduction of disulphide bridges and its implication in the polymeric structure. *Biochem. J.*, **197**, 155–162

27. Allen, A. (1978). Structure of gastrointestinal mucus glycoproteins and the viscous and gel-forming properties of mucus. *Br. Med. Bull.*, **34**, 28–33

28. Mantle, M., Mantle, D. and Allen, A. (1981). Polymeric structure of pig small intestine mucus glycoprotein: dissociation by proteolysis or by reduction of disulphide bridges. *Biochem. J.*, **195**, 227–285

29. Fahim, R.E.F., Forstner, G.G. and Forstner, J.F. (1983). Heterogeneity of rat goblet-cell mucin before and after reduction. *Biochem. J.*, **209**, 117–124

30. Mantle, M., Forstner, G.G. and Forstner, J.F. (1984). Antigenic and structural features of goblet-cell mucin of human small intestine. *Biochem. J.*, **217**, 159–167

31. Marshall, T. and Allen, A. (1978). The isolation and characterization of the high-molecular-weight glycoprotein from pig colonic mucus. *Biochem. J.*, **173**, 569–578

32. Pearson, J.P., Kaura, R., Taylor, W.H. and Allen, A. (1983). The composition and polymeric structure of mucus glycoprotein from human gallbladder bile. *Biochim. Biophys. Acta*, **706**, 221–228

33. Slayter, H.S., Cooper, A.G. and Brown, M.C. (1974). Electron microscopy and physical parameters of human blood group i, A, B and H antigens. *Biochemistry*, **13**, 3365

34. Slayter, H.S., Lamblin, G., le Trent, A., Galabert, C., Houdret, N., Degrand, P. and Roussel, P. (1984). Complex structure of human bronchial mucus glycoprotein. *Eur. J. Biochem.*, **142**, 209–218

35. Sheehan, J., Oakes, K., Carlstedt, I. (1986). Electron microscopy of cervical, gastric and bronchial mucus glycoproteins. *Biochem. J.*, **239**, 147–153

36. Sellers, L.A., Allen, A., Morris, E. and Ross-Murphy, S.B. (1983). Rheological studies on pig gastrointestinal mucus secretions. *Trans. Biochem. Soc.*, **11**, 763–764

37. Allen, A., Hutton, D.A., Leonard, A.J., Pearson, J.P. and Sellers, L.A. (1986). The role of mucus in protection of the gastroduodenal mucosa. *Scand. J. Gastroenterol.*, **21** (Suppl. 125), 71–77

38. Hollander, F. (1954). The two-component mucus barrier. *Arch. Intern. Med.*, **93**, 107–128

39. Florey, H. (1955). Mucin and the protection of the body. *Proc. Roy. Soc. Lond.*, **143**, 144–158

40. Heatley, N.G. (1959). Mucosubstance as a barrier to diffusion. *Gastroenterology*, **37**, 313–318

41. Ross, I.N., Bahari, H.M.M. and Turnberg, L.A. (1981). The pH gradients across mucus adherent to rat fundic mucosa *in vivo* and the effect of potential damaging agents. *Gastroenterology*, **81**, 713–718

42. Takeuchi, K.D., Magee, D., Critchlow, J., Mathew, S. and Silen, W. (1983). Studies of the pH gradient and thickness of frog gastric mucus gel. *Gastroenterology*, **84**, 331–340

43. Flemström, G. and Kivilaakso, E. (1983). Demonstration of a pH gradient at the luminal surface of rat duodenum *in vivo* and its dependence on mucosal alkaline secretion. *Gastroenterology*, **84**, 787–794

44. Flemström, G. and Garner, A. (1982). Gastroduodenal HCO_3 transport: characteristics and proposed role in acidity regulation and mucosal protection. *Am. J. Physiol.*, **242**, G183–93

45. Allen, A. and Garner, A. (1980). Gastric mucus and bicarbonate secretion and their possible role in mucosal protection. *Gut*, **21**, 249–262

46. Lacy, E.R. (1985). Gastric mucosal resistance to a repeated ethanol insult. *Scand. J. Gastroenterol.*, **20**, 63–72

47. Younan, F., Pearson, J.P., Allen, A. and Venables, C.W. (1982). Gastric mucus degradation in vivo in peptic ulcer patients and the effects of vagotomy. In Chantler, E.N., Elder, J.B. and Elstein, M. (eds.) *Mucus in Health and Disease II*, pp. 235–237. (New York: Plenum Press)

48. Allen, A. (1981). The structure and function of gastrointestinal mucus. In Harmon, J.W. (ed.) *Basic Mechanisms of Gastrointestinal Mucus*, pp. 351–357. (Baltimore and London: Wilkins and Wilkins)

49. Younan, F., Pearson, J.P., Allen, A. and Venables, C.W. (1982). Changes in the structure of the mucous gel on the mucosal surface of the stomach in association with peptic ulcer disease. *Gastroenterology*, **82**, 827–831

50. Pearson, J.P., Ward, R., Allen, A., Roberts, N.B. and Taylor, W.H. (1986). Mucus degradation

by pepsin comparison of mucolytic activity of human pepsin 1 and pepsin 3: implications in peptic ulceration. *Gut*, **27**, 243–248

51. Taylor, W.H. (1982). Biochemistry and pathological physiology of pepsin 1. *Adv. Clin. Enzymol.*, **2**, 79–91
52. Lipkin, M. (1981). Proliferation and differentiation of gastrointestinal cells in normal and disease states. In Johnson, L.R. (ed.) *Physiology of the Gastrointestinal Tract*, pp. 617–639. (New York: Raven Press)
53. Sanders, M.J., Ayalon, A., Roll, M. and Soll, A.H. (1985). The apical surface of canine chief cell monolayers resists H$^+$ back diffusion. *Nature*, **313**, 82–84
54. Allen, A. and Carroll, N.J.H. (1985). Adherent and soluble mucus in the stomach and duodenum. *Dig. Dis. Sci.*, **30**, 55S–62S
55. Domschke, W., Domschke, S., Hornig, D. and Demling, L. (1978). Prostaglandin-stimulated gastric mucus secretion in man. *Acta Hepato-gastroenterol.*, **25**, 292–294
56. Johansson, C. and Kollberg, B. (1979). Stimulation by intragastrically administered E$_2$ prostaglandin of human gastric mucus output. *Eur. J. Clin. Invest.*, **9**, 229–232
57. Quadros, E., Ramsamooj, E., Rajapaksa, T. and Wilson, D.E. (1984). Cytoprotective effects of prostaglandin E$_1$ (PGE$_1$) analogue: relationship to mucus synthesis and release in man and the rat. *Gastroenterology*, **86**, (5) 1214
58. Teo, P., Scruggs, W. and Wilson, D.E. (1979). The effects of prostaglandin endoperoxide analogue on canine gastric acid and mucus secretion. *J. Dig. Dis. Sci.*, **24**, 449
59. Bolton, J.P., Palmer, D. and Cohen, M.M. (1978). Stimulation of mucus and nonparietal cell secretion by the E$_2$ prostaglandins. *Am. J. Dig. Dis.*, **23**, 359
60. Nezamis, J.E. and Robert, A. (1980). Gastric mucus may mediate the cytoprotective effect of prostaglandins. *Gastroenterology*, **78**, 1228
61. Mahoney, J.M. and Waterbury, L.D. (1981). The effect of orally administered prostaglandins on gastric mucus secretions in the rat. *Prostagl. Med.*, **7**, 101
62. Lamont, T., Ventola, A.S., Maull, E.A. and Szabo, S. (1983). Cysteamine and prostaglandin F$_2$ stimulated rat gastric mucin release. *Gastroenterology*, **84**, 306
63. Waterbury, L.D., Mahoney, J.M. and Garay, G.L. (1984). Effect of enprostil, an anti-ulcer prostaglandin on gastric mucus secretion. *Gastroenterology*, **86** (5) 1294
64. Bersimbaev, R.I., Tairov, M.M. and Salganik, R.I. (1985). Biochemical mechanisms of regulation of mucus secretion by prostaglandin E$_2$ in rat gastric mucosa. *Eur. J. Pharmacol.*, **115**, 259–266
65. McQueen, S., Hutton, D.A., Allen, A. and Garner, A. (1983). Gastric and duodenal surface mucus gel thickness in rat: effect of prostaglandins and damaging agents. *Am. J. Physiol.*, **8**, 388–394
66. Sellers, L.A., Carroll, N.J.H. and Allen, A. (1986). Misoprostil-induced increases in adherent gastric mucus thickness and luminal mucus output. *Dig. Dis. Sci.*, **31**, 91S–95S
67. Bickel, M. and Kauffman, G.L. (1981). Gastric mucus gel thickness: effects of distension, 16-16-dimethyl prostaglandin E$_2$ and carbenoxolone. *Gastroenterology*, **80**, 770–775
68. Keogh, J.P., McQueen, S., Allen, A. and Garner, A. (1985). Secretion of adherent mucus gel by amphibian gastric mucosa *in vitro*. *Gut*, **26**, A1109
69. Metsa-Ketela, T., Parantainen, J. and Vapaatalo, H. (1980). Effects of prostaglandins on gastric acid and mucus secretion. *Adv. Prostgl. Thromboxane Res.*, **8**, 153
70. Allen, A., Hutton, D., McQueen, S. and Garner, A. (1983). Dimensions of gastro-duodenal surface pH gradients exceed those of adherent mucus gel layers. *Gastroenterology*, **85**, 463–466
71. Schacter, H. (1978). Glycoprotein biosynthesis. In Horowitz, M.I. and Pigman, W. (eds.) *The Glycoconjugates*, Vol. II, pp. 87–181. (New York: Academic Press)
72. Jentjens, T., Smits, A.L. and Strong, G.J. (1984). 16,16-dimethyl prostaglandin E$_2$ stimulates galactose and glucosamine but not serine incorporation in rat gastric mucous cells. *Gastroenterology*, **87**, 409–416
73. Tao, P. and Wilson, D.E. (1984). Effects of prostaglandin E$_2$, 16,16-dimethyl prostaglandin E$_2$ and a prostaglandin endoperoxide analogue (U46619) on gastric secretory volume, [H$^+$], and mucus synthesis and secretion in the rat. *Prostaglandins*, **28**, (3) 353–365
74. Terano, A., Hiraishi, H., Ohta, S. *et al.* (1984). Stimulation of mucus production by arachidonicacid in rat gastric monolayer culture. *Gastroenterology*, **86** (5) 1279
75. Allen, A., Flemström, G., Garner, A., Silen, W. and Turnberg, L. (eds.) (1983). *Mechanisms of Mucosal Protection in the Upper Gastrointestinal Tract*. (New York: Raven Press)

75. Allen, A., Flemström, G., Garner, A., Silen, W. and Turnberg, L. (eds.) (1983). *Mechanisms of Mucosal Protection in the Upper Gastrointestinal Tract.* (New York: Raven Press)
76. Allen, A. (1981). The structure and function of gastrointestinal mucus. In Harmon, J.W. (ed.) *Basic Mechanisms of Gastrointestinal Mucosal Cell Injury and Protection*, pp. 351–357. (London: Williams and Wilkins)
77. Machen, T.E. and Paradiso, A.M. (1987). Regulation of intracellular pH in the stomach. *Ann. Rev. Physiol.*, **49**, 21–35
78. Robert, A., Nezamis, J.E., Lancaster, C. and Hanchar, A.J. (1979). Cytoprotection by prostaglandins in rats. Prevention of gastric necrosis produced by alcohol, HCl, NaOH, hypertonic NaCl, and thermal injury. *Gastroenterology*, **77**, 433–443
79. Pihan, G., Majzoubi, D., Hauderischild, C., Trier, J.S. and Szabo, S. (1986). Early microcirulatory stasis in acute gastric mucosal injury in the rat and prevention by 16,16-dimethyl PGE$_2$. *Gastroenterology*, **91**, 1415–1426
80. Silen, W. and Ito, S. (1985). Mechanisms for rapid re-epithelialization of the gastric mucosal surface. *Ann. Rev. Physiol.*, **47**, 217–229
81. Sellers, L.A., Allen, A. and Bennett, M.K. (1987). Formation of a fibrin based gelatinous coat over repairing rat gastric epithelium following acute ethanol damage: interaction with adherent mucus. *Gut*, **28**, 835–843

Index

218